DEDICATION

This Smoking and Tobacco Control Monograph is dedicated to the
hundreds of community volunteers who served on community Boards
or task forces or otherwise contributed to the implementation of the
Community Intervention Trial for Smoking Cessation (COMMIT) project.
Without their unstinting energy and enthusiasm, this project could not
have been accomplished. We also wish to pay tribute to the extraordinary
community directors and their staffs who gave more of themselves to this
project than anyone could have expected. They are the real heroes of
COMMIT.

Foreword

The first great "public health revolution" in developed countries involved measures to control infectious disease, and now we are in the midst of the second revolution: the massive attack on chronic disease. In this revolution, the dramatic decline in cigarette smoking in the United States since 1964 stands out as the most striking success story, which is especially remarkable considering the fact that antismoking advocates play the part of David against the Goliath of the tobacco industry. Antitobacco forces, including public advocacy groups, have made steady advances in controlling the smoking epidemic despite the tobacco industry's greater expenditures to expand tobacco use. The industry's counterattacks continue with steadily increasing intensity; this points to a clear need to increase the scope and effectiveness of all existing educational and regulatory antitobacco strategies. This monograph on the Community Intervention Trial for Smoking Cessation (COMMIT) field experience meets this need extraordinarily well because organizing, activating, and empowering communities to take action against smoking surely stands as the most important strategy for use in public health campaigns that emphasize control of tobacco use.

This monograph, *Community-Based Interventions for Smokers: The COMMIT Field Experience*, is one of an excellent series on various aspects of tobacco and health published since 1991 by the National Cancer Institute and the first to deal with community-based approaches. It reports exciting victories: (1) a modest decrease in smoking rates in light-to-moderate smokers, especially in the hard-to-reach categories of individuals of low educational attainment and (2) an impressive accomplishment in community empowerment.

Many monographs and most scientific articles either confine themselves to a description of health problems or concentrate on the final results of interventions designed to solve these problems. It is indeed rare to find a document that tells *how* a problem was addressed: which methods were used, what resources and training were needed, what barriers were found, how the barriers were overcome, and how the intervention could have been improved.

This attention to process is long overdue. Given that eight previous community-based research studies on cardiovascular disease risk factors (including smoking) from the United States, Finland, Australia, South Africa, and Switzerland have been reported since 1972 (see Chapter 2), it is striking to note the absence of reporting on the *process* of achieving change. The responsibility for this absence can be laid at the door of the scientific journals, whose policy is to focus on results rather than methods, thereby excluding information with the greatest potential to help those who could attempt such programs.

COMMIT, with its 22 communities comprising 11 treatments and 11 controls, furnishes excellent opportunities for providing information on process, thanks to the diversity of experience it obtained and the excellence of its recordkeeping. These factors allow for good estimates of effort expended and results achieved for multiple intervention strategies carried out in varied settings, such as the media, health care venues, worksites, community organizations, and schools.

The authors deserve great praise for putting together 14 chapters of such value and usefulness. The resultant state-of-the-art compendium will serve policymakers and practitioners who wish to attempt community-based programs for virtually any health problem that requires broad community participation. That COMMIT was organized as a research project gives it the credibility needed to promote it as a blueprint for success. Both successes and failures are described, and programs in both the United States and Canada are described in enough detail to let us appreciate not only the logic of planning and methods of intervention but also the human drama involved.

Jane Farquharson, a community health specialist from Dalhousie University, Nova Scotia, Canada, has said, "Scientists learn from data, people learn from stories." Stories in this case are the monograph's details of process, as mentioned earlier. Lest scientists become offended, one can add that scientists interpret data as well, but it is only as activists that they, together with the people they help, can create community change. The stories of Chapters 5 through 13 are the how-to section of this document and give the information and inspiration needed to plan and implement simple or complex community intervention programs.

These chapters, whose stories are rich with lessons that will guide future community work, are the "trees" of the monograph. The "forest" is the ability of COMMIT to demonstrate the power of the people to better their lives by collaborating toward a shared goal. In the 19th century, the French writer and politician Alexis de Tocqueville labeled this country a "nation of joiners"—a trait he found admirable. COMMIT illustrates this American characteristic more than 100 years later, showing how members of the 11 treatment communities joined in a common cause for health.

De Tocqueville's symbolic nation of joiners was demonstrated in the community Boards and their task forces, which were created early in the 11 COMMIT communities. As organized events proceeded and gained recognition, community involvement increased manyfold. COMMIT's successes in creating community events ("magnet events") tell the world how ferment from "below" (from the people of a community) can change their local world. For example, imagine the excitement in Bellingham, WA, as COMMIT staff members paraded in giant turkey costumes, or during an annual parade, in giant cigarette costumes!

Each element of COMMIT's multicomponent campaign represented an innovation—as so often happens when pioneering efforts are made. Many barriers were encountered along the way, sometimes to be overcome by luck, sometimes by ingenuity and perseverance, sometimes not at all.

COMMIT staff members encountered a dramatic barrier as they worked toward adoption of smoke-free school policies in two communities. In each instance, a single school board member who was a smoker blocked the policy change. The obstacle was overcome in only one of these communities, after intense public discussion sparked by a COMMIT Board member's letter to the editor of the local newspaper. Thus, a committed Board member bore out the wisdom inherent in this quote from anthropologist, Margaret Mead, "Never doubt the ability of a few dedicated individuals to change the world, indeed, it is the only way it ever has." COMMIT, as a laboratory, teaches us how to create many such dedicated individuals whose talents were enhanced, for example, during service on the task forces.

The story of many examples of barriers overcome during the COMMIT trial is a heartening antidote to the undercurrent of cynicism, fear, and alienation that exists in the United States today. The ultimate power of the COMMIT monograph will manifest itself when this message of hope (we can improve our lives if we work together in common cause) and suggestions of how to accomplish change are disseminated widely to those who need encouragement.

One community was remarkably successful in "stirring the pot" and putting the hazards of smoking at the top of the community's agenda through skillful use of media advocacy. As such experts in social marketing as Drs. June Flora and Craig Lefebvre have pointed out, a successful message often can be grafted onto a topic that already has captured the public's attention. At the height of the great public debate over the possibility of harmful contaminants in a shipment of Chilean grapes, the COMMIT staff in Medford/Ashland, OR, was able to show that the cyanide content of inhaled cigarette smoke was potentially much more toxic than the grape's pesticide content.

Another COMMIT success was the finding that young people were surprisingly effective as catalysts for change. This observation highlights another tenet of social marketing: Messages should be delivered by highly credible people. COMMIT interventionists discovered that many young people were eager to help and were often remarkably successful in garnering the public's attention. An exciting example occurred during an attempt by COMMIT to decrease illegal sales of cigarettes to minors in Raleigh, NC. Three months earlier, the city council had rejected COMMIT's proposal to restrict vending machine cigarette sales, but after one adolescent's testimony council members rapidly approved the new legislation. The testimony in part simply stated, "You can't educate vending machines."

Community empowerment, including use of volunteers, perhaps the most important COMMIT result, is evident from all community stories but was carefully quantified as well; 94 percent of seven categories of process objectives were achieved and 99 percent for the category "Mobilization of Boards and Task Forces."

Given the impressive success in community empowerment, which also can be called a "bottom-up" approach, a major question is how best to harness the power of newly activated members of any community. First is the potential for the COMMIT monograph to be the country's current best creative and adaptable "cookbook" for change and thus a vehicle for wide adaptation. However, as described in the monograph's last chapter, one answer to the question of how to channel this "power" is to ask for "top-down" assistance from all levels of government and other policymakers. As Canada, Australia, and the States of California and Massachusetts have shown, increasing taxes on tobacco is the single most effective way to decrease tobacco use in a country or State. Nationally supported antismoking media campaigns also are needed to interact with and magnify the effect of community actions. Enforcement of existing laws in tobacco sales to minors, policies on vending machines, and restrictions and bans on advertising are also governmental responsibilities.

Adding these governmental activities to countrywide community-based activities could result in a synergistic interaction that would strengthen and propel a national movement toward a truly smoke-free society. This also might help us gain the courage, wisdom, and moral force to mobilize a nation of joiners and stem the ruthless expansion of tobacco companies into developing countries.

The COMMIT field experience, as described in this pioneering monograph, supplies powerful lessons and important tools for the public health movement by demonstrating the simple truth: Comprehensive community interventions do make a difference.

John W. Farquhar, M.D.
Professor of Medicine
Professor of Health Research
  and Policy
Stanford University

Acknowledgments

Community-Based Interventions for Smokers:The COMMIT Field Experience was developed under the general editorship of the Smoking and Tobacco Control Program (STCP), National Cancer Institute (NCI), **Donald R. Shopland**, Coordinator.

The senior scientific editor for the Community Intervention Trial for Smoking Cessation (COMMIT) monograph was **Beti Thompson, Ph.D.**, Associate Member, Cancer Prevention Research Unit, Fred Hutchinson Cancer Research Center, Seattle, Washington. Contributing editors were **David M. Burns, M.D.**, Professor of Medicine, University of California at San Diego Medical Center, San Diego, California, and **William R. Lynn**, COMMIT Project Officer, Cancer Control Science Program, Division of Cancer Prevention and Control, National Cancer Institute, National Institutes of Health, Bethesda, Maryland.

The editors and STCP staff members would like to express their sincere appreciation to **Terry F. Pechacek, Ph.D.**, for the energy he brought to the COMMIT project, especially during the early stages of the trial, and for the leadership, direction, and support he gave to COMMIT. Dr. Pechacek served as the NC1 Program Director for COMMIT from 1987 to 1991; he is currently with the Department of Social and Preventive Medicine, State University of New York at Buffalo, Buffalo, New York.

The STCP staff members gratefully acknowledge the COMMIT field directors, staff members and volunteers, and authors who made this monograph possible. The organizational/institutional affiliations listed below represent the authors principal affiliation during the COMMIT trial. At the end of each chapter, each author's current organizational affiliation with complete address is provided. Individual chapter attributions follow:

Chapter 1.   **Smoking Control and the COMMIT Experience— Summary and Overview**

Donald R. Shopland
National Cancer Institute
Bethesda, MD

David M. Burns, M.D.
University of California at San Diego
    Medical Center
San Diego, CA

Beti Thompson, Ph.D.
Fred Hutchinson Cancer Research Center
Seattle, WA

William R. Lynn
National Cancer Institute
Bethesda, MD

Len C. Stanley, M.P.H.
Research Triangle Institute
Research Triangle Park, NC

Juliet Thompson
Fred Hutchinson Cancer Research Center
Seattle, WA

Kitty K. Corbett, Ph.D., M.P.H.
Division of Research
Kaiser Permanente Medical Care Program
Oakland, CA

Chapter 6. Activities To Involve the Smoking Public in Tobacco Control in COMMIT

Russell C. Sciandra
Roswell Park Memorial Institute
Buffalo, NY

Lawrence Wallack, Dr.P.H.
Division of Research
Kaiser Permanente Medical Care Program
Oakland, CA

Carolyn L. Johnson, R.N.
Oregon Research Institute
Eugene, OR

Janine Sadlik
Roswell Park Memorial Institute
Buffalo, NY

Juliet Thompson
Fred Hutchinson Cancer Research Center
Seattle, WA

Chapter 7. Changing Public Policy Around Tobacco Control in the COMMIT Communities

David S. Carrell, Ph.D.
University of Washington
Seattle, WA

Carolyn L. Johnson, R.N.
Oregon Research Institute
Eugene, OR

Len C. Stanley, M.P.H.
Research Triangle Institute
Research Triangle Park, NC

Juliet Thompson
Fred Hutchinson Cancer Research Center
Seattle, WA

Sandy Tosti, M.A.
Division of Research
Kaiser Permanente Medical Care Program
Berkeley, CA

Edward Lichtenstein, Ph.D.
Oregon Research Institute
Eugene, OR

Paul R. Pomrehn, M.D.
University of Iowa
Iowa City, IA

Russell C. Sciandra
Roswell Park Memorial Institute
Buffalo, NY

Elizabeth A. Lindsay, Ph.D.
University of Waterloo
Waterloo, Ontario
CANADA

Norman Hymowitz, Ph.D.
University of Medicine and Dentistry of
    New Jersey Medical School
Newark, NJ

Robert E. Mecklenburg, D.D.S., M.P.H.
R.O.W. Sciences, Inc.
Rockville, MD

Linda C. Churchill, M.S.
University of Massachusetts Medical
    School
Worcester, MA

Blake Poland, Ph.D.
University of Waterloo
Waterloo, Ontario
CANADA

Linda Nettekoven, M.A.
Oregon Research Institute
Eugene, OR

Russell E. Glasgow, Ph.D.
Oregon Research Institute
Eugene, OR

Robert H. Shipley, Ph.D.
Research Triangle Institute
Research Triangle Park, NC

A.J. Roy Cameron, Ph.D.
University of Waterloo
Waterloo, Ontario
CANADA

Lesa T. Dalton
American Health Foundation
New York, NY

Aleena Erickson
University of Iowa
Iowa City, IA

Sharon Ann Rankins-Burd
Roswell Park Memorial Institute
Buffalo, NY

Sandy Tosti, M.A.
Division of Research
Kaiser Permanente Medical Care Program
Oakland, CA

Glorian Sorensen, Ph.D., M.P.H.
University of Massachusetts Medical
    School
Worcester, MA

Kitty K. Corbett, Ph.D., M.P.H.
Division of Research
Kaiser Permanente Medical Care Program
Oakland, CA

Chapter 11. Involving Diverse Community Organizations in Tobacco Control Activities

Kitty K. Corbett, Ph.D., M.P.H.
Division of Research
Kaiser Permanente Medical Care Program
Oakland, CA

Linda Nettekoven, M.A.
Oregon Research Institute
Eugene, OR

Linda C. Churchill, M.S.
University of Massachusetts Medical
    School
Worcester, MA

Lesa T. Dalton
American Health Foundation
New York, NY

Carolyn L. Johnson, R.N.
Oregon Research Institute
Eugene, OR

Lysha Dickinson
Division of Research
Kaiser Permanente Medical Care Program
Oakland, CA

Glorian Sorensen, Ph.D., M.P.H.
University of Massachusetts Medical
    School
Worcester, MA

Beti Thompson, Ph.D.
Fred Hutchinson Cancer Research Center
Seattle, WA

Chapter 12. Promoting Communitywide Tobacco Control Activities by Involving Schools

Deborah Bowen, Ph.D.
Fred Hutchinson Cancer Research Center
Seattle, WA

Lesa T. Dalton
American Health Foundation
New York, NY

Rosemary Walker, M.Sc.
Research Triangle Institute
Research Triangle Park, NC

Susan Crystal
University of Washington
Seattle, WA

Mario A. Orlandi, Ph.D., M.P.H.
American Health Foundation
New York, NY

Chapter 13. Involving Youth in Awareness of, Promotion of, and Political Activities for Tobacco Control

Robert J. McGranaghan, M.P.H.
Division of Research
Kaiser Permanente Medical Care Program
Oakland, CA

Sharon Ann Rankins-Burd
Roswell Park Memorial Institute
Buffalo, NY

Ted Purcell
University of Massachusetts Medical
    Center
Worcester, MA

Chapter 14. What Have We Learned and Where Do We Go From Here?

Beti Thompson, Ph.D.
Fred Hutchinson Cancer Research Center
Seattle, WA

William R. Lynn
National Cancer Institute
Bethesda, MD

Donald R. Shopland
National Cancer Institute
Bethesda, MD

The editors would like to acknowledge with sincere appreciation the following distinguished scientists, researchers, and others who contributed critical reviews:

Glen Bennett, M.P.H.
Coordinator
Advanced Technologies Applications
   in Health Education Programs
National Heart, Lung, and Blood Institute
National Institutes of Health
Bethesda, MD

Richard A. Carleton, M.D.
Professor of Medicine
Brown University School of Medicine
Chief of Cardiology
Memorial Hospital of Rhode Island
Pawtucket, RI

Michael P. Eriksen, Sc.D.
Director
Office on Smoking and Health
National Center for Chronic Disease Prevention
   and Health Promotion
Centers for Disease Control and Prevention
Atlanta, GA

John W. Farquhar, M.D.
Director
Stanford Center for Research
   in Disease Prevention
Stanford University
Palo Alto, CA

Terry F. Pechacek, Ph.D.
Associate Professor
Department of Social and Preventive Medicine
State University of New York at Buffalo
Buffalo, NY

Cheryl L. Perry, Ph.D.
Professor
Division of Epidemiology
University of Minnesota School of Public Health
Minneapolis, MN

THE COMMIT RESEARCH GROUP

The COMMIT Research Group comprises NCI staff members, advisers, and contractors responsible for the overall design and implementation of the COMMIT trial and is composed of the following individuals:

National Cancer Institute

Division of Cancer Prevention and Control (DCPC), Cancer Control Science Program (CCSP)

CCSP Acting Associate Director, Thomas J. Glynn, Ph.D.; Coordinator, Smoking and Tobacco Control Program, Donald R. Shopland

Public Health Applications Research Branch, DCPC, CCSP. Chief, Marc Manley, M.D., M.P.H.; COMMIT Program Director, William R. Lynn

Biometry Branch, DCPC. Acting Chief, Laurence S. Freedman; Lead Research Investigator, Sylvan B. Green, M.D.; Computer Systems Analyst, Donald K. Corle, MS.; Mathematical Statisticians, Barry Graubard, Ph.D., Stuart Baker, Ph.D.

Prevention and Control Extramural Research Branch, DCPC, CCSP. Acting Chief, Sherry L. Mills, M.D., M.P.H.; Public Health Adviser, Daria A. Chapelsky, M.P.H.

Division of Cancer Etiology

Biostatistics Branch. Head, Epidemiologic Methods Section, Mitchell Gail, M.D., Ph.D.; Medical Statistician, Steven Mark, M.D., Sc.D.

Chair, COMMIT Steering Committee

Erwin Bettinghaus, Ph.D., M.A., Michigan State University

Collaborating Research Institutions

American Health Foundation (New York, New York)

Principal Investigator: Mario A. Orlandi, Ph.D., M.P.H.; Co-Principal Investigator: Alfred McAlister, Ph.D.; Co-Investigators: Jacqueline Royce, Ph.D.; Eugene Lewit, Ph.D.; Project Director: Lesa T. Dalton, B.A.; Field Director: Avril Dawkins, B.A.; Community Analyst: Bonnie Edelman, B.S.

Fred Hutchinson Cancer Research Center (Seattle, Washington)

    Principal Investigator: Beti Thompson, Ph.D.; Co-Investigators: Maureen
Henderson, M.D., Dr.P.H.; Deborah Bowen, Ph.D.; Community Analyst:
K. Mark Leek, M.A.; Field Director: Juliet Thompson, B.A.

Kaiser Permanente Medical Care Program, Northern California Region,
Division of Research (Oakland, California)

    Principal Investigator: Lawrence Wallack, Dr.P.H.; Co-Investigator:
Kitty K. Corbett, Ph.D., M.P.H.; Project Director: Robert J. McGranaghan,
M.P.H.; Field Director: Sandy Tosti, M.A.; Field Director (until 1/90):
Joan Bennett, M.A.

Lovelace Medical Foundation (Albuquerque, New Mexico)

    Principal Investigator: Neil1 F. Piland, Dr.P.H.; Project Director:
Lawrence R. Berger, M.D., M.P.H.; Community Analyst: Annette M.
Phillipp, M.P.H.; Field Director: Aile Shebar, R.N.

Oregon Research Institute (Eugene, Oregon)

    Principal Investigator: Edward Lichtenstein, Ph.D.; Co-Principal
Investigator: Russell E. Glasgow, Ph.D.; Project Coordinator: Linda
Nettekoven, M.A.; Field Director: Carolyn L. Johnson, R.N.; Community
Analyst: Shari Reyna, M.A.

Research Triangle Institute (Research Triangle Park, North Carolina)

    Principal Investigator: Tyler D. Hartwell, Ph.D.; Co-Principal
Investigator: Robert H. Shipley, Ph.D.; Project Director: David Austin,
M.S., M.P.H.; Project Director (until 9/89): Elizabeth T. Walker, B.S.;
Field Director: Len C. Stanley, M.P.H.; Community Analyst: Bonnie
Veaner, M.P.H.; Community Organizer: Carol Stephenson, B.S.

Roswell Park Memorial Institute (Buffalo, New York)

    Principal Investigator:K. Michael Cummings, Ph.D., M.P.H.; Co-
Principal Investigator: Terry F. Pechacek, Ph.D.; Project Director: Russell
C. Sciandra, M.A.; Community Analyst: Eva Anderson Sciandra, B.S;
Field Directors: Janine Sadlik, B.S., Sharon Ann Rankins-Burd.

University of Iowa (Jowa City, Iowa)

    Principal Investigator: Paul R. Pomrehn, M.D., M.S.; Project Director:
John E. Ferguson, Ph.D.; Co-Investigators: Kristi J. Ferguson, Ph.D.;
Robert B. Wallace, M.D., M.S.; Samuel L. Becker, Ph.D.; Harry A. Lando,
Ph.D. (University of Minnesota); Community Analyst: Virginia
Daughety, Ph.D.; Community Analyst (until 2/92): Kelly O'Berry, B.S.;
Field Director: Aleena Erickson, B.A.

University of Massachusetts Medical School (Worcester, Massachusetts)

> Principal Investigator: Judith K. Ockene, Ph.D.; Co-Principal Investigator: Glorian Sorensen, Ph.D., M.P.H.; Project Coordinator: Linda C. Churchill, M.S.; Field Director: Barbara Silva; Community Organizers: Philip Merriam, M.S.P.H.; Gary Donnelly, M.P.H.; Community Analyst: Edward Purcell, B.S.; Community Analyst (until 7/89): Kristine Sanden, B.S.

University of Medicine and Dentistry of New Jersey (Newark, New Jersey)

> Principal Investigator: Norman Hymowitz, Ph.D.; Co-Principal Investigators: Lawrence Meinert, M.D.; Lee B. Reichman, M.D.; Norman L. Lasser, M.D., Ph.D.; John Slade, M.D.; Project Director: Karel Campbell, B.A.; Co-Project Director: Janice Marshall, R.N., M.S.N.; Field Director: Sharon Jones Rudolph, B.S.; Community Analyst: Connie Strickland Farrakhan, M.A.

University of Waterloo (Waterloo, Ontario) and McMaster University (Hamilton, Ontario, Canada)

> Principal Investigator: J. Allan Best, Ph.D.; Co-Investigators: A.J. Roy Cameron, Ph.D.; Charles H. Goldsmith, Ph.D.; Elizabeth A. Lindsay, Ph.D., M.S.; Blake Poland, Ph.D.; Nancy A. Ross, M.A.; Edward Smith, Dr.P.H. (until (6/89); S. Martin Taylor, Ph.D.; Leslie Van Dover, Ph.D., R.N.; Norman F. White, M.D.; Douglas M.C. Wilson, M.D.; Mark P. Zanna, Ph.D.; Project Director: Rosemary Walker, M.Sc.; Community Analyst: Terri Finch, B.A.; Field Director: Dianne Ferster

COMMIT Coordinating Center

Information Management Services, Inc. (Silver Spring, Maryland)

> Principal Investigator: Janis A. Beach, A.A.; Co-Principal Investigator: Carol A. Giffen, D.V.M.; Project Director: Marie A. Topor, B.S.; Senior Information Specialists: Jerome L. Felix, M.A.; Lauren E. Rich, B.S.; Systems Analysts: James J. Rovan, B.S.; Rusty Shields, B.S.; Survey Statistician: Charles D. Palit, Ph.D.; Biostatistician: David Pee, M. Phil.; Project Coordinator: Mary L. Lamb, B.A.

Policy Advisory Committee (PAC)

> Chair: Virginia L. Ernster, Ph.D.; Karl Bauman, Ph.D.; David M. Burns, M.D.; Richard A. Carleton, M.D.; William 'I'. Friedewald, M.D.; Charles Hennekens, M.D., Dr.P.H.; Donald Iverson, Ph.D. (also served as Chair [1987-1988]); Kenneth E. Warner, Ph.D.

Finally, the editors would like to acknowledge the significant contributions of the following staff members of R.O.W. Sciences, Inc., Rockville, MD, who provided technical and editorial assistance in the preparation of this monograph. In particular, the editors would like to acknowledge the contribution of

Richard H. Amacher, MS., R.O.W. Project Director, who served as Project Manager for the contract under which this publication was produced.

Douglas Bishop, Art Director

Rebecca A. Charton, Senior Librarian

Faye Grant, Administrative Secretary

Catherine Hageman, Word Processing Supervisor

Sabrina Hinton, Administrative Secretary

James R. Libbey, Managing Editor

Frances Nebesky, Senior Copyeditor

Donna Selig, Proofreader

Barbara Shine, Proofreader

Donna Tharpe, Quality Control Proofreader

Ruth Thompson, Word Processing Specialist

Keith W. Stanger, Graphics Services Coordinator

Sonia Van Putten, Word Processing Specialist

COMMIT MONOGRAPH DEVELOPMENT PROCESS

This represents the sixth volume in the smoking and tobacco control monograph series. The compilation process for this volume was slightly different from those generally followed in the past.

In 1993, the STCP Coordinator and COMMIT Program Director presented a concept for the volume to the COMMIT Printing and Publications Committee (P & P). The committee was established as one of several mechanisms to help prioritize manuscripts generated from the trial and to develop a process for coordinating and accessing trialwide data. In addition to offering helpful suggestions for the content and overall approach to the volume, the committee asked Dr. Beti Thompson to serve as one of the volume's scientific editors. In addition to Dr. Thompson, editors included Dr. David M. Burns and Mr. William R. Lynn.

STCP staff members, in consultation with the volume's scientific editors, developed a detailed outline for the volume along with a list of potential authors who represented COMMIT Principal Investigators and COMMIT field staff. The inclusion of the latter was critical given the primary purpose of the volume was to document the COMMIT intervention field experience-both positive and negative. Although individual chapters were generally written by a COMMIT Principal Investigator, the experience of the COMMIT field staff members formed the basis of what occurred at the community level. This hands-on experience was documented by COMMIT's extensive collection of program records and case studies. A meeting of authors and editors was held to help guide the effort, answer questions, develop a working outline, and make writing assignments. Several iterations of each chapter were usually necessary before a final draft was submitted to NCI.

Once a "final" draft of the entire volume was completed, NCI sent copies to a small group of experts who were asked to critically review the volume. These reviewers, acknowledged above, were chosen for their specific knowledge and expertise in community-based health programs. Comments received from these individuals were sent to the scientific editors for their consideration and possible integration into the volume.

This monograph, *Community-Based Interventions for Smokers: The COMMIT Field Experience,* is the work of dozens of individuals-STCP trial investigators and staff, smoking control experts, and outside scientists and experts. The monograph is organized into 14 separate chapters within 3 sections as laid out in the "Contents," which immediately follows.

Contents

Smoking Control and the COMMIT Experience—Summary and Overview

Donald R. Shopland, David M. Burns, Beti Thompson, and William R. Lynn

INTRODUCTION   Tobacco use, especially the practice of cigarette smoking, remains the largest preventable cause of death and disability in the United States, producing more than $50 billion in health care costs in 1993 (Bartlett et al., 1994). This continuing disease burden overshadows the substantial progress made in reducing the prevalence of smoking in the past 40 years (Burns et al., in preparation; Shopland, 1995). In 1955, nearly 60 percent of adult men and nearly 30 percent of adult women were regular cigarette smokers (Haenszel et al., 1956). Currently, 25 percent of adults in the United States are cigarette smokers, but only 20.4 percent, one in every five, report they smoke on a daily basis (Centers for Disease Control and Prevention, 1994).

Changes in smoking behavior have occurred with, and been partially driven by, gradually evolving efforts to influence smoking behavior (U.S. Department of Health and Human Services, 1991). Initial efforts in public information and education were followed by the development of behavioral and pharmacologic approaches to assist smokers to achieve and maintain a nonsmoking status. The limited success of these efforts with individual smokers eventually led to an understanding of smoking as an addictive process in which social forces played a critical role in both initiation and maintenance of the behavior. The potential of broadly structured community-based interventions providing persistent and inescapable messages to quit smoking was recognized and formed the scientific foundation for the Community Intervention Trial for Smoking Cessation (COMMIT) discussed in this volume.

As the content of this monograph clearly demonstrates, a great deal has been learned about mobilizing communities and organizing their efforts to change smoking behavior. The impact of COMMIT's community organization approach on smokers' behavior was modest, at least for the first 4 years of the intervention. Although no change was noted in the target group of heavy smokers, there was a statistically significant difference in the quit rates between intervention and comparison communities among light-to-moderate smokers (COMMIT Research Group, 1995a and 1995b). Light-to-moderate smokers, it should be emphasized, comprise 80 percent of the U.S. adult smoking population (Giovino et al., 1994).

Although COMMIT did not accelerate the quit rate among heavy smokers, the larger-than-expected percentage of smokers who quit throughout the communities demonstrated that many aspects of the national effort were working. It remains to be determined the extent to which broad policy-based interventions, other alternative tobacco control strategies, or a longer duration of community-based interventions will substantially alter smoking behavior, particularly among heavy smokers.

One clear result of the approaches described in this volume was successful mobilization and organization of communities around an externally defined public health objective. All the communities were successful in developing an organizational structure and using that structure to accomplish a defined set of objectives contained in the COMMIT protocol. This success is the focus of this monograph. A better understanding of what works and what does not work in efforts to mobilize a community around a public health goal is one of the most valuable results of COMMIT.

The findings in the intervention vs. comparison communities in COMMIT need to be placed in an appropriate perspective. There was no difference between intervention and comparison communities among smokers consuming 25 or more cigarettes daily (heavy smokers), but 18 percent of those smokers in both communities quit smoking during the 4 years of the trial. Similarly, 30.6 percent of smokers of fewer than 25 cigarettes per day (light-to-moderate smokers) quit smoking in the intervention communities vs. only 27.5 percent in the comparison communities (COMMIT Research Group, 1995a and 1995b). These data clearly demonstrate that substantial rates of cessation occurred among light-to-moderate and heavy smokers. The results of the trial do not demonstrate that it is difficult to get smokers to quit; large numbers of both light-to-moderate and heavy smokers did so. The results of the trial do demonstrate that it is difficult to use many of the traditional public health approaches to tobacco control, delivered by means of a community organization structure, to dramatically accelerate the already high rates of cessation occurring in the population.

In addition, the intervention approach did demonstrate an effect that has significant public health implications among the light-to-moderate smokers in the trial, especially compared with the general difficulty in changing other addictive behaviors. Furthermore, this effect was greatest among those smokers with a high school education or less, a group in which cessation rates have been relatively low and on whom other intervention approaches have had little effect. This effort, produced by means of a public health mode of delivery, shows the great potential of such prevention efforts to provide additional years of quality life to the population in a more cost-effective fashion than disease treatments by the health care delivery system.

TRENDS IN THE MAGNITUDE OF SMOKING AS A PUBLIC HEALTH PROBLEM

The focus of any public health intervention should be reduction of incidence and prevalence rates in the entire population, and it is useful to measure tobacco control efforts by this yardstick. Figure 1 demonstrates that during the past 40 years the prevalence of smoking among white males has been cut in half, from nearly 60 percent in 1955 to less than 30 percent in 1993 (Haenszel et al., 1956; Centers for Disease Control and Prevention, 1994). The figure shows that the change in prevalence among white females is more modest, dropping from approximately 30 percent in 1955 to 22.5 percent in 1993, but the absolute prevalence remains lower among females than among males.

Figure 1
Prevalence of cigarette smoking among adults by race and gender, United States, 1955-93

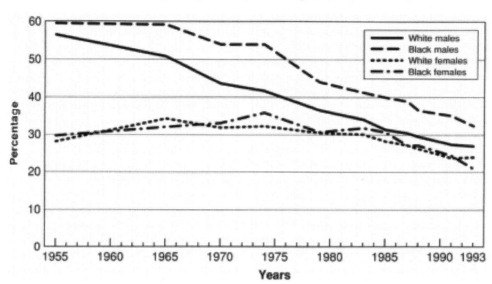

Source: *Shopland, 1995.*

Figure 1 shows that the change in smoking prevalence among blacks is only slightly less successful, with rates among black males falling from 60 percent in 1955 to 32.4 percent in 1993. Smoking prevalence changes among black females are nearly identical to those in white females.

Slowing the rate at which adolescents become smokers has proven more difficult than convincing older smokers to quit. About one-third of high-school-age adolescents use some form of tobacco (Giovino et al., 1994). Initiation rates among older adolescents have declined steadily (Burns et al., in press; Pierce et al., 1994), but changes among younger adolescents have been far less positive (Cummings et al., 1995).

Initiation rates among younger age adolescents (14 to 17 years old) decreased slightly from 1980 to 1984 but increased between 1985 and 1989 (Cummings et al., 1995). The largest annual increase occurred in 1988, the year the R.J. Reynolds Tobacco Company introduced its now famous "Joe the Camel" cartoon character. Had initiation rates from 1985 to 1989 remained at the 1984 level, there would have been more than 500,000 fewer adolescent smokers in the United States during this time. In comparison, among young adults (ages 18 to 21), initiation rates decreased slightly during the 1980's (Cummings et al., 1995).

Smoking prevalence rates among black adolescents have declined (Institute of Medicine, 1994), whereas rates among white adolescents have

3

Figure 2
Prevalence of daily smoking among white and black high school seniors in the United States

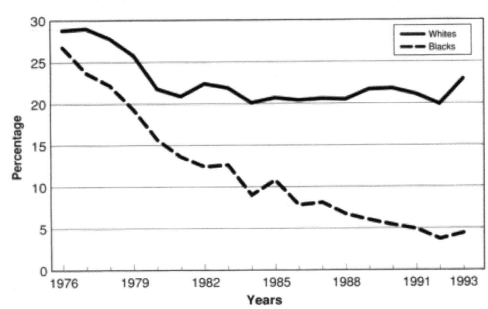

Source: *Johnston et al., 1994.*

changed little (Figure 2). Although current estimates of smoking initiation rates for adolescents are not available, smoking prevalence increased among 8th- and 10th-grade students nationally between 1991 and 1993 (Johnston et al., 1994). These trends coincided with aggressive new marketing practices by the cigarette industry, many of which are reaching children (U.S. Department of Health and Human Services, 1994).

The effort to alter the public health problem of tobacco use has clearly made substantial progress over the past 40 years; however, we have had greater success in aiding smokers to break their addiction than we have had in preventing children from becoming addicted. In understanding this differing response by adults who are already addicted and children who have not yet become smokers, it is critical to examine the activities of the tobacco industry during the period of these tobacco control efforts.

ACTIVITIES OF THE TOBACCO INDUSTRY Over the past four decades, the tobacco industry has aggressively responded to each major public health initiative directed at reducing smoking with a combination of efforts intended to undermine these initiatives. The industry introduced a series of new product modifications, including filtered cigarettes in the 1950's and low-tar cigarettes in the 1970's, to allay the public's concern about the health risks of smoking and to convince people that whatever risks existed had been either reduced drastically or eliminated. More important, during the past 40 years, cigarette manufacturers have conducted massive, annual, multibillion dollar advertising campaigns to convince smokers and potential smokers to smoke.

During the time COMMIT interventions were in the field (midfall 1988 through 1992), outlays for all cigarette advertising and promotional expenditures *almost equaled the amount spent the previous 10 years* (Federal Trade Commission, 1995). Expenditures increased 60 percent during the relatively brief COMMIT intervention period, from $3.28 billion in 1988 to more than $5.3 billion in 1992 (unadjusted for inflation) (Figure 3).

The most recent data from the Federal Trade Commission show that cigarette manufacturers spent more than $6 billion for advertising and promotional expenditures in 1993, the last year complete data are available (Federal Trade Commission, 1995). This represents more than a 15-percent increase over 1992 (Table 1).

Significant changes also have occurred in the types and categories of advertising and promotional activities conducted. When the U.S. Congress banned cigarette advertising on electronic media in 1971, the bulk of cigarette advertising shifted to print media and outdoor and transit advertising. Until the early 1980's, these categories accounted for the preponderance of all cigarette advertising and promotional expenditures.

Figure 3
Domestic cigarette advertising and promotional expenses, 1963-93*

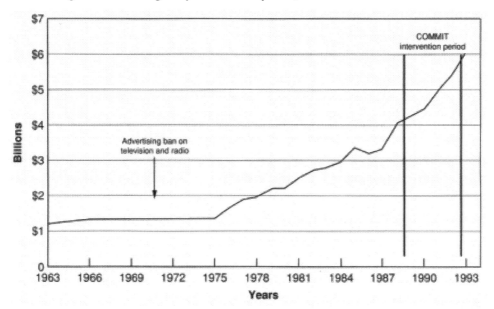

* All expenditures were converted to 1993 dollars.
Source: Federal Trade Commission, 1995.

Table 1

Domestic cigarette advertising and promotional expenditures, by type and category, United States 1992 and 1993 (in thousands of dollars)

Type of Advertising	1992 ($)	% of Total	1993 ($)	% of Total	% Change From 1992
Newspapers	35,467	.7	36,204	.6	+2.0
Magazines	237,061	4.5	235,195	3.9	-.08
Outdoor	295,657	5.7	231,450	3.8	-21.7
Transit	53,293	1.0	39,113	.6	-26.6
Point of Sale	366,036	7.0	400,909	6.6	+9.5
Promotional Allowances	1,514,026	28.9	1,557,505	25.8	+2.9
Sampling Distribution	49,315	.9	40,190	.7	-18.5
Specialty Item Distribution	339,997	6.5	755,761	12.5	+122.0
Public Entertainment	89,739	1.7	84,275	1.4	-6.1
Direct Mail	34,345	.7	31,463	.5	-8.3
Coupons and Retail Value-Added Promotions	2,175,373	41.6	2,559,170	42.4	+15.0
All Others	41,608	.8	63,915	1.2	+53.6
Total	5,231,917	100.0	6,034,915	100.0	+15.4

Source: Federal Trade Commission, 1995.

However, from the early 1980's onward, the cigarette industry increasingly began to emphasize promotional activities, and each year the industry has committed a larger share of its total advertising and promotional budgets to these types of activities. Promotional allowances and coupons and retail value added accounted for nearly 70 percent of all expenditures in 1993. Less than 10 percent of all expenditures were devoted to advertising in newspapers, magazines, and outdoor and transit advertising. Nonetheless, the dollar amount allocated for these categories was nearly $542 million for 1993, a sum that exceeded the total spent for all domestic cigarette advertising in 1975 (unadjusted for inflation) (Federal Trade Commission, 1995).

Promotional allowances, which accounted for approximately one-quarter of the $6 billion spent in 1993, are various incentives and fees paid by a manufacturer to wholesalers and retailers to stock and promote a company's products. By far the single largest amount spent in 1993 was for coupons and value-added promotions—more than $2.5 billion—an increase of nearly $400 million from the previous year.

Specialty item distribution accounted for more than $755 million in expenditures for 1993—more than double the amount spent in 1992—and now accounts for nearly 12 percent of all advertising expenditures. This category includes the practice of putting a brand's logo on such things as T-shirts, caps, sunglasses, sporting goods, and so forth that either are sold to the consumer or can be ordered from catalogs in exchange for package premiums or coupons. Recent studies have shown that tobacco company advertising of promotional activities is reaching adolescents. Among persons ages 12 to 17 in 1992, 25 percent of nonsmoking adolescents reported having received promotional items from tobacco companies; nearly 50 percent of smoking teens reported having received such items (U.S. Department of Health and Human Services, 1994). Another study (Biener et al., 1994) found 52 percent of Boston 12- to 17-year-olds reported having seen a tobacco company catalog, and 54 percent reported knowing someone younger than 18 years who owned a tobacco promotional item.

During the interval that public health efforts to reduce tobacco use have been increasing, there has been a disproportionate increase in advertising and promotional activity by the tobacco industry, and this increased activity has been accompanied by a shift to promotional activities that may have a greater attraction for adolescents than for adults (Institute of Medicine, 1994). This enormous allocation of resources by the tobacco industry undoubtedly has slowed the rates of positive changes in smoking behavior over the past 40 years, and all current and future tobacco control efforts should be examined in the context of this growing industry effort to keep smokers smoking and recruit adolescents to the smoking ranks.

COMMIT AND THE EVOLUTION OF THE NATIONAL CANCER INSTITUTE'S SMOKING AND TOBACCO CONTROL PROGRAM
Tobacco use research at the National Cancer Institute (NCI) began in the early 1950's when cigarette smoking was first linked with lung cancer (U.S. Congress, 1957). Over the next decades, NCI funded hundreds of millions of dollars in basic and applied research on smoking and health (U.S. Department of Health and Human Services, 1990). NCI's early research concentrated on the areas of tobacco use epidemiology; the chemistry, pharmacology, and toxicology of tobacco and tobacco smoke; autopsy studies; and experimental tobacco carcinogenesis. During the early 1970's, NCI shifted its research focus to identify hazardous substances in tobacco smoke and ways to reduce or eliminate their presence (National Cancer Institute and National Heart, Lung, and Blood Institute, 1978). In the late 1970's, NCI's smoking research focus shifted again to include an examination of behavioral issues related to why people smoked.

In 1982, coincident with the release of the Surgeon General's report on cancer (U.S. Department of Health and Human Services, 1982), NCI began a major planning effort to reduce the national prevalence of tobacco use and thereby attain a significant reduction in those cancers most associated with tobacco consumption. NCI initiated a research program to identify effective approaches to reach individual smokers and persuade them to quit and to encourage adolescents not to start.

Priorities for targeting intervention research were identified from a systematic approach that used consensus development involving hundreds of scientists and other experts (Greenwald et al., 1987). The resulting consensus was a two-pronged strategy, the first of which included:

- physician and dentist interventions to reduce patient smoking prevalence;

- self-help and minimal interventions to provide materials and strategies to individuals who wish to quit on their own; and

- mass media interventions using electronic and print media to encourage cessation and prevention of tobacco use initiation.

The second prong of the strategy targeted populations with needs for specific interventions or (as with youth) primary targets for prevention of initiation. These strategies included:

- population interventions, including people of color, women, and ethnic populations, to develop appropriate smoking prevention and cessation programs;

- school-based programs to develop curricula to prevent the onset of tobacco use among adolescents; and

- interventions to prevent the initiation of spitting tobacco use and promote cessation.

Results from nearly 60 controlled trials helped guide the COMMIT effort and efforts by other Institutes within the National Institutes of Health as well as other Public Health Service (PHS) and non-PHS agencies. For example, the National Heart, Lung, and Blood Institute has funded community risk-factor-reduction projects (Farquhar et al., 1984; Lasater et al., 1984; Blackburn et al., 1984) as well as clinical interventions directed at individuals considered at high risk for heart disease (Multiple Risk Factor Intervention Trial Research Group, 1982), all involving adult smokers. These efforts, like COMMIT, were designed during the 1970's and early 1980's and were based on what, at that time, was considered the state of the art in smoking cessation interventions, especially for reaching heavy smokers. Cessation results from U.S.-based cardiovascular risk reduction trials, although mixed generally, have been positive. For example, the Stanford Five-City Project observed a greater decline in smoking prevalence in their treatment communities than in controls, based on their cohort survey, with a larger treatment effect in men than women (Fortmann et al., 1993); the Minnesota Heart Health Program reported a modest intervention effect on prevalence of smoking among women but not men in their cross-sectional analysis but reported no effect for either in their cohort sample (Lando et al., 1995; Luepker et al., 1994); and the Pawtucket Heart Health Program reported no significant intervention effect (Carleton et al., 1995). Similar findings have been observed from studies in other countries. (See Chapter 2 for further discussion.)

Recently, it has become clear that policy interventions aimed at changing the social context and general environment in which tobacco is purchased and consumed are as or more important than delivery of cessation and prevention services (U.S. Department of Health and Human Services, 1991). Smoking control policy interventions need to be integrated with community-based service delivery efforts if they are to be considered comprehensive, and many of these policy changes often require change at a higher social and political level than the local community (e.g., tax increases).

COMMIT did not attempt to change communitywide policies but rather worked within the policy framework that existed within each community at the time the interventions were implemented. Although it was not the intent of the COMMIT protocol to change communitywide laws and regulations, effort was put into increasing the influence of existing policies and economic factors that discourage smoking (COMMIT Research Group, 1995a and 1995b). COMMIT actively emphasized the benefits of policies such as smoke-free environments for worksites, health care facilities, and other community organization sites, but these policies were accomplished primarily through individual consultations or group seminars. No systematic effort was made to implement change throughout the community either through communitywide ordinances or regulations.

Scientific evidence continues to accumulate to demonstrate the potential for policy interventions to modify cigarette smoking behavior among adults and children (U.S. Department of Health and Human Services, 1991; Tobacco Control, 1992; Institute of Medicine, 1994). Implementation of tobacco policy change is best accomplished at the State and local levels through community and coalition support for policies in several important areas: smoke-free indoor air, implementation and enforcement of laws and ordinances limiting minors' access to tobacco products, cigarette tax increases, and reduction or elimination of certain cigarette advertising and promotional activities.

PURPOSE OF THIS MONOGRAPH   The purpose of this monograph is to present a synthesis of the operational and process lessons learned from COMMIT. The monograph is specifically intended to provide detailed information about the COMMIT intervention process in a manner not possible in scientific journals. The writers and editors have attempted to distill this information in a format that is particularly useful to individuals interested in a community-based approach to smoking control and that describes how to effectively organize, develop, and implement a comprehensive program aimed at adult smokers at the local level.

The overall lessons learned from the COMMIT field experience are discussed in more detail in Chapter 14. Briefly, they include these findings:

- It is possible to establish a partnership with communities so that they will organize around a community problem.

- It is possible to promote a research agenda even when that agenda is not the primary problem facing a community.

- Community volunteers are willing and able to plan intervention activities that are congruent with an intervention protocol.

- Community volunteers are willing to implement intervention activities.

- The COMMIT model of community organization and structure of Boards and task forces was well received and is relevant for use with other community problems.

- Community volunteers would have liked outcome data during the trial so that they could make midcourse corrections, if necessary.

- Communities were interested in continuing tobacco control activities. An earlier planning period for transition and assistance in obtaining additional resources would have been useful.

- Resources are important in maintaining tobacco control; however, organized groups can effectively take on tobacco control with few external resources.

Operational experience with what works and does not work at the programmatic level frequently provides the core for interventions tested in controlled scientific investigations. Current concepts of what constitutes effective approaches to tobacco control frequently outstrip both the tools needed to evaluate them and the data needed to definitively prove their impact.

The focus of this monograph is a description of how COMMIT was conducted rather than the outcome results. While the experience is fresh, the monograph attempts to present to the larger public health community the best judgments of the COMMIT research team about what constitutes a comprehensive, community-based approach to tobacco control for reaching adult smokers. It is hoped that this description will aid both those currently designing and implementing programs and those creating the next generation of scientific studies in tobacco control.

The monograph is organized to follow the research channels used in the COMMIT communities. Each chapter contains a brief rationale for intervening through a particular channel and then describes experiences across the trial. The monograph is intended to be descriptive. Toward that end, chapters conclude with a section on lessons learned or what could have been done differently.

The monograph may be read as a unit or in sections of particular interest. Chapters 2 through 4 provide descriptions of the project and are included for those who wish to understand the research aspects as well as applications from the field. Chapter 2 provides a context for community studies. Chapter 3 describes COMMIT and the evaluation plan for the trial, and Chapter 4 focuses on the development of the intervention.

Chapter 5 describes the process of understanding communities and mobilizing them to participate in tobacco control.

Chapters 6 through 13 cover individual channels of intervention used in COMMIT. Chapter 6 focuses on public education in COMMIT and includes information on media campaigns, communitywide campaigns, and contests to help smokers quit. Chapter 7 describes public policy changes in COMMIT communities and how community Boards and task forces worked for such changes. Chapter 8 describes how COMMIT sought to build the capacity of communities' cessation resources and services. Chapter 9 reviews the tobacco control activities of health care providers. Chapter 10 specifies how worksites were brought into intervention activities and encouraged to make policy changes. Chapter 11 reviews attempts made to draw community organizations into participating in intervention activities. Chapter 12 describes interventions conducted in schools, and Chapter 13 demonstrates how youth can become involved in tobacco control outside the school. Finally, Chapter 14 presents the overall lessons learned and the implications for future community-based tobacco control initiatives.

COMMIT INTERVENTION MATERIALS   The authors especially would like to call the readers' attention to the numerous samples of COMMIT resource materials located throughout the monograph. These materials represent a mere fraction of all intervention materials used and are presented to provide a better understanding of the range of materials developed. Of note is the variation of materials across the 11 geographically and ethnically diverse communities. Although the COMMIT sites implemented a standard protocol, the diversity of materials—from unique logos to culturally specific materials—reflects the adaptation of the protocol by individual communities. The community-specific aspect of the intervention materials also is an important indicator of the true community ownership of the COMMIT project.

Unfortunately, it was never the intention of NCI or the COMMIT research team to produce sufficient quantities of these materials for general distribution. *We regret that we are unable to honor requests for COMMIT resource materials.*

REFERENCES

Bartlett, J.C., Miller, L.S., Rice, D.P., Max, W.B. Medical care expenditures attributable to smoking—United States, 1993. *MMWR. Morbidity and Mortality Weekly Report* 43: 469-472, 1994.

Biener, L., Fowler, F.J., Roman, A.M. *Tobacco Advertising and Promotions: The Impact on Massachusetts Teens*. Boston: Massachusetts Department of Health, 1994.

Blackburn, H., Luepker, R.V., Kline, F.G., Bracht, N., Carlaw, R., Jacobs, D., Mittelmark, M., Stauffer, L., Taylor, H.L. The Minnesota Heart Health Program: A research and demonstration project in cardiovascular disease prevention. In: *Behavioral Health: A Handbook of Health Enhancement and Disease Prevention*, J.D. Matarazzo, S.M. Weiss, J.A. Herd, N.E. Miller, and S.M. Weiss (Editors). New York: John Wiley & Sons, 1984, pp. 1171-1178.

Burns, D.M., Lee, L., Shen, L.Z., Gilpin, E., Tolley, D., Vaughn, J., Shanks, T.G. Cigarette smoking behavior in the United States. In: *Changes in Cigarette-Related Disease Risks and Their Implication for Prevention and Control*. Smoking and Tobacco Control Monograph No. 7. Rockville, MD: U.S. Department of Health and Human Services, Public Health Service, National Institutes of Health, National Cancer Institute, in preparation.

Burns, D.M., Lee, L., Vaughn, J.W., Chiu, Y.K., Shopland, D.R. Rates of smoking initiation among adolescents and young adults, 1907-1981. *Tobacco Control: An International Journal*, in press.

Carleton, R.A., Lasater, T.M., Assaf, A.R., Feldman, H.A., McKinlay, S., and the Pawtucket Heart Health Program Writing Group. The Pawtucket Heart Health Program: Community changes in cardiovascular risk factors and projected disease risk. *American Journal of Public Health* 85(6): 777-785, 1995.

Centers for Disease Control and Prevention. Cigarette smoking among adults—United States, 1993. *MMWR. Morbidity and Mortality Weekly Report* 43: 925-930, 1994.

COMMIT Research Group. Community Intervention Trial for Smoking Cessation (COMMIT): I. Cohort results from a four-year community intervention. *American Journal of Public Health* 85: 183-192, 1995a.

COMMIT Research Group. Community Intervention Trial for Smoking Cessation (COMMIT): II. Changes in adult cigarette smoking prevalence. *American Journal of Public Health* 85: 193-200, 1995b.

Cummings, K.M., Shah, D., Shopland, D.R. Trends in smoking initiation among adolescents and young adults—United States, 1980-1989. *MMWR. Morbidity and Mortality Weekly Report* 44(28): 521-525, 1995.

Farquhar, J.W., Fortmann, S.P., Maccoby, N., Wood, P.D., Haskell, W.L., Taylor, C.B., Flora, J.A., Solomon, D.S., Rogers, T., Adler, E., Breitrose, P., Weiner, L. The Stanford Five City Project: An overview. In: *Behavioral Health: A Handbook of Health Enhancement and Disease Prevention*, J.D. Matarazzo, S.M. Weiss, J.A. Herd, N.E. Miller, and S.M. Weiss (Editors). New York: John Wiley & Sons, 1984, pp. 1154-1165.

Federal Trade Commission. *Federal Trade Commission Report to Congress for 1993. Pursuant to the Federal Cigarette Labeling and Advertising Act.* Washington, DC: Federal Trade Commission, 1995.

Fortmann, S.P., Taylor, C.B., Flora, J.A., Jatulis, D.E. Changes in adult cigarette smoking prevalence after 5 years of community health education: The Stanford Five-City Project. *American Journal of Epidemiology* 137: 82-96, 1993.

Giovino, G., Schooley, M.W., Zhu, B.-P., Chrismon, J.H., Tomar, S.L., Peddicord, J.P., Merritt, R.K., Husten, C.G., Eriksen, M.P. Surveillance for selected tobacco-use behaviors—United States, 1900-1994. *MMWR. Morbidity and Mortality Weekly Report* 43: 1-43, 1994.

Greenwald, P., Cullen, J.W., McKenna, J.W. Cancer prevention and control: From research through applications. *Journal of the National Cancer Institute* 79: 389-400, 1987.

Haenszel, W., Shimkin, M.B., Miller, H.P. *Tobacco Smoking Patterns in the United States. Public Health Monograph No. 45.* Public Health Service Publication No. 463. Rockville, MD: U.S. Department of Health, Education, and Welfare, Public Health Service, 1956.

Institute of Medicine. *Growing Up Tobacco Free. Preventing Nicotine Addiction in Children and Youths.* B.S. Lynch and R.J. Bonnie (Editors). Washington, DC: National Academy Press, 1994.

Johnston, L.D., O'Malley, P.M., Bachman, J.G. *National Survey Results on Drug Use From the Monitoring the Future Study, 1975-1993: Vol. I. Secondary School Students.* Rockville, MD: National Institutes of Health, National Institute on Drug Abuse, 1994.

Lando, H.A., Pechacek, T.F., Pirie, P.L., Murray, D.M., Mittlemark, M.B., Lichtenstein, E., Nothwehr, F., Gray, C. Changes in adult cigarette smoking in the Minnesota Heart Health Program. *American Journal of Public Health* 85(2): 201-208, 1995.

Lasater, T., Abrams, D., Artz, L., Beaudin, P., Cabrera, L., Elder, J., Ferreira, A., Knisley, P., Peterson, G., Rodrigues, A., Rosenberg, P., Snow, R., Carleton, R. Lay volunteer delivery of a community-based cardiovascular risk factor change program: The Pawtucket experiment. In: *Behavioral Health: A Handbook of Health Enhancement and Disease Prevention*, J.D. Matarazzo, S.M. Weiss, J.A. Herd, N.E. Miller, and S.M. Weiss (Editors). New York: John Wiley & Sons, 1984, pp. 1166-1170.

Luepker, R.V., Murray, D.M., Jacobs, D.R., Mittelmark, M.B., Bracht, N., Carlaw, R., Crow, R., Elmer, P., Finnegan, J., Folsom, A.R., Grimm, R., Hannan, P.J., Jeffrey, R., Lando, H., McGovern, P., Mullis, R., Perry, C.L., Pechacek, T., Pirie, P., Sprafka, J.M., Weisbrod, R., Blackburn, H. Community education for cardiovascular disease prevention: Risk factor changes in the Minnesota Heart Health Program. *American Journal of Public Health* 84(9): 1383-1393, 1994.

Multiple Risk Factor Intervention Trial Research Group. Multiple risk factor intervention trial. Risk factor changes and mortality results. *Journal of the American Medical Association* 248(12): 1465-1477, 1982.

National Cancer Institute and National Heart, Lung, and Blood Institute. *Smoking and Health. A Program To Reduce the Risk of Disease in Smokers. Status Report.* Bethesda, MD: National Institutes of Health, 1978.

Pierce, J.P., Lee, L., Gilpin, E.A. Smoking initiation by adolescent girls, 1944 through 1988. An association with targeted advertising. *Journal of the American Medical Association* 271: 608-611, 1994.

Shopland, D.R. Effect of smoking on the incidence and mortality of lung cancer. Chapter 1. In: *Lung Cancer*, B.E. Johnson and D.H. Johnson (Editors). New York: John Wiley & Sons, 1995, pp. 1-14.

Tobacco Control: An International Journal. Policy research: Strategic directions. *Tobacco Control: An International Journal* 1(suppl): S1-S56, 1992.

U.S. Congress. "False and Misleading Advertising (Filter-Tip Cigarettes)." Hearings before a Subcommittee of the Committee on Government Operations. Washington, DC: U.S. House of Representatives, 85th Congress, First Session, July 18, 19, 23-26, 1957.

U.S. Department of Health and Human Services. *The Health Consequences of Smoking: Cancer. A Report of the Surgeon General*. DHHS Publication No. (PHS) 82-50179. Rockville, MD: U.S. Department of Health and Human Services, Public Health Service, Office on Smoking and Health, 1982.

U.S. Department of Health and Human Services. *Smoking, Tobacco, and Cancer Program. 1985-1989 Status Report*. NIH Publication No. 90-3107. Bethesda, MD: U.S. Department of Health and Human Services, Public Health Service, National Institutes of Health, 1990.

U.S. Department of Health and Human Services. *Strategies To Control Tobacco Use in the United States: A Blueprint for Public Health Action in the 1990's*. Smoking and Tobacco Control Monographs—1. NIH Publication No. 92-3316. Bethesda, MD: U.S. Department of Health and Human Services, Public Health Service, National Institutes of Health, National Cancer Institute, 1991.

U.S. Department of Health and Human Services. *Preventing Tobacco Use Among Young People. A Report of the Surgeon General*. Atlanta, GA: U.S. Department of Health and Human Services, Public Health Service, Centers for Disease Control and Prevention, National Center for Chronic Disease Prevention and Health Promotion, Office on Smoking and Health, 1994.

AUTHORS

Donald R. Shopland
Coordinator
Smoking and Tobacco Control Program
National Cancer Institute
National Institutes of Health
Executive Plaza North, Room 241
6130 Executive Boulevard, MSC-7337
Bethesda, MD 20892-7337

David M. Burns, M.D.
Professor of Medicine
University of California at San Diego
  Medical Center
200 West Arbor Drive
San Diego, CA 92103-8375

Beti Thompson, Ph.D.
Associate Professor
University of Washington School of Public
Health and Community Medicine
Associate Member
Fred Hutchinson Cancer Research Center,
  MP-702
1124 Columbia Street
Seattle, WA 98104

William R. Lynn
COMMIT Project Officer
Public Health Applications Research Branch
Cancer Control Science Program
National Cancer Institute
National Institutes of Health
Executive Plaza North, Room 241
6130 Executive Boulevard, MSC-7337
Bethesda, MD 20892-7337

Background for a Comprehensive Community-Based Trial for Smoking Control

Norman Hymowitz, Michael D. Mueller, William R. Lynn, and
Beti Thompson

INTRODUCTION   Americans suffer greatly from diseases that are not the inevitable consequence of being born or growing old. Diseases that were rare in society prior to the 20th century, such as coronary heart disease (CHD), lung cancer, and chronic obstructive pulmonary disease (COPD), now have reached epidemic proportions (U.S. Department of Health and Human Services, 1989). The dramatic increase in these chronic diseases reflects changes in 20th-century American culture and lifestyle, including changes in dietary and exercise habits and the explosive increase in cigarette smoking during the first half of this century. Former U.S. Surgeon General C. Everett Koop considers cigarette smoking to be the single most important preventable cause of premature death and disability in society today (U.S. Department of Health and Human Services, 1988). It is sobering to note that this mass phenomenon was unknown in America prior to this century.

By the time of the first Surgeon General's Report in 1964, more than 50 percent of adult males and nearly 30 percent of adult females smoked cigarettes. The prevalence among men ages 20 to 30 was 70 percent (Warner, 1986). Since that landmark Surgeon General's Report, considerable progress has been made in the nonsmoking arena. By 1993, the prevalence of smoking in the United States dropped to 27.7 percent for males and 22.2 percent for females. The relatively small drop in prevalence for females has been attributed variously to the changing role of women in today's society and the marketing strategies of tobacco companies (Fiore et al., 1989). Most Americans, smokers as well as nonsmokers, are aware of the harmful effects of cigarettes (U.S. Department of Health and Human Services, 1989 and 1991); furthermore, most adult smokers say they would like to stop smoking (U.S. Department of Health and Human Services, 1990).

The dangers of environmental tobacco smoke (ETS) are now well established, and the U.S. Environmental Protection Agency has labeled secondhand smoke as a Class A carcinogen (U.S. Department of Health and Human Services, 1993a). Legislation and policies curtailing and even banning smoking in public places have increased dramatically in recent years (U.S. Department of Health and Human Services, 1993b).

Despite these positive signs, there remains much work ahead. Young people continue to acquire the smoking habit at an alarming rate (Pierce et al., 1989; U.S. Department of Health and Human Services, 1994); more than 46 million Americans continue to smoke (U.S. Department of Health and Human Services, 1990); and progress in the antismoking field is uneven.

African-Americans respond less well to antismoking campaigns than whites (Centers for Disease Control, 1990); the poor and least educated continue to smoke at a high rate (Pierce et al., 1989); and high smoking rates among women have boosted lung cancer past breast cancer as the number one cause of cancer death among American women (American Cancer Society, 1992).

INDIVIDUAL ORIENTATIONS TO TOBACCO CONTROL
Research focusing on tobacco control began in the 1970's. A quick review of the smoking control research literature indicates that most research has focused on individual-oriented strategies (U.S. Department of Health and Human Services, 1991). Such interventions usually take place in clinics and involve labor-intensive treatments, often administered by professional therapists. The objective of such research is to identify interventions that produce high rates of smoking cessation. Unfortunately, the effects are limited to the relatively few patients or clients who can participate in such clinics. For example, multicomponent group intervention programs (Pechacek, 1979) are among the most effective clinical strategies available. They feature a synthesis of motivational, educational, and behavioral approaches to smoking cessation and use several behavioral strategies to help smokers acquire skills that will enable them to stop smoking and remain abstinent (Pechacek, 1979). Although multicomponent group intervention programs may yield impressive initial and long-term quit rates (Pechacek, 1979), their effectiveness suffers from the limited availability of skilled therapists, the limited numbers of smokers who can be accommodated, the cost of the treatment, and often, the reluctance of smokers to participate in intensive group or individual programs. However, most smokers stop on their own without the aid of a specific program, perhaps reflecting an environment that increasingly favors nonsmokers.

In an attempt to broaden the reach of clinical interventions, strategies have been "repackaged" for use in other settings. If the successful ingredients of the multicomponent programs can be packaged into a self-help manual or videotape that can be used by many smokers with minimal or no professional supervision, the potential public health effect of the intervention can be vastly expanded. During the past decade, research interest has shifted from the search for more effective clinical treatments to an exploration of ways to repackage existing treatments to enhance their public health impact (Hymowitz, 1992; Lichtenstein and Glasgow, 1992; Cohen et al., 1989), and the National Cancer Institute Smoking and Tobacco Control Program has supported numerous studies in this area. This interest has led to research on bibliotherapy and self-help manuals (Glasgow et al., 1981), computer-assisted cessation technologies (Schneider and Benya, 1984), quit-smoking contests and lotteries (Glasgow et al., 1985), hot lines (Ossip-Klein et al., 1991), and imaginative use of print (Cummings et al., 1987) and electronic (Flay et al., 1988) media.

Another relatively new emphasis is the focus on different channels for reaching smokers and delivering interventions. Nontraditional settings, such as worksites (Sorensen et al., 1990-91; Hymowitz et al., 1991; Glasgow and Terborg, 1988), hospitals (Hudzinski and Frohlich, 1990), physician offices (Ockene, 1987; Cummings et al., 1989), religious organizations (Lasater et al., 1986; Eng et al., 1985), and health clinics (Mayer et al., 1990) provide opportunities to reach many smokers from all segments of society, many of whom are missed by more traditional group-help or clinical approaches. Moreover, these settings often provide excellent opportunities for long-term intervention and followup, thereby increasing the likelihood of long-term success.

PUBLIC HEALTH MODEL OF TOBACCO CONTROL
In the past 15 years, the perceptions of smoking behavior have changed. Increasingly, it is seen as a public health problem as well as an individual problem. The public health model is based on the relationship among three factors: (1) the host or recipient of a disease, (2) the agent or cause of the disease, and (3) the environment or setting in which the disease occurs. Smoking fits this model. The agent of the disease is tobacco, the recipient is the smoker, and the environment includes all those cues and constraints within an individual's world that promote or inhibit the use of tobacco. Tobacco control efforts can be built around this model. Instead of intervening between the agent and the host, activities can be directed toward the environment that promotes the agent of the disease. For example, the tobacco companies spend more than $4 billion annually to promote their products and increase the companies' legitimacy (Warner, 1986), despite the fact that cigarette smoking claims the lives of more than 400,000 Americans each year (U.S. Department of Health and Human Services, 1989). Policies that prohibit tobacco promotion and advertising, or keep it to a minimum, can have a large effect on smoking onset among youngsters. Similarly, as demonstrated in California, taxation of tobacco can fund counterpromotion activities (U.S. Department of Health and Human Services, 1989).

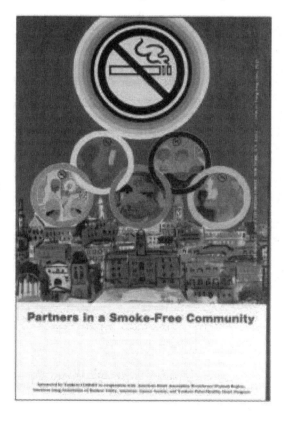

Partners in a Smoke-Free Community

Societal norms—shared rules and expectations for behavior—produce a complex system of formal and informal guidelines for the appropriateness of behaviors (Robertson, 1977). The most effective strategies for tobacco control are those that strike at the heart of the social mores and norms that support the smoking epidemic. However, norms vary by time, social network, and locality; thus, to produce large-scale changes in smoking behavior, intervention must target large social entities. To this end, health promotion researchers now are focusing on the community as the target of intervention.

Community-based interventions have both advantages and disadvantages over traditional individual-based interventions. As many researchers have observed, smoking is promoted through the social and physical environment of the community; thus, it is embedded in the smoker's way of life. Large-scale efforts to change this environment have the potential to affect many smokers at a lower cost per person. Some disadvantages of community-based programs, from a research perspective, are the broad secular trends in smoking behavior that are intertwined with program effect, the quasi-experimental and often complicated designs of studies that make it difficult to sort out cause-and-effect relationships, and the lack of long-term followup (Farquhar et al., 1984).

For these reasons, the mounting national and international experience in community control of smoking over the past 20 years has not produced conclusive evidence that these programs bring about either broad or long-term change in smoking behavior in target populations. However, the evidence is sometimes compelling and offers much value to designers of other large-scale studies. A brief review of this literature provides a good backdrop to the Community Intervention Trial for Smoking Cessation (COMMIT).

PAST COMMUNITY-BASED STUDIES OF TOBACCO CONTROL Experience with community intervention for health promotion derives largely from a host of multifactor studies of heart disease prevention (Hymowitz, 1987). Several excellent reviews of the community intervention literature are available (Hymowitz, 1987; Thompson and Pertschuk, 1992; U.S. Department of Health and Human Services, 1991 and 1987). A few of these are described below.

The Stanford Three Community Study was the first major community intervention trial. It began in 1972, with three communities randomized to mass media, mass media plus intensive face-to-face intervention, or control. Only the community with mass media and intensive face-to-face intervention showed a substantial decrease in the mean number of cigarettes smoked per day, with the high-risk group identified for the individual interactions showing a large and meaningful decrease (–42.3 percent) (Farquhar et al., 1977). However, the control city showed a decrease of 17 percent for a net reduction of –25 percent (Farquhar et al., 1977).

The North Karelia Project in Finland was also an initial major community intervention trial; it focused on the control of cardiovascular disease (CVD) in one county, with another county selected for control. This demonstration project, initiated in 1972, was a response to a request of the North Karelians for assistance in dealing with the high rate of CVD in their population.

Smoking was one component of the intervention (Puska et al., 1976). By 1982, 36 percent of North Karelian men ages 30 to 59 were current smokers compared with 42 percent in the reference community, a statistically significant difference (Puska et al., 1983 and 1989). The interpretation of the trial is difficult given that the community requested the intervention and that national legislative changes also may have contributed to the change in prevalence.

The Stanford Three Community Study described above was followed by three similar studies funded by the National Heart, Lung, and Blood Institute. These studies, the Stanford Five-City Project, the Minnesota Heart Health Program, and the Pawtucket Heart Health Program, further investigated the possibility of changing behavior at the community level. Final results of the Stanford Five-City Project, conducted in two treatment communities, showed a statistically significant 13-percent decrease in smoking in a cohort sample but no significant differences in a cross-sectional sample (Fortmann et al., 1993). The Minnesota project used three pairs of communities, and within each pair, one community was nonrandomly assigned to intervention and one to control. Both cohort and cross-sectional surveys showed no difference in smoking for males; however, the cross-sectional survey indicated a decline in smoking for females (Luepker et al., 1994). The Minnesota project also implemented interventions in schools and found that, in the intervention communities, 14.6 percent of students were smokers at graduation, compared with 24.1 percent in the comparison communities (Perry et al., 1992). Potential weaknesses of this study include the diversity among the communities, the lack of randomization, and evidence of a strong secular trend for smoking cessation that may have made it difficult to see any intervention effects. The Pawtucket project initially focused on social networks, such as worksites, schools, religious organizations, and other organizations, to spread an antismoking intervention but later added social marketing and communitywide activities. A "Quit and Win" contest showed good participation and good long-term results (Elder et al., 1986). Overall results from the Pawtucket project showed downward, symmetrical, and secular trends in smoking prevalence (Carleton et al., 1995).

The Australian North Coast Healthy Lifestyle Programme: Quit for Life used a social marketing approach to community intervention (Egger et al., 1983). Professional media and advertising techniques were used to prepare messages. The media included organizations from television, radio, and print, and stickers, posters, T-shirts, balloons, and self-help quit kits were among other advertising techniques used. In addition to the media campaign, a variety of community antismoking programs were offered in the community receiving media plus community programs. These programs included a 5-day plan, commercial quit-smoking groups, a quit club, a quit 1-day workshop, a quit 5-day clinic, hypnotherapy, and doctor's kits. The results of prevalence surveys taken at baseline and during years 2 and 3 suggest that the Australian North Coast Healthy Lifestyle Programme: Quit for Life was effective in reducing the prevalence of smoking in the experimental communities compared with the reference community

(Egger et al., 1983). The biggest change in the prevalence of smoking occurred in Lismore, the mass media and specific intervention community. Of the specific quit-smoking programs offered, the most popular were those that did not require face-to-face contact (kits, informational brochures, factsheets, and so forth) (Egger et al., 1983). Among smokers who reported quitting, most reported that they quit smoking on their own, a finding that emphasizes the importance of creating a social milieu that encourages and supports self-initiated quit-smoking attempts.

The National Research Program in Switzerland also focused on CVD prevention. This project involved two pairs of communities, with one community per pair randomized to intervention. The observed decrease in smoking prevalence was statistically significant. It also was found that light and moderate smokers were more likely to quit than heavy smokers (Gutzwiller et al., 1985). The major weakness of this study was low response rates to the outcome surveys.

Another Australian study, the Sydney Quit for Life Anti-Smoking Campaign, used mass media to reduce smoking prevalence in two Australian cities, Sydney and Melbourne. The remainder of Australia was used as a control area. The intervention was phased into the two cities, first in Sydney and a year later in Melbourne. The combined effect of the program was statistically significant in both intervention cities (Dwyer et al., 1986). Long-term effects of the trial were most dramatic for men in Sydney, where smoking prevalence dropped 2.5 percent in the first 6 months of the intervention and continued at a decline of 1.12 percent per year; similar trends were seen in Melbourne. However, after an initial decline, women did not continue to decrease their smoking prevalence rates (Pierce et al., 1989).

Several other important community or large-scale intervention studies have revealed positive effects on prevalence of cigarette smoking. Among them are the Community Hypertension, Atherosclerosis, and Diabetes (CHAD) program in Israel (Gofin et al., 1981 and 1986), the Cardiovascular Disease Prevention Program in an Austrian community (Rhomberg, 1991), and the Coronary Risk Factor Study in South Africa (Steenkamp et al., 1991). In addition, several community studies are under way in Germany, Ireland, Sweden, and the Netherlands that also target general risk factors related to health, including smoking.

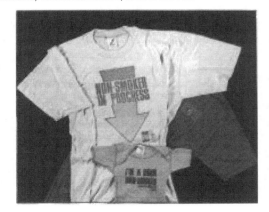

LESSONS FROM PREVIOUS STUDIES

The review of studies suggests several lessons on smoking.

- The recognition that behavior occurs within a social environment has implications for each level of the social environment. Although communities can be extremely influential in shaping that environment, communities exist within broader systems, including Federal and State systems, both of which are likely to have a great impact on smoking behavior. For example, the annual Surgeon General reports alert health care professionals about new findings in tobacco use and control. The Federal Government imposes regulations on the sale of tobacco; it also collects taxes on tobacco. Every State government in the United States has placed restrictions on youth access to tobacco. Most recently, one State, California, has experimented with dedicating State taxes on tobacco products to antismoking media campaigns. This "top down" support of the greater entities within which communities operate can be a powerful contributor to community change, as suggested by North Karelia legislative changes that came during the intervention period. The recent Canadian and California experiences with increased taxes and the subsequent greater decrease in smoking prevalence compared with the United States overall also emphasize the importance of support from the larger systems.

- It is important to recognize that cigarette smoking and associated adverse health consequences are community problems that require community solutions. Individual and clinical interventions have an important place in the antismoking arena, but true success will not be obtained until communities and their concerned citizens let it be known that "enough is enough." Communities should take a stand to protect their youth from lung cancer, CHD, COPD, and the many other ill effects of smoking. Also, it is up to communities to implement rules and regulations that protect their citizens from the affliction of ETS. Communities can help create a social climate in which cigarette smoking is viewed as an unacceptable behavior.

- It is noteworthy that in both the North Karelia and the Australian studies intervention effects continued to be observed throughout the 10 years of the study. This finding documents the importance of long-term commitment. Community intervention studies are unique public health endeavors, and often, a considerable amount of time is needed to organize the community, mobilize diverse intervention channels, and introduce comprehensive social marketing and behavioral programs that not only lead to the prevention of smoking onset and the modification of existing smoking behavior but also contribute to changes in social norms and mores.

- An advantage of community interventions is that the effect of specific interventions is enhanced by their presentation within the context of an "enriched" milieu. Hence, coordination of several different interventions in communities may enhance the effectiveness of all.

- Prior community intervention studies underscore the importance of the considerable thought and attention required for coordination and planning to maximize community resource and intervention effects. Together, systematic programming can contribute to a change in the social milieu, so necessary for the long-term modification of smoking behavior.

- Although community-based smoking cessation and prevention approaches are likely to be less efficacious than individual or clinical programs, they are designed to be more cost-effective and to reach larger numbers of smokers, thus producing a larger public health effect.

- There can be little question that Federal, State, community, and individual approaches to smoking cessation have an important place in the antismoking arena. Smokers who desire clinical treatment and support ought to be able to obtain the help they need. However, in view of the magnitude of the smoking problem in the United States, the great numbers of smokers in need of assistance, and the terrible toll that cigarette smoking continues to take on the health of this Nation, it is also necessary to implement effective public health strategies.

REFERENCES

American Cancer Society. *Cancer Facts and Figures 1992.* Atlanta, GA: American Cancer Society, Inc., 1992.

Carleton, R.A., Lasater, T.M., Assaf, A.R., Feldman, H.A., McKinlay, S., and the Pawtucket Heart Health Program Writing Group. The Pawtucket Heart Health Program: The community changes in cardiovascular risk factors and projected disease risk. *American Journal of Pulic Health.* 85: 777-785, 1995.

Centers for Disease Control. Cigarette smoking cessation—United States, 1989. *MMWR. Morbidity and Mortality Weekly Report* 39: 676-680, 1990.

Cohen, S., Lichtenstein, E., Prochaska, J.O., Rossi, J.S., Gritz, E.R., Carr, C.R., Orleans, T.R., Schoenbach, V.J., Biener, L., Abrams, D., DiClemente, C., Curry, S., Marlatt, G.A., Cummings, K.M., Emont, S.L., Giovino, G., Ossip-Klein, D. Debunking myths about self-quitting: Evidence from 10 prospective studies of persons who attempt to quit smoking by themselves. *American Psychologist* 44: 1355-1365, 1989.

Cummings, K.M., Sciandra, R., Markello, S. Impact of a newspaper mediated quit smoking program. *American Journal of Public Health* 77: 1452-1453, 1987.

Cummings, S.R., Richard, R.J., Duncan, C.L., Hansen, B., Vander Martin, R., Gilbert, B., Coates, T.J. Training physicians about smoking cessation: A controlled trial in private practices. *Journal of General Internal Medicine* 4: 482-489, 1989.

Dwyer, T., Pierce, J.P., Hannam, C.D., Burke, N. Evaluation of the Sydney "Quit for Life" anti-smoking campaign: Part 2. Changes in smoking prevalence. *The Medical Journal of Australia* 144: 344-347, 1986.

Egger, G., Fitzgerald, W., Frape, G., Monaem, A., Rubenstein, P., Tyler, C., McKay, B. Results of large scale media antismoking campaign in Australia: North Coast "Quit For Life" programme. *British Medical Journal* 287: 1125-1128, 1983.

Elder, J.P., McGraw, S.A., Abrams, D.B., Ferreira, A., Lasater, T.H., Longpre, H., Peterson, G.S., Schwertfeger, R., Carleton, R.A. Organizational and community approaches to community-wide prevention of heart disease: The first two years of the Pawtucket Heart Health Program. *Preventive Medicine* 15: 107-117, 1986.

Eng, E., Hatch, J., Callan, A. Institutionalizing social support through the church and into the community. *Health Education Quarterly* 12(1): 81-92, 1985.

Farquhar, J.W., Maccoby, N., Solomon, D.S. Community applications of behavioral medicine. In: *Handbook of Behavioral Medicine*, W.D. Gentry (Editor). New York: Guilford, 1984, pp. 437-478.

Farquhar, J.W., Maccoby, N., Wood, P.D., Breitrose, H., Haskell, W.L., Meyer, A.J., Alexander, J.K., Brown, B.W., Jr., McAlister, A.L., Nash, J.D., Stern, M.P. Community education for cardiovascular health. *The Lancet* 1: 1192-1195, 1977.

Fiore, M.C., Novotny, T.E., Pierce, J.P., Hatziandreu, E.J., Patel, K.M., Davis, R.M. Trends in cigarette smoking in the United States: The changing influence of gender and race. *Journal of the American Medical Association* 261: 49-55, 1989.

Flay, B.R., Brannon, B.R., Johnson, C.A., Hansen, W.B., Ulene, A.L., Whitney-Saltiel, D.A., Gleason, L.R., Sussman, S., Gavin, M.D., Glowacz, K.M., Sobol, D.F., Spiegel, D.C. The television school and family smoking prevention and cessation project. *Preventive Medicine* 17: 585-607, 1988.

Fortmann, S.P., Taylor, C.B., Flora, J.A., Jatulis, D.E. Changes in adult cigarette smoking prevalence after 5 years of community health education: The Stanford Five-City Project. *American Journal of Epidemiology* 137: 82-96, 1993.

Glasgow, R.E., Klesges, R.C., Mizes, J.S., Pechacek, T.F. Quitting smoking: Strategies used and variables associated with success in a stop-smoking contest. *Journal of Consulting and Clinical Psychology* 53: 905-912, 1985.

Glasgow, R.E., Schafer, L., O'Neill, K. Self-help books and amount of therapist contact in smoking cessation programs. *Journal of Consulting and Clinical Psychology* 49: 659-667, 1981.

Glasgow, R.E., Terborg, J. Occupational health promotion programs to reduce cardiovascular risk. *Journal of Consulting and Clinical Psychology* 56: 365-373, 1988.

Gofin, J., Kark, E., Mainemer, N., Kark, S.L., Abramson, J.H., Hopp, C., Epstein, L.M. Prevalence of selected health characteristics of women and comparisons with men: A community health survey in Jerusalem. *Israel Journal of Medical Sciences* 17: 145-159, 1981.

Gofin, J.R., Gofin, J.H., Abramson, J.H., Ban, R. Ten-year evaluation of hypertension, overweight, cholesterol, and smoking control: The CHAD program in Jerusalem. *Preventive Medicine* 15: 304-312, 1986.

Gutzwiller, F., Nater, B., Martin, J. Community-based primary prevention of cardiovascular disease in Switzerland: Methods and results of the National Research Program (NRP 1A). *Preventive Medicine* 14: 482-491, 1985.

Hudzinski, L.G., Frohlich, E.D. One-year longitudinal study of a no-smoking policy in a medical institution. *Chest* 97: 1198-1202, 1990.

Hymowitz, N. Community and clinical trials of disease prevention: Effects on cigarette smoking. *Public Health Reviews* 15: 45-81, 1987.

Hymowitz, N. Smoking modification: Research and clinical application. In: *Handbook for Assessing and Treating Addictive Disorders*, C.E. Stout, J.L. Levitt, and D.H. Ruben (Editors). New York: Greenwood, 1992, pp. 145-164.

Hymowitz, N., Campbell, K., Feuerman, M. Long-term smoking intervention at the worksite: Effects of quit-smoking groups and an "enriched milieu" on smoking cessation in adult white-collar employees. *Health Psychology* 10: 366-369, 1991.

Lasater, T.M., Wells, B.L., Carleton, R.A., Elder, J.P. The role of churches in disease prevention research studies. *Public Health Reports* 101: 125-131, 1986.

Lichtenstein, E., Glasgow, R.E. Smoking cessation: What have we learned over the past decade? *Journal of Consulting and Clinical Psychology* 60: 518-527, 1992.

Luepker, R.V., Murray, D.M., Jacobs, D.K., Jr., Mittelmark, M.B., Bracht, N., Carlaw, R., Crow, R., Elmer, P., Finnegan, J., Folsom, A.R., Mullis, R., Perry, C.L., Pechacek, T., Pirie, P., Sprafka, J.M., Weisbrod, R., Blackburn, H. Community education for cardiovascular disease prevention. *American Journal of Public Health* 84(9): 1383-1393, 1994.

Mayer, J.P., Hawkins, B., Todd, R. A randomized evaluation of smoking cessation interventions for pregnant women at a WIC clinic. *American Journal of Public Health* 80: 76-78, 1990.

Ockene, J.K. Physician delivered interventions for smoking cessation: Strategies for increasing effectiveness. *Preventive Medicine* 7: 723-737, 1987.

Ossip-Klein, D.J., Giovino, G.A., Megahed, N., Black, P.M., Emont, S.L., Stiggins, J. Effects of a smokers' hotline: Results of a 10-county self-help trial. *Journal of Consulting and Clinical Psychology* 59: 325-332, 1991.

Pechacek, T.F. Modification of smoking behavior. In: *Smoking and Health: A Report of the Surgeon General*. DHEW Publication No. (PHS) 79-50066. Rockville, MD: U.S. Department of Health and Human Services, Public Health Service, Office of the Assistant Secretary for Health, Office on Smoking and Health, 1979, pp. 19-1–19-63.

Perry, C.L., Kelder, S.H., Murray, D.M., Klepp, K.I. Community wide smoking prevention: Long-term outcomes of the Minnesota Heart Health Program and the Class of 1989 Study. *American Journal of Public Health* 82(9): 1210-1216, 1992.

Pierce, J.P., Fiore, M.C., Novotny, T.E., Hotziandreu, E.J., Davis, R.M. Trends in cigarette smoking in the United States: Projections to the Year 2000. *Journal of the American Medical Association* 261: 61-65, 1989.

Puska, P., Koskela, K., Pakarinen, H., Puumalainen, P., Soininen, V., Tuomilehto, J. The North Karelia Project: A programme for community control of cardiovascular disease. *Scandinavian Journal of Social Medicine* 4: 57-60, 1976.

Puska, P., Nissinen, A., Salonen, J.T., Toumilehto, J. Ten years of the North Karelia Project: Results with community-based prevention of coronary heart disease. *Scandinavian Journal of Social Medicine* 11: 65-68, 1983.

Puska, P., Tuomilehto, J., Nissinen, A., Salonen, J.T., Vartiainen, E., Pietinen, P., Koskela, K., Korhonen, H.J. The North Karelia Project: 15 years of community-based prevention of coronary heart disease. *Annals of Medicine* 21: 169-173, 1989.

Rhomberg, H.P. Ten years' experience in a cardiovascular disease prevention program in Austria. *Cor Vasa* 33: 103-106, 1991.

Robertson, I. *Sociology.* New York: Worth Publishers, 1977.

Schneider, S.J., Benya, A. Computerized direct mail to treat smokers who avoid treatment. *Computers and Biomedical Research* 17: 409-418, 1984.

Sorensen, G., Glasgow, R.E., Corbett, K. (for the COMMIT Research Group). Promoting smoking control through worksites in the Community Intervention Trial for Smoking Cessation (COMMIT). *International Quarterly of Community Health Education* 11(3): 239-257, 1990-91.

Steenkamp, H.J., Jooste, P.L., Jordaan, P.C., Swanepoel, A.S., Rossouw, J.E. Changes in smoking during a community-based cardiovascular disease intervention programme. *South African Medical Journal* 79: 250-253, 1991.

Thompson, B., Pertschuk, M. Community intervention and advocacy. In: *Prevention of Coronary Heart Disease,* J.K. Ockene and I.S. Ockene (Editors). Boston: Little, Brown, 1992, pp. 493-515.

U.S. Department of Health and Human Services. *Smoking and Health: A National Status Report.* DHHS Publication No. (CDC) 87-8396. Rockville, MD: U.S. Department of Health and Human Services, Public Health Service, Centers for Disease Control, Office on Smoking and Health, 1987.

U.S. Department of Health and Human Services. *The Health Consequences of Smoking: Nicotine Addiction. A Report of the Surgeon General, 1988.* DHHS Publication No. (CDC) 88-8406. Rockville, MD: U.S. Department of Health and Human Services, Public Health Service, Centers for Disease Control, Center for Health Promotion and Education, Office on Smoking and Health, 1988.

U.S. Department of Health and Human Services. *Reducing the Health Consequences of Smoking: 25 Years of Progress. A Report of the Surgeon General, 1989.* DHHS Publication No. (CDC) 89-8411. Rockville, MD: U.S. Department of Health and Human Services, Public Health Service, Centers for Disease Control, Center for Chronic Disease Prevention and Health Promotion, Office on Smoking and Health, 1989.

U.S. Department of Health and Human Services. *The Health Benefits of Smoking Cessation: A Report of the Surgeon General, 1990.* DHHS Publication No. (CDC) 90-8416. Rockville, MD: U.S. Department of Health and Human Services, Public Health Service, Centers for Disease Control, Center for Chronic Disease Prevention and Health Promotion, Office on Smoking and Health, 1990.

U.S. Department of Health and Human Services. *Strategies To Control Tobacco Use in the United States: A Blueprint for Public Health Action in the 1990's.* Smoking and Tobacco Control Monographs-1. NIH Publication No. 92-3316. Rockville, MD: U.S. Department of Health and Human Services, Public Health Service, National Institutes of Health, National Cancer Institute, 1991.

U.S. Department of Health and Human Services. *Respiratory Health Effects of Passive Smoking: Lung Cancer and Other Disorders. The Report of the U.S. Environmental Protection Agency.* Smoking and Tobacco Control Program Monograph No. 4. NIH Publication No. 93-3605. Rockville, MD: U.S. Department of Health and Human Services, Public Health Service, National Institutes of Health, National Cancer Institute, 1993a.

U.S. Department of Health and Human Services. *Major Local Tobacco Control Ordinances in the United States.* Smoking and Tobacco Control Monograph No. 3. NIH Publication No. 93-3532. Rockville, MD: U.S. Department of Health and Human Services, Public Health Service, National Institutes of Health, National Cancer Institute, 1993b.

U.S. Department of Health and Human Services. *Preventing Tobacco Use Among Young People: A Report of the Surgeon General.* Atlanta, GA: U.S. Department of Health and Human Services, Public Health Service, Centers for Disease Control and Prevention, National Center for Chronic Disease Prevention and Health Promotion, Office on Smoking and Health, 1994.

Warner, K.E. *Selling Smoke: Cigarette Advertising and Public Health.* Washington, DC: American Public Health Association, 1986.

AUTHORS

Norman Hymowitz, Ph.D.
Professor of Clinical Psychiatry
Department of Psychiatry and Mental
  Health Services
University of Medicine and Dentistry of
  New Jersey Medical School
Newark, NJ 07103

Michael D. Mueller, M.S.
Senior Technical Writer
R.O.W. Sciences, Inc.
Suite 400
1700 Research Boulevard
Rockville, MD 20850-3142

William R. Lynn
COMMIT Project Officer
Public Health Applications Research Branch
Cancer Control Science Program
National Cancer Institute
National Institutes of Health
Executive Plaza North, Room 241
6130 Executive Boulevard, MSC-7337
Bethesda, MD 20892-7337

Beti Thompson, Ph.D.
Associate Professor
University of Washington School of Public
  Health and Community Medicine
Associate Member
Fred Hutchinson Cancer Research Center,
  MP-702
1124 Columbia Street
Seattle, WA 98104

Community Intervention Trial for Smoking Cessation: Description and Evaluation Plan

William R. Lynn and Beti Thompson

INTRODUCTION   The Community Intervention Trial for Smoking Cessation (COMMIT) was a large-scale undertaking that incorporated virtually all key features of past community trials. It was the largest National Cancer Institute (NCI) effort to test methods to help people stop smoking. COMMIT used many methods and strategies developed in smaller NCI-funded trials conducted in the early 1980's (U.S. Department of Health and Human Services, 1990) and incorporated many of these methods into a community-based approach, which involved community groups, institutions, and organizations in confronting the smoking problem in their community.

COMMIT focused on heavy smokers (those smoking more than 25 cigarettes per day). At the time of trial development, heavy smokers represented about one-third of all adult smokers. Heavy smokers account for nearly half the lung and other smoking-related cancers, and the risk of disease and death from heart and lung diseases dramatically increases as the number of cigarettes smoked per day increases (U.S. Department of Health and Human Services, 1982 and 1989).

Heavy smokers appear to face special problems in quitting. Several large prospective studies have indicated that spontaneous quit rates are lower among heavy smokers than among light-to-moderate smokers. Data from the Multiple Risk Factor Intervention Trial (MRFIT) special intervention group indicate that even when fairly intensive smoking cessation interventions are offered on a continuous basis for up to 6 years, heavy smokers have more difficulty quitting and maintaining abstinence (Hughes et al., 1981). Similarly, some community-based studies (Gutzwiller et al., 1985; Steenkamp et al., 1991) suggest that light and moderate smokers have less difficulty quitting than heavy smokers. Thus, it was appropriate to target this group of hard-to-reach smokers who account for much of the excess morbidity and mortality related to smoking.

TRIAL COMMUNITIES   In response to a request for proposals from NCI, several investigators competed for participation in a community-based trial aimed at reducing smoking rates in heavy smokers. Major criteria for being selected for participation were the ability to recruit two similar communities that agreed to be randomized to receive either active intervention or control surveillance and having experience in smoking control and community studies. For purposes of the study, a community was broadly defined and could include a well-defined portion of a major metropolitan area or two small cities in the same geographic region. Communities within matched pairs were required to have some boundary separation to maintain independence of intervention activities and to prevent contamination. Within each pair, communities were matched for general sociodemographic factors, including population size, age distribution, demographic profile (ethnicity, proportion female, age distribution, educational distribution, and mean family income level), mobility and migration patterns, extent of urbanization, estimated smoking prevalence rates, and access to a variety of intervention channels.

Criteria for selecting the pair of communities varied by research institution; however, they were required to fall within certain size parameters. The communities were later examined for characteristics thought to be related either to cigarette smoking behavior or access to channels that had been defined for intervention. Some of the latter characteristics included whether community residents received their health care within the community, whether they worked within the community, the availability of media resources, and baseline smoking prevalence. The research institutions and their associated community pairs are identified in Table 1.

Table 1
List of the 22 COMMIT communities

Contracting Organization	Community Sites
Waterloo Research Institute Waterloo, Ontario, Canada	Brantford[a] Peterborough
Kaiser Foundation Research Institute Oakland, CA	Vallejo[a] Hayward
Roswell Park Memorial Institute Buffalo, NY	Utica[a] Binghamton/Johnson City
Research Triangle Institute Research Triangle, NC	Raleigh[a] Greensboro
Fred Hutchinson Cancer Research Center Seattle, WA	Bellingham[a] Longview/Kelso
University of Medicine and Dentistry of New Jersey Newark, NJ	Paterson[a] Trenton
Oregon Research Institute Eugene, OR	Medford/Ashland[a] Albany/Corvallis
University of Massachusetts Medical School Worcester, MA	Fitchburg/Leominster[a] Lowell
The Lovelace Institutes Albuquerque, NM	Santa Fe[a] Las Cruces
University of Iowa Iowa City, IA	Cedar Rapids/Marion[a] Davenport
American Health Foundation New York, NY	Yonkers[a] New Rochelle

[a] *Community randomized to receive intervention.*

The community populations ranged from 49,421 to 251,208 with comparable statistical means for the pooled intervention and comparison communities. Overall, the intervention and comparison communities were well matched with regard to general sociodemographic variables (see Table 2). A cluster analysis was performed using census data for eight demographic variables on which the pairs could demonstrate agreement: racial distribution, Hispanic ethnicity, gender by age, gender by marital status, general occupational category, educational attainment, family income, and years resident in the current household. This analysis verified the comparability of the households in the community pairs.

Table 2

Sociodemographic characteristics of community pairs

Community/Area	Population	White (%)	Female (%)	Ages 25-64 (%)	High School Graduate (%)	Low Income (%)
Vallejo, CA	120,060	52.1	50.2	51.1	80.7	17.1
Hayward, CA	141,893	63.5	50.8	53.9	75.3	16.3
Cedar Rapids/Marion, IA	144,243	96.3	51.7	52.1	85.0	20.6
Davenport, IA	125,593	91.0	52.1	50.5	81.5	24.9
Fitchburg/Leominster, MA	79,339	91.3	51.8	49.8	72.0	24.2
Lowell, MA	103,439	81.2	51.4	47.5	65.8	27.9
Paterson, NJ	141,431	41.3	52.1	49.3	54.9	28.2
Trenton, NJ	91,688	42.0	51.3	49.9	58.2	29.7
Santa Fe, NM	68,092	81.3	52.3	55.7	83.4	22.0
Las Cruces, NM	69,015	88.8	51.0	48.2	78.4	34.3
Yonkers, NY	61,698	68.3	53.6	53.0	72.9	22.5
New Rochelle, NY	49,421	70.9	53.5	52.7	72.5	21.3
Utica, NY	76,967	87.8	53.1	46.8	68.8	37.1
Binghamton/Johnson City, NY	73,632	93.2	53.1	47.8	74.2	35.8
Raleigh, NC	232,652	70.8	51.5	54.8	86.5	18.9
Greensboro, NC	251,208	71.1	52.7	53.4	79.0	21.0
Medford/Ashland, OR	66,832	94.7	52.4	49.1	83.4	29.8
Albany/Corvallis, OR	77,323	92.2	50.4	45.6	87.5	31.4
Bellingham, WA	76,908	92.9	51.3	48.4	85.4	24.9
Longview/Kelso, WA	62,433	95.0	50.9	50.3	77.5	28.2
Brantford, Ontario, Canada	88,525	a	51.5	50.7	56.3	14.9
Peterborough, Ontario, Canada	91,075	a	52.2	49.7	63.4	15.0
Mean for Intervention Sites	105,159	74.6	51.8	51.4	76.2	22.7
Mean for Comparison Sites	103,338	76.6	51.8	50.6	74.5	24.6

[a] *Data not available.*

TRIAL TIMELINE   The COMMIT trial was initiated in September 1986 and was implemented in three phases. Phase I (October 1986 through October 1988) focused on the development of a standard intervention protocol, an evaluation plan, and the baseline assessment, randomization, and mobilization of communities. During Phase II (October 1988 through December 1992) the intervention was implemented in the 11 intervention communities. During Phase III (January 1993 through March 1995) final surveys were conducted, and data from the trial continue to be analyzed.

OVERALL   The study's evaluation plan measures changes in community smoking
EVALUATION   patterns and allows for testing the assumptions that have guided the
PLAN   development of the intervention strategies. Evaluation strategies are organized into four components: (1) outcome evaluation, which measures changes in smoking behavior; (2) impact evaluation, which measures changes in factors thought to be important in facilitating communitywide smoking behavior changes (including social norms about smoking, tobacco intervention activities by health care providers, and media coverage of tobacco issues); (3) process evaluation, which documents the extent of intervention implementation; and (4) economic evaluation, which estimates the costs of the COMMIT interventions.

OUTCOME   The primary hypothesis to be tested in the trial was that the
EVALUATION   implementation of a defined intervention protocol, delivered through multiple community groups and organizations and using limited external resources, would result in a quit rate in heavy smokers that was at least 10 percentage points greater (e.g., 25 versus 15 percent) than that observed in the comparison communities. Outcome evaluation was designed to measure the effect of the COMMIT intervention on (1) smoking cessation rates among cohorts of heavy smokers, (2) smoking cessation rates among cohorts of light-to-moderate smokers, (3) the prevalence of overall smoking among adults, and (4) smoking onset among adolescents. The primary outcome measure was the smoking cessation rate of a representative cohort of heavy smokers; a secondary outcome measure was the smoking cessation rate of a representative cohort of light-to-moderate smokers.

Endpoint and   To identify residents to be tracked as cohort members and to
Evaluation Cohorts provide baseline prevalence estimates, a telephone survey was performed at baseline (January 1988) prior to randomization of communities. The baseline telephone survey provided information on smoking prevalence and recent quit rates for adults between ages 25 and 64 in the paired communities. The overall estimated prevalence of cigarette smoking was about 28 percent, which was comparable with national estimates of 30 percent, as reported in the 1984 National Health Interview Survey (Kovar and Poe, 1985). The specific estimates for the 22 communities (shown in Table 3) demonstrate that the community pairs were well matched not only on demographic characteristics but also on smoking prevalence and recent cessation behavior.

Table 3

Estimated smoking prevalence (by percent) and quit rates (by percent) in the COMMIT communities

Community/Area	Smoking Prevalence 1988	Quit Rate		
		Rate for 2.5 Years, 1983-85	Rate for 2.5 Years, 1986-88	Rate for 5 Years, 1983-88
Vallejo, CA	26.06	11.8	18.4	28.0
Hayward, CA	24.90	10.6	18.9	27.5
Cedar Rapids/Marion, IA	22.35	14.0	18.8	30.1
Davenport, IA	26.22	14.2	16.3	28.2
Fitchburg/Leominster, MA	26.27	12.2	17.5	27.6
Lowell, MA	29.08	11.1	16.9	26.1
Paterson, NJ	26.49	7.0	14.5	20.5
Trenton, NJ	28.76	9.9	13.3	21.9
Santa Fe, NM	21.96	16.0	22.5	34.9
Las Cruces, NM	19.54	13.6	21.0	31.7
Yonkers, NY	24.76	11.8	18.4	28.0
New Rochelle, NY	24.87	14.0	16.9	28.5
Utica, NY	26.49	11.9	16.9	26.8
Binghamton/Johnson City, NY	25.54	11.4	17.0	26.5
Raleigh, NC	22.84	12.4	19.7	29.6
Greensboro, NC	25.67	11.8	16.9	26.6
Medford/Ashland, OR	21.05	13.5	20.1	30.9
Albany/Corvallis, OR	18.29	13.2	19.2	29.8
Bellingham, WA	20.10	13.1	22.6	32.8
Longview/Kelso, WA	25.53	12.7	18.3	28.7
Brantford, Ontario, Canada	32.02	11.2	13.2	22.9
Peterborough, Ontario, Canada	28.06	10.3	17.0	25.6
Mean for Intervention Sites	24.45	12.3	18.4	28.4
Mean for Comparison Sites	25.44	12.1	17.4	27.4

Source: COMMIT Research Group, 1991.

The baseline telephone survey was conducted centrally using a modified random-digit-dialing technique with community-specific geographic screening to identify households within the target areas. Questions about gender, age, name, and smoking status of each adult household member (age 18 or older) were asked of an eligible proxy. This roster was used to identify potential members of the cohorts and to provide the basis for community smoking prevalence and quit-rate estimates. The response rate for this survey was 88.1 percent, with an average of 6,000 households listed in each of the 22 communities.

From this roster, current smokers and recent quitters were interviewed to determine the quantity and duration of cigarette smoking, quit attempts, desire to quit, and demographic and socioeconomic characteristics and to obtain tracking information. Groups of about 500 heavy smokers and 500 light-to-moderate smokers between ages 25 and 64 were identified in each community. (A smoker was defined as one who has smoked at least 100 cigarettes and who smokes currently; a heavy smoker was defined as one who smokes 25 or more cigarettes per day.) The response rate for this extended interview was 86.4 percent. The group of approximately 500 heavy and 500 light-to-moderate smokers was then subdivided into an endpoint cohort and evaluation cohort.

A randomly chosen 80-percent sample was drawn from each heavy and light-to-moderate smoker group to form the endpoint cohorts. Cohort members were not explicitly notified of their status; however, respondents were informed that annual contacts would occur. The endpoint cohorts were contacted briefly by telephone each year to determine smoking status and to update tracking information. To minimize reactivity, these cohorts were resurveyed indepth only at the end of the study. Figure 1 gives information on cohort size and smoking habits and shows the timing of cohort surveys. Attrition within cohorts was anticipated; the initial cohort sample sizes were selected so that sufficient statistical power would exist for the cohorts at the end of the trial.

The remaining 20 percent (approximately 100 individuals) of each heavy and light-to-moderate smoker group, along with approximately 100 recent quitters (who had quit within the previous 5 years) were identified to be part of the evaluation cohort. In 1989, an additional 100 nonsmokers (who never smoked or had quit more than 5 years earlier) per community were added to this cohort. At the beginning of the intervention (1989), members of this cohort were asked questions to assess three elements related to intermediate trial goals: the population impact of COMMIT on intervention program awareness, receptivity, and participation; recognition that smoking is a public health problem; and change in the social acceptability of smoking (see Figure 1). Questions also were asked at the midpoint (1991) and the end (1993) of the intervention. Members of the evaluation cohort also were contacted in 1990 and 1992 to update smoking status and tracking information.

The primary analysis compared quit rates among cohorts of heavy smokers in the pooled intervention and comparison communities. Other analyses compared quit rates among cohorts of light-to-moderate smokers, changes in prevalence of smoking, and changes in norms and attitudes about smoking. To ensure that the cohorts remained as representative as possible of their communities, no intervention activities were directed at individual cohort members; trial investigators and local program staff members had no knowledge of which smokers had been selected for the COMMIT cohorts. Population-based surveys were conducted centrally by

Figure 1

Surveys to assess smoking status (endpoint) and surveys to assess communitywide changes (evaluation)

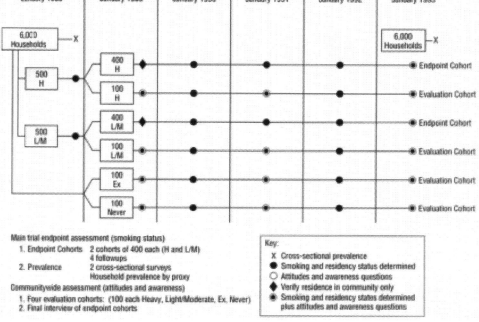

Main trial endpoint assessment (smoking status)
1. Endpoint Cohorts   2 cohorts of 400 each (H and L/M)
                       4 followups
2. Prevalence   2 cross-sectional surveys
                       Household prevalence by proxy
Communitywide assessment (attitudes and awareness)
1. Four evaluation cohorts: (100 each Heavy, Light/Moderate, Ex, Never)
2. Final interview of endpoint cohorts

Key:
X   Cross-sectional prevalence
●   Smoking and residency status determined
○   Attitudes and awareness questions
◆   Verify residence in community only
◉   Smoking and residency states determined
    plus attitudes and awareness questions

Key: H = heavy; L/M = light-to-moderate; Ex = ex-smoker; Never = never-smoker.

Source: COMMIT Research Group, 1991.

independent contractors. All surveys were identified as being sponsored by the U.S. Public Health Service and were not linked to local COMMIT activities.

Definition of Trial Endpoints
At the end of the trial, smoking status among individuals in the heavy smoker cohort was determined and compared for the intervention and comparison communities. A "quitter" was defined as a smoker who did not smoke for at least 6 months prior to the final followup survey in 1993. The quit rates were selected as the primary endpoint and—because an estimated 6,000 households in each community would have to be contacted to identify the heavy smokers—community members' change in smoking prevalence served as a secondary endpoint. The two endpoints provided different but complementary information. The cohorts gave information on individuals followed over time, but the data might have been complicated by loss to followup and reactivity. The community was the unit of analysis, and the community quit rates and prevalence of smoking were also valid indicators of community change.

Because the community was the unit of analysis, the power calculations for the cohort endpoint depend mainly on the number of communities and the estimates of variance in quit rates between communities. The power was less sensitive to the number of individuals in the cohort in each community. Using an estimate of the intercommunity variance based on data from the MRFIT and assuming that matching was completely ineffective, a cohort of 250 heavy smokers in each community yields a power of about 90 percent for detecting a 10-percent difference in the quit rate among heavy smokers, using a one-sided test, with the probability of a Type I error set at .05. The power to detect a difference of 10 percent among all smokers is also about 90 percent (Gail et al., 1992).

Matching Communities
COMMIT was a randomized study employing a matched-pairs design. Matching was not necessary for evaluation plan efficiency; however, because the study consisted of matched pairs of communities, efficiency was increased (Freedman et al., 1990). Pairs of communities were selected on the basis of their geographical proximity and were later matched on variables strongly expected to relate to the outcome variable—the smoking quit rate. The matching variables ideally would be related to the smoking quit rates, but quantitative data on the gain in efficiency from the matching were not available. Therefore, before randomization, the baseline survey of each community was conducted to determine the prevalence of smoking and, of great relevance, the smoking quit rate over the previous 5 years. When this sequence (initial matching, acquisition of baseline information, randomization) was utilized, it was possible, even before the study began, to estimate the gains in efficiency from the matching. With the use of the baseline quit rates as surrogates for the quit rates to be observed over the 5 years of the study, an efficiency gain resulting from matching is predicted. The power for the cohort analyses may be as high as 98 percent, if the matching is as effective as findings indicate (Freedman et al., 1990).

IMPACT EVALUATION
Impact evaluation was conducted by special population surveys to monitor whether changes in the channels of intervention that were hypothesized to reach the smokers were occurring. These included surveys of physicians and dentists, physicians' and dentists' office staffs, worksites, schools, cessation resources and services providers, and religious organizations. Hypotheses also were suggested that youth would be affected by a community trial; thus, youth also were surveyed. Each population is briefly described below; for more detail, see Mattson and colleagues (1990-91).

Physicians and Dentists
Surveys of physicians and dentists within the communities were conducted to assess the impact of interventions on patients' counseling. Questionnaire items corresponded to the practice behaviors that were included in the intervention protocol. Information also was collected on office environments (smoke-free or not) and opportunities for training in smoking cessation counseling.

Physicians' and Dentists' Office Staffs   Surveys of physicians' and dentists' office staff were conducted to determine office environments, availability of smoking cessation assistance for patients, signage regarding nonsmoking, and presence of chart reminder systems for smoking patients.

Worksites   Worksite surveys focused on the presence of restrictive smoking policies, the presence or absence of employer motivational or incentive programs, and the availability of worksite smoking cessation programs.

Schools   Surveys in schools focused on restrictive smoking policies, including identification of groups to whom restrictions applied (e.g., students, staff).

Cessation Resources and Services Providers   This survey assessed the number of cessation resources and services available in the communities and the extent to which such services were used.

Religious Organizations   This group was surveyed for the presence of restrictive smoking policies as well as the availability of smoking cessation resources.

Youth   The COMMIT intervention targeted adult heavy smokers, but it was likely that a communitywide campaign against smoking would also affect the smoking behavior of adolescents. For this reason, the COMMIT evaluation included assessments of the smoking habits and attitudes of representative samples of ninth-grade students in intervention and comparison communities in 1990 and 1993. A random sample of approximately 18 ninth-grade classrooms per community, involving approximately 450 students, was surveyed in 1990 and again in 1993. The sample size of the youth survey was designed to permit detection of a 5-percent net change (e.g., from 10 to 15 percent) in surveyed adolescent smoking prevalence between intervention and comparison matched communities.

PROCESS EVALUATION   Another level of evaluation revolved around the activities that were developed to meet the impact objectives. The activities had process objectives attached to them that were designed to achieve the impact goals. Process objectives specified what was considered to be the minimal amount of intervention change required to contribute to the achievement of the overall trial goal. Information was collected on the implementation of each protocol activity, including when events were held, number of attendees, materials distributed, and miscellaneous information. This information was collected through a computerized tracking system developed for this project (Corbett et al., 1990-91).

The COMMIT Program Records System (PRS) was a computerized relational database that had two major purposes: (1) data collection of activities and participation by local groups and individuals and regular updating of the denominators for the various process objectives; and (2) provision of an efficient system to capture, retrieve, display, and report information both locally and trialwide. Centralized quality control procedures were followed.

The data collection process was based on standard forms completed by field staff members as specific activities were initiated, planned, and implemented. The data from the forms were then entered into the system, using preexisting screens and prompts. During the initial stages of the local operations, field staff members also entered the names, addresses, and other contact information for the various groups that were the targets for intervention (e.g., physicians and dentists, hospitals and clinics, worksites, schools, cessation resources and services providers, and religious organizations). These files were named the "affiliate" files and were used to produce sampling frames for surveys and mailing labels and to provide the denominators, updated annually, for each of the targeted groups. The system also allowed recording of data related to other trial objectives, such as monitoring of media (newspapers, billboards, and some electronic media) and optional activities conducted by the community.

The system produced, on request, a status report for process objective attainment. Summary scores of process objectives attained were calculated by community, intervention channel, and the overall trial.

Another part of process evaluation was the development of a method to collect regular qualitative data on trial activities, which was done through a quarterly report that described various interactions with the community volunteers working on the trial, monitored legislative events, kept track of changes in the community context, and documented case studies within the communities (Corbett et al., 1990-91).

ECONOMIC EVALUATION   The final level of evaluation for the trial was an economic analysis to estimate the costs of the trial. The primary outcome of this analysis would be the estimated marginal societal costs of increased smoking cessation (Mattson et al., 1990-91). The analysis also would examine the resources provided by the funding agency and estimate the extent to which those agency resources generated additional community resources for smoking cessation.

SUMMARY   The COMMIT evaluation was as ambitious as the trial. Trial investigators developed a multilevel approach to the project evaluation. Each level down from the outcome evaluation in the cohort of heavy smokers provided a richer and more indepth understanding of what happened in the trial. In a symposium held more than a decade ago, researchers acknowledged that community interventions presented unique problems for assessment of results because the interventions were designed to reach further than the individuals being evaluated (Hulley, 1978; Syme, 1978). Using the multilevel evaluation plan described here will allow researchers to ascertain the "dose" of intervention delivered to each community, the association between the dose and the intermediary agents that were expected to change their activities and behavior to encourage smokers to quit (e.g., policies advocated by physicians and dentists, worksite policies), the receipt of the interventions by individuals (change in attitudes and community norms around smoking), and the change in behavior (smoking cessation).

REFERENCES

COMMIT Research Group. Community Intervention Trial for Smoking Cessation (COMMIT): Summary of design and intervention. *Journal of the National Cancer Institute* 83(22): 1620-1628, 1991.

Corbett, K., Thompson, B., White, N., Taylor, M. (for the COMMIT Research Group). Process evaluation in the Community Intervention Trial for Smoking Cessation (COMMIT). *International Quarterly of Community Health Education* 11(3): 291-309, 1990-91.

Freedman, L.S., Green, S.B., Byar, D.P. Assessing the gain in efficiency due to matching in a community intervention study. *Statistics in Medicine* 9: 943-952, 1990.

Gail, M.H., Byar, D.P., Pechacek, T.F. (for the COMMIT Research Group). Aspects of statistical design for the Community Intervention Trial for Smoking Cessation (COMMIT). *Controlled Clinical Trials* 13: 6-21, 1992.

Gutzwiller, F., Nater, B., Martin, J. Community-based primary prevention of cardiovascular disease in Switzerland: Methods and results of the National Research Program (NRP 1A). *Preventive Medicine* 14: 482-491, 1985.

Hughes, G.H., Hymowitz, N., Ockene, J.K., Simon, N., Vogt, T.F. (for the MRFIT Group). The Multiple Risk Factor Intervention Trial (MRFIT) V. Intervention on smoking. *Preventive Medicine* 10: 476-500, 1981.

Hulley, S.B. Symposium on CHD prevention trials: Design issues in testing life style intervention. *American Journal of Epidemiology* 108(2): 85-86, 1978.

Kovar, M.G., Poe, G.S. *The National Health Interview Survey: Design, 1973-84, and Procedures, 1975-83. A National Probability Sample Survey of the Civilian Noninstitutionalized Population of the United States.* National Center for Health Statistics. Washington, DC: Supt. of Docs., U.S. Govt. Print. Off., 1985.

Mattson, M., Cummings, K.M., Lynn, W., Giffen, C., Corle, D., Pechacek, T.F. (for the COMMIT Research Group). Evaluation plan for the Community Intervention Trial for Smoking Cessation (COMMIT). *International Quarterly of Community Health Education* 11(3): 271-289, 1990-91.

Steenkamp, H.J., Jooste, P.L., Jordaan, P.C., Swanepoel, A.S., Rossouw, J.E. Changes in smoking during a community-based cardiovascular disease intervention programme. *South African Medical Journal* 79(5): 250-253, 1991.

Syme, S.L. Life style intervention in clinic-based trials. *American Journal of Epidemiology* 108(2): 87-91, 1978.

U.S. Department of Health and Human Services. *The Health Consequences of Smoking: Cancer. A Report of the Surgeon General.* DHHS Publication No. (PHS) 82-50179. Rockville, MD: U.S. Department of Health and Human Services, Public Health Service, Office on Smoking and Health, 1982.

U.S. Department of Health and Human Services. *Reducing the Health Consequences of Smoking: 25 Years of Progress: A Report of the Surgeon General.* DHHS Publication No. (CDC) 89-8411. Rockville, MD: U.S. Department of Health and Human Services, Public Health Service, Centers for Disease Control, Center for Chronic Disease Prevention and Health Promotion, Office on Smoking and Health, 1989.

U.S. Department of Health and Human Services. *Smoking, Tobacco, and Cancer Program: 1985-1989 Status Report.* NIH Publication No. 90-3107. Rockville, MD: U.S. Department of Health and Human Services, Public Health Service, National Institutes of Health, National Cancer Institute, 1990.

AUTHORS

William R. Lynn
COMMIT Project Officer
Public Health Applications Research Branch
Cancer Control Science Program
National Cancer Institute
National Institutes of Health
Executive Plaza North, Room 241
6130 Executive Boulevard, MSC-7337
Bethesda, MD 20892-7337

Beti Thompson, Ph.D.
Associate Professor
University of Washington School of Public
   Health and Community Medicine
Associate Member
Fred Hutchinson Cancer Research Center,
   MP-702
1124 Columbia Street
Seattle, WA 98104

Community Intervention Trial for Smoking Cessation: Development of the Intervention

William R. Lynn, Beti Thompson, and Terry F. Pechacek

INTRODUCTION The Community Intervention Trial for Smoking Cessation (COMMIT) intervention protocol was developed by collaborating trial investigators during a 24-month planning phase. To select the specific intervention methods included in the COMMIT protocol, the investigators used a wide variety of data from controlled and demonstration trials of smoking control strategies as well as advice from public health experts and their own experience in large-scale behavior change efforts. The protocol took into account several theoretical perspectives on health behavior change, including social learning theories (Bandura, 1977 and 1986; Abrams et al., 1986; Elder et al., 1986), persuasion models for communication and social influences (Bandura, 1977; Flay et al., 1983; McAlister et al., 1982; Rogers, 1973), the health belief model (Green et al., 1980; Rosenstock, 1974), action research models for community organization and innovation diffusion (Rothman, 1979; Grusky and Miller, 1981; Gusfield, 1962; Rogers and Shoemaker, 1971), and others.

In evaluating smoking control literature, it was obvious that the vast majority of the published literature had focused on individual-oriented strategies as discussed in Chapter 2 of this monograph. Although these interventions were viewed as efficacious in many settings, especially clinical settings, most COMMIT investigator team members saw them as inefficient and inconsistent with the overall intervention philosophy of this trial, which is intended to achieve large-scale change within the community. In addition, enhancement of traditional cessation services (i.e., quit-smoking programs and self-help materials) was deemed as supportive of the overall goals of the trial but insufficient to achieve the breadth of change desired. The consensus of the investigators was that other primary intervention strategies were needed to reach large portions of the smokers in the community; furthermore, such strategies needed a high potential of increasing both the frequency and success rate of self-initiated quit-smoking attempts.

The investigators were guided in the development of the COMMIT protocol by the fundamental assumption that a community approach to smoking control must focus on the social and environmental factors that influence smokers' contemplation of quitting, efforts to initiate quitting behaviors, and ability to maintain abstinence on a permanent basis (Farquhar, 1978; Farquhar et al., 1981; Blackburn and Pechacek, 1986; Thompson and Kinne, 1990). It also was expected that communitywide intervention strategies would be more effective because they would provide a sustained intervention effect on a large segment of the smoking population, as opposed

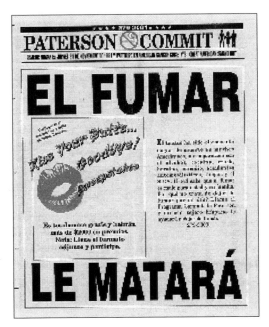

to sporadic higher intensity intervention contacts with only the small segment of smokers willing to attend or participate in more traditional smoking cessation interventions (Leventhal et al., 1980; Schwartz, 1991). A significant portion of the trial intervention effort was expected to focus on changing the community's social norms regarding smoking as well as the overall informational environment so that it would be difficult for any smokers in the community to escape the consistent and repeated messages about the benefits of cessation; simultaneously, they would be provided with ongoing cues and opportunities to initiate quitting behaviors (Lichtenstein et al., 1990-91; Thompson and Kinne, 1990; Thompson et al., 1990-91).

Nevertheless, it also was recognized that few tried-and-tested interventions existed that were not individual oriented. A few community studies, such as the North Karelia Project (Puska et al., 1983), the Australian North Coast Healthy Lifestyle Programme: Quit for Life (Egger et al., 1983), and others discussed in Chapter 2, targeted smoking cessation as one of their endpoints. The projects used several strategies, including mass media and skills training, which were examined in the development of the COMMIT interventions. However, the COMMIT interventions were developed primarily from existing programs within the Smoking and Tobacco Control Program of the National Cancer Institute (NCI). The trial investigators selected the best individual or small-group interventions that existed and grouped them together in an intervention package that was expected to reach all facets of the community. Channels of intervention that were thought to be key for reaching heavy smokers were identified and provided an organizing structure for specific activities. The interventions were designed to be delivered through a community-organization approach so that they would become an integral part of the everyday lives of the community's smokers.

INTERVENTION GOALS AND OBJECTIVES   The evaluation of COMMIT specified one primary outcome goal—an increased cessation rate by heavy smokers in the intervention communities. However, for that goal to be reached, several other community changes had to occur. Using a public health perspective and a community focus of intervention, the investigators defined four general intervention goals to guide the COMMIT effort:

1. *Increase the priority of smoking as a public health issue.* As previously discussed, most intervention efforts have focused on smoking as

an individual's problem behavior, resulting in primarily clinically oriented cessation methods rather than interventions that involved the broad social and environmental networks in which a smoker lives and smokes. The COMMIT intervention defined smoking as a community problem that requires public health action by the community at large. Although the COMMIT intervention was focused primarily on adult smoking cessation, smoking prevention also must be addressed; hence, activities focusing on youth and prevention were incorporated into many trial interventions.

2. *Increase the community capacity to modify smoking behavior.* When smoking has been viewed as an individual problem, community resources to assist smokers have tended to be relatively sparse. In conjunction with efforts to meet the first goal, it is acknowledged that individual smokers who seek assistance need to have an adequate system of resources and services available. These resources and services need to be fully integrated into community institutions and groups so that the logistical barriers to their use can be reduced and delivery of these services by the community can increase the overall capacity to address the smoking problem. The investigators recognized that traditional clinical programs are used by a small minority of smokers and that the community resources and services promoted by COMMIT need to include any and all methods that may interest smokers. Furthermore, mechanisms must be in place to remind smokers of the available opportunities to seek help with cessation.

3. *Increase within a community the influence of existing policy and economic factors that discourage smoking.* Local and State laws and ordinances controlling smoking in public places and limiting tobacco sales have become common in the United States and Canada (U.S. Department of Health and Human Services, 1993). It is clear that such policies and economic factors can be an important part of the social environment of smokers and their decisions to attempt cessation. Factors that

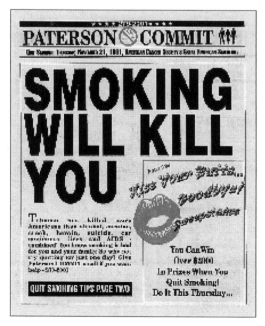

can influence smoking rates include cigarette taxes; constraints on advertising and promotion of tobacco products; policies related to the sale and distribution of cigarettes, especially to minors; and restrictions on smoking in public places, worksites, organizations, and other settings where smokers tend to congregate.

4. *Increase social norms and values supporting nonsmoking.* The social acceptability of smoking is steadily declining in the United States and Canada (U.S. Department of Health and Human Services, 1989). Although a social norm supporting nonsmoking is emerging, progress in many communities is still hampered by the prevailing perception that smoking is a problem of an individual. As intervention efforts attempt to highlight smoking as a public health and community problem, opportunities will arise to strengthen the perception that nonsmoking is normative and to be valued and that smoking is harmful to the community at large. As the social acceptability of smoking declines, the negative social consequences of smoking increase and further reinforce both quitting behaviors and maintenance of abstinence in recent quitters.

These four overall trial goals led to the establishment of several objectives that, if reached, could be expected to help meet the goals. Similarly, the identification of trial activities was predicated on the relationship between those activities and the objectives they were intended to attain. The philosophy that a hierarchical association exists between the overall trial goal, intermediate trial goals, impact objectives, mandated intervention activities, and process objectives led to a systematic development of goals and objectives.

Intermediate goals were directed at the various channels of intervention identified as being critical to achieving community change. The channels contained intermediary agents that were likely to come into regular and repeated contact with smokers. In addition, the intermediary agents also were thought to be amenable to new practices that would encourage smoking cessation. An example is found in the health care provider channel. Because the majority of smokers see a health care provider annually, a relatively simple change on the part of providers—reminding smokers to stop or setting quit dates with smokers—may be sufficient to lead many smokers to attempt cessation. The intermediate goal, then, is to build a critical mass of health care providers who give such regular encouragement. To achieve that goal, several impact objectives were established; for example, 80 percent of community physicians and 65 percent of community dentists should receive training in basic smoking cessation practices, and 30 percent of physicians' offices should receive training in setting up office systems to track smokers and document that cessation encouragement was given.

Similar impact objectives were established for each of the four major channels of intervention (i.e., health care providers, worksites and organizations, cessation resources and services, and public education), plus a fifth overarching channel of community mobilization. Attempts also were made to quantify the degree to which objectives had to change to achieve the trial goals. Through the use of existing literature, previous intervention experience, and advice from experts in the smoking field, consensus was reached among the trial investigators concerning the quantification of the impact objectives (Wallack and Sciandra, 1990-91; Ockene et al., 1990-91; Sorensen et al., 1990-91; Pomrehn et al., 1990-91).

Impact objectives, in turn, led to the mandated activities required by the protocol. The extant literature, experience of investigators, and much discussion resulted in the identification of a set of activities for each intervention channel considered likely to lead to realization of the impact objectives. Assessment of the implementation of intervention activities was accomplished through the completion of process objectives that documented various components of the activities. A computerized system for tracking process objective achievement also was developed (Corbett et al., 1990-91).

INTERVENTION AREAS   The intervention protocol was divided into five major sections corresponding to the channels of intervention: Community Mobilization, an overarching section to organize the community around tobacco control; Health Care Providers; Worksites and Organizations; Cessation Resources and Services; and Public Education. Each of the five channels was selected for its potential contribution toward achieving the trial outcome. Most mandated intervention activities within each channel area had proved efficacious in other settings, and the investigators believed that combining such intervention activities would result in a synergism that would lead to change. Each channel is described below.

Community Mobilization Channel   COMMIT's overall goal of community mobilization was to build the capacity of communities to address smoking control issues. Community mobilization also was intended to facilitate the implementation of smoking control activities and ensure maintenance of these activities.

Achieving citizen participation and community partnership requires mobilization of a community. Mobilization is a process through which community members become aware of a problem, identify the problem as a high priority for community action, and institute steps to resolve the problem (Thompson and Pertschuk, 1992). Each community has its own structures, history, and resources necessitating some variation between communities in the process of mobilization. The logic and philosophy of the trial provided each community, through standard mobilization features, with some discretion in local trial management. The basic mobilization model was designed to provide scientific integrity while allowing some local flexibility to establish structures and implement activities in a manner congruent with local practice.

The mobilization plan began with a strong understanding of the community gained through a community analysis designed to yield a systematic understanding of community history, social climate, culture, structures, resources, organizations, and key individuals. Research staff identified several key individuals as candidates for an initial planning group, where members were introduced to the trial's rationale, design, and protocol. Depending on their enthusiasm and availability, they were asked to serve on a short-term Community Planning Group charged with developing a more comprehensive and long-lasting community Board. Each intervention community had to form a new community Board, which was required to provide project legitimacy, access, and overall management support to the community; to represent the key sectors considered to be important in all communities (i.e., health care, business and labor, health voluntary organizations, media, education); and to accurately represent the community. Rules were established to maximize community involvement in intervention planning and implementation. Wherever local groups or organizations existed that could conduct an intervention activity, they were given highest priority to do so, even if required training of staff or enhancing the resources that were already dedicated to the activity was required. Similarly, rules were established for resource allocation in accordance with the philosophy that the resources available through the trial were by themselves insufficient to implement the protocol but should be perceived as "seed" resources to develop existing or new community mechanisms for smoking control.

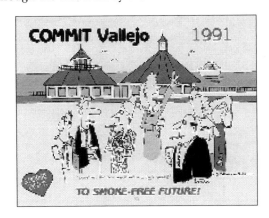

The trial protocol was developed by the investigators before the communities were randomized; therefore, the community had no input into the content of the protocol. However, communities were expected to develop their own plans, consistent with the protocol, to achieve a social climate that would support non-use of tobacco. To maximize the potential of communities to make a permanent change, external resources (NCI funded), both fiscal and human, were limited and considered seed resources. Limiting resources would encourage the communities to contribute some of their own resources and thereby eventually incorporate some tobacco control activities into their own organizational structures.

Health Care Providers Channel
Health care providers and the settings in which they work are important to reaching heavy smokers in the community (Ockene et al., 1990-91). Targeted health care providers included physicians and dentists, although it also was considered desirable to involve pharmacists, nurses, respiratory therapists, and other health care providers. The mandated intervention activities focused on involving community health professionals in smoking cessation intervention activities in their practices and in their roles as community leaders. Each community identified key influential health

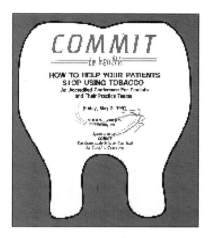

professionals who were interested and able to play leadership roles in the COMMIT intervention. National training equipped these influentials to persuade their colleagues indirectly through discussions at meetings and social events and directly through presentation of types of training events to make smoking cessation counseling part of their regular practice. An important component of this task force was the policy change expected to take place in all health care facilities in the communities. Intervention objectives included smoke-free hospitals, medical offices, nursing homes, and substance abuse treatment centers. Enhancing the availability of cessation information and antismoking promotional messages was also an important goal of this channel.

Worksites and Organizations Channel

Worksites are an ideal location for promotion and support of smoking cessation efforts, including both programs and policies. Seventy percent of adults between the ages of 18 and 65 are employed (Sorensen et al., 1990-91). Worksites and community organizations are opportune places to publicize project activities, offer quit-smoking programs, promote policy changes, and foster environments supportive of successful quitting. They also are important as sources for personnel and local resources to support project activities, particularly large-scale community events. Intervention activities described for worksites and organizations were to be offered widely in the community; however, activities were targeted particularly to sites in which heavy smokers could be reached most effectively. Worksites offered great potential for reaching less educated and less motivated heavy smokers who might not volunteer for or be reached by other community antismoking activities. Restrictive smoking policies were seen as having much to contribute to the social environment; therefore, many COMMIT intervention activities in this channel were oriented to presentations and consultations with worksites to assist them in implementing policies.

Other organizations also were targeted for intervention. Fraternal organizations, civic groups, religious organizations, and so forth were used both for promotion of smoking cessation policies and activities and as targets for such interventions. The protocol called for intervention activities such as presentations to encourage more restrictive policies, provide information to such groups, and attempt to involve these groups in promotion activities.

Cessation Resources and Services Channel

In addition to the powerfully addictive nature of tobacco, there are many barriers that contribute to the continuing high smoking rate among adults. Although knowledge of the hazards of smoking and the benefits of quitting provide reasons for cessation, barriers to quitting include willingness to take a risk, paucity of cues to quit smoking, difficulty in obtaining self-help materials, low awareness and use of existing smoking cessation services, high relapse rates among smokers trying to quit, and inadequate social support for smokers who are motivated to quit. A wealth of information exists regarding methods and techniques that can aid smokers who are trying to quit (Schwartz, 1991; Thompson and Hopp, 1991). Much is available in self-help formats, including books, pamphlets, audiotapes, and videotapes, and most of these materials are available from voluntary health agencies free or at minimal cost. Numerous programs to help smokers have been developed and refined over the past three decades. Programs offered by the major health voluntary organizations, local hospitals, and other community agencies have benefited from the thousands of research projects on smoking cessation conducted in recent years.

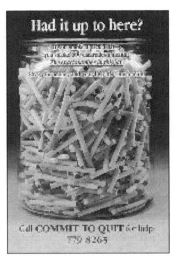

A fundamental assumption underlying COMMIT intervention activities was that an increase in cessation rates requires a change in the social circumstances surrounding smokers' decisions to quit, to initiate quitting, and to maintain abstinence (Pomrehn et al., 1990-91). The aim of COMMIT was not to provide cessation services; rather, the aim was to increase the demand for cessation resources and services as smokers became more willing to attempt cessation. Thus, activities in this channel were limited to those that provided the regular, inescapable messages about opportunities for cessation. Specific intervention activities, such as a voluntary smokers' registry, newsletters, and publication of guides promoting cessation resources and services, were undertaken to increase the quantity and utilization of existing services. Those activities also were designed to enhance the efforts of other trial interventions, particularly worksite, organizational, and health care provider interventions.

Public Education Channel
Communitywide public education efforts were central to the trial's activities to meet overall intervention goals. Educational efforts focused on mass media campaigns promoting smoking as a public health problem, smoking prevention, and communitywide cessation activities. The media contribute significantly to the overall context in which personal decisions about initiating, continuing, or quitting smoking occur. The media are a key source of social-environmental cues regarding nonsmoking behavior (Wallack and Sciandra, 1990-91). An important function of this channel was to establish and maintain the visibility and credibility of COMMIT in the communities.

Mass communication plays a significant role in the ongoing effort to control smoking. The media can perform an important agenda-setting function, they can confer status and legitimacy, and they can activate public discussion. In addition, the media can reinforce nonsmoking behavior (among both smokers and nonsmokers), generating further help-seeking behavior (e.g., calling a toll-free number) and recruiting smokers into treatment programs, and can advertise and promote opportunities for cessation. The media also can promote norms that are supportive of nonsmoking and quitting.

Smoking prevention among youth was not a primary program focus in COMMIT. However, activities targeted at youth have the potential for increasing the community's awareness of smoking and health issues and for shifting social norms. Health promotion through educational, policy, and regulatory activities aimed at youth have traditionally been noncontroversial and can provide leverage for community organizing efforts. Tobacco education activities for youth were used to enhance the visibility, credibility, and acceptability of COMMIT. Although school-based, tobacco use education was not emphasized in COMMIT, it is hypothesized that the overall intervention can decrease the prevalence of adolescent smoking, can have an effect on smokeless tobacco use among adolescents, and will modify the precursors of adolescent smoking behavior.

SPECIAL CONSIDERATIONS OF THE INTERVENTION DESIGN

An important factor in the COMMIT intervention was the necessity to constrain the intervention to relatively small communities so that a rigorously designed trial could be implemented. However, it is important to note that communities are not independent social systems. They exist also in a larger social context, and external events or changes in the broad social system can have a substantial effect on the local community. As a conceptual framework, a system's perspective provides a useful model. In such a perspective, the community is made up of many different components, including political, economic, and health sectors (Thompson and Kinne, 1990). Changes in any part of the system or changes external to the system reverberate throughout the system and result in adjustments or responses that will ultimately affect the entire system. Social norms change along with the system to provide new rules of conduct (Robertson, 1977).

Just as the North Karelia Project showed that an implemented national policy could affect smoking behavior nationally (Puska, 1983) and just as the Minnesota Heart Health Program indicated a large secular trend that may have overwhelmed any intervention effect (Luepker et al., 1994), several external factors were present during the COMMIT trial that could have had an impact on the communities involved. For example, California passed Proposition 99, which released huge amounts of resources for antismoking activities, including mass media campaigns that directed attention to minorities, members of low socioeconomic groups, and other subgroups of smokers. Another example is Canada's passing an excise tax that raised the price of a package of cigarettes to new highs and resulted in a decrease in the prevalence of smoking. Within New York State, policies on smoking in public places, including worksites, were strengthened.

Nationally, the U.S. Environmental Protection Agency classified secondhand smoke as a Class A carcinogen (U.S. Environmental Protection Agency, 1992), making employers think more seriously about the liability associated with smoking in the workplace. National fast-food restaurant chains became at least particially smoke-free to to project an image of protecting youth. In short, the broad social environment within which the pairs of communities were located may have changed substantially, making it difficult to determine what the effects of the COMMIT intervention alone were.

The COMMIT interventions initially were formulated to provide synergy between the various activities. Synergy is the cooperation among various parts of the system or the way the components of a system act together. When activities are oriented toward a common goal, synergy makes the net effect of the forces greater than the sum of its parts. Synergy makes it impossible to separate out the contribution to the outcome of the various parts of the COMMIT intervention. The investigators had to be satisfied that the package they developed produced synergy, which meant that no channel could be emphasized over another and that subsequent analyses to account for the contribution of specific channels were not possible. This approach was further complicated by issues of measurement. Only the achievement of process objectives was measurable; it was not possible to assess the interaction between various activities or process objectives.

Another key consideration involved the group of investigators involved in the project. Because the individuals came from a variety of disciplines, backgrounds, and experience levels, there was initially considerable controversy over the approach to take. The options were reduced to two basic approaches: In one approach, the 11 intervention communities would simply be given resources to design their own studies, whereas a standardized protocol would be followed in the other. The first approach would produce a purer community study but would likely result in many different interventions. This could not be regarded as a rigorous randomized controlled trial. The second approach fulfilled the requirements of scientific rigor but greatly constrained the role of the community in designing interventions. The limited time for planning and discussion of these issues made it difficult for investigators to come to consensus. The design process of the trial alienated various "stakeholders," and this resulted in wasted effort and time.

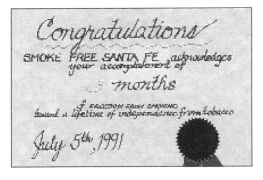

SUMMARY   The theoretical base for COMMIT used existing knowledge, state-of-the-art interventions, and the wisdom of investigators in the field to develop an intervention strategy and protocol oriented to meet the trial's overall goals and impact and process objectives. Mandated activities were intended to lead to achievement of the impact objectives, which in turn would lead to attainment of the intermediate and overall trial goals. A number of lessons were learned in the development of the protocol.

1. The intervention strategies implemented in COMMIT were designed to have a large effect on the communities' attitudes to and behaviors regarding cigarette smoking, yet there was little in the literature to provide insights on how best to do this. Even media studies that had been conducted previously showed only marginal changes in knowledge and attitudes.

2. Although the COMMIT protocol was built on the best knowledge available from randomized clinical trials in the area of smoking control, it is not clear how those experiences can be extrapolated to a randomized community trial.

3. A unique feature of COMMIT was that the diverse and extensive interventions were combined in such a manner that a communitywide effect was anticipated. Based on the supposition that people are more likely to stop smoking when the policies regulating smoking, the opportunities for cessation, and the messages about the dangers of smoking for both smokers and nonsmokers are predominant within a community, COMMIT wished to create a social environment in the intervention communities where smoking was nonnormative. Despite these ambitious goals, it was unclear how best to change policies and get messages to the target group of heavy smokers.

4. It was assumed that implementation of the mandated activities through the five intervention channels would make it difficult for any smoker to avoid messages about or opportunities for smoking cessation. Again, there was not strong evidence from the results of other trials to support the assumption.

5. The community is not an entity in and of itself; rather, it exists in a broader social context that also may be changing. When a community rides the secular trend, it is difficult to judge the effects of an intervention; it may have been better to build more flexibility into the protocol so that different tactics could have been used when the external environment changed.

6. Synergy is an excellent construct but was impossible to measure in this trial. That may not be completely negative, but if efficient trials or interventions are to be devised, it would be helpful to be able to identify the components of the intervention.

7. Lack of attention to stakeholders in the development of the protocol led to considerable controversy. More time should have been allowed to reach consensus in a trial of this magnitude.

REFERENCES

Abrams, D.B., Elder, J.P., Carleton, R.A., Lasater, T.M., Artz, L.M. Social learning principles for organizational health promotion: An integrated approach. In: *Health and Industry: A Behavioral Medicine Perspective*, M.F. Cataldo and T.J. Coates (Editors). New York: Wiley-Interscience, 1986, pp. 28-51.

Bandura, A. *Social Learning Theory*. Englewood Cliffs, NJ: Prentice-Hall, 1977.

Bandura, A. *Social Foundations of Thought and Action: A Social Cognitive Theory*. Englewood Cliffs, NJ: Prentice-Hall, 1986.

Blackburn, H., Pechacek, T.F. Smoking cessation and the Minnesota Heart Health Program. In: *Proceedings of the Fifth World Conference on Smoking and Health*, W.F. Forbes, R.C. Frecker, and D. Nostbakken (Editors). Ottawa, Canada: Canadian Council on Smoking and Health, 1986, pp. 159-164.

Corbett, K., Thompson, B., White, N., Taylor, M. (for the COMMIT Research Group). Process evaluation in the Community Intervention Trial for Smoking Cessation (COMMIT). *International Quarterly of Community Health Education* 11(3): 291-309, 1990-91.

Egger, G., Fitzgerald, W., Frape, G., Monaem, A., Rubenstein, P., Tyler, C., McKay, B. Result of large scale media antismoking campaign in Australia: North Coast "Quit for Life" Programme. *British Medical Journal* 286: 1125-1128, 1983.

Elder, J.P., McGraw, S.A., Abrams, D.B., Ferreira, A., Lasater, T.M., Longpre, H., Peterson, G.S., Schwertfeger, R., Carleton, R.A. Organizational and community approaches to community-wide prevention of heart disease: The first two years of the Pawtucket Heart Health Program. *Preventive Medicine* 15: 107-117, 1986.

Farquhar, J. The community-based model of life style intervention trials. *American Journal of Epidemiology* 108: 103-111, 1978.

Farquhar, J.W., Magnus, P.F., Maccoby, N. The role of public information and education in cigarette smoking control. *Canadian Journal of Public Health* 72: 412-420, 1981.

Flay, B.R., Hansen, W.B., Johnson, C.A., Sobel, J.L. "Involvement of Children in Motivating Smoking Parents To Quit Smoking With a Television Program." Paper presented at the Fifth World Conference on Smoking and Health, Manitoba, Canada, 1983.

Green, L.W., Kreuter, M.W., Deeds, S.G., Partridge, K.B. *Health Education Planning: A Diagnostic Approach*. Palo Alto, CA: Mayfield, 1980.

Grusky, O., Miller, G.A. (Editors). *The Sociology of Organizations: Basic Studies*. (2nd ed.) New York: Free Press, 1981.

Gusfield, J.R. Mass society and extremist politics. *American Sociological Review* 27: 19-30, 1962.

Leventhal, H., Cleary, P.D., Safer, M.A., Gutman, M. Cardiovascular risk factor modification by community-based programs for life-style changes: Comments on the Stanford study. *Journal of Consulting and Clinical Psychology* 48: 150-158, 1980.

Lichtenstein, E., Wallack, L., Pechacek, T. (for the COMMIT Research Group). Introduction to the Community Intervention Trial for Smoking Cessation (COMMIT). *International Quarterly of Community Health Education* 11(3): 173-185, 1990-91.

Luepker, R.V., Murray, D.M., Jacobs, D.K., Jr., Mittelmark, M.B., Bracht, N., Carlaw, R., Crow, R., Elmer, P., Finnegan, S., Folsom, A.R., Grimm, R., Hannan, P.J., Jeffrey, R., Lando, H., McGovern, P., Mullis, R., Perry, C.L., Pechacek, T., Pirie, P., Sprafka, J.M., Weisbrod, R., Blackburn, H. Community education for cardiovascular disease prevention: Risk factor changes in the Minnesota Heart Health Program. *American Journal of Public Health* 84(9): 1383-1393, 1994.

McAlister, A., Puska, P., Salonen, J.T., Toumilehto, J., Koskela, K. Theory and action for health promotion: Illustrations from the North Karelia Project. *American Journal of Public Health* 72: 43-50, 1982.

Ockene, J.K., Lindsay, E., Berger, L., Hymowitz, N. (for the COMMIT Research Group). Health care providers as key change agents in the Community Intervention Trial for Smoking Cessation (COMMIT). *International Quarterly of Community Health Education* 11(3): 223-237, 1990-91.

Pomrehn, P., Sciandra, R., Shipley, R., Lynn, W., Lando, H. (for the COMMIT Research Group). Enhancing resources for smoking cessation through community intervention: COMMIT as a prototype. *International Quarterly of Community Health Education* 11(3): 259-269, 1990-91.

Puska, P., Nissinen, A., Salonen, J.T., Tuomilehto, J. Ten years of the North Karelia Project. Results with community-based prevention of coronary heart disease. *Scandinavian Journal of Social Medicine* 11(3): 65-68, 1983.

Robertson, I. *Sociology*. New York: Worth, 1977.

Rogers, E. *Communication Strategies for Family Planning*. New York: Free Press, 1973.

Rogers, E.M., Shoemaker, F.F. *Communication of Innovations: A Cross-Cultural Approach*. (2nd ed.) New York: Free Press, 1971.

Rosenstock, I. Historical origins of the health belief model. *Education Monographs* 2: 328-335, 1974.

Rothman, J. Three models of community organization practice. In: *Strategies of Community Organization: A Book of Readings*, F.M. Cox, J.L. Erlich, J. Rothman, and J.E. Tropman (Editors). Itasca, IL: Peacock Publishers, 1979, pp. 86-102.

Schwartz, J.L. Methods for smoking cessation. *Clinics in Chest Medicine* 12(4): 737-768, 1991.

Sorensen, G., Glasgow, R.E., Corbett, K. (for the COMMIT Research Group). Promoting smoking control through worksites in the Community Intervention Trial for Smoking Cessation (COMMIT). *International Quarterly of Community Health Education* 11(3): 239-257, 1990-91.

Thompson, B., Hopp, H. Community-based programs for smoking cessation. *Clinics in Chest Medicine* 12: 801-818, 1991.

Thompson, B., Kinne, S. Social change theory: Applications to community health. In: *Health Promotion at the Community Level*, N. Bracht (Editor). Newbury Park, CA: Sage, 1990, pp. 45-65.

Thompson, B., Pertschuk, M. Community intervention and advocacy. In: *Prevention of Coronary Heart Disease*, J.K. Ockene and I.S. Ockene (Editors). Boston: Little, Brown, 1992, pp. 493-515.

Thompson, B., Wallack, L., Lichtenstein, E., Pechacek, T. (for the COMMIT Research Group). Principles of community organization and partnership for smoking cessation in the Community Intervention Trial for Smoking Cessation (COMMIT). *International Quarterly of Community Health Education* 11(3): 187-203, 1990-91.

U.S. Department of Health and Human Services. *Reducing the Health Consequences of Smoking: 25 Years of Progress. A Report of the Surgeon General.* DHHS Publication No. (CDC) 89-8411, Rockville, MD: U.S. Department of Health and Human Services, Public Health Service, Centers for Disease Control, Center for Disease Prevention and Health Promotion, Office on Smoking and Health, 1989.

U.S. Department of Health and Human Services. *Major Local Tobacco Ordinances in the United States.* Smoking and Tobacco Control Monograph No. 3. NIH Publication No. 93-3532. Rockville, MD: U.S. Department of Health and Human Services, Public Health Service, National Institutes of Health, National Cancer Institute, 1993.

U.S. Environmental Protection Agency. *Respiratory Health Effects of Passive Smoking: Lung Cancer and Other Disorders.* EPA/600/6-90/006F. Washington, DC: Office of Research and Development, Office of Health and Environmental Assessment, 1992.

Wallack, L., Sciandra, R. (for the COMMIT Research Group). Media advocacy and public education in the Community Intervention Trial for Smoking Cessation (COMMIT). *International Quarterly of Community Health Education* 11(3): 205-221, 1990-91.

AUTHORS

William R. Lynn
COMMIT Project Officer
Public Health Applications Research Branch
Cancer Control Science Program
National Cancer Institute
National Institutes of Health
Executive Plaza North, Room 241
6130 Executive Boulevard, MSC-7337
Bethesda, MD 20892-7337

Beti Thompson, Ph.D.
Associate Professor
University of Washington School of Public
  Health and Community Medicine
Associate Member
Fred Hutchinson Cancer Research Center,
  MP-702
1124 Columbia Street
Seattle, WA 98104

Terry F. Pechacek, Ph.D.
Coinvestigator
Department of Social and Preventive
  Medicine
State University of New York at Buffalo
  School of Medicine and Biomedical
  Services
270 Sarber Hall
Buffalo, NY 14214-3000

Mobilizing the COMMIT Communities for Smoking Control

Beti Thompson, Linda Nettekoven, Dianne Ferster, Len C. Stanley, Juliet Thompson, and Kitty K. Corbett

INTRODUCTION   Twenty years of community intervention studies have taught us much about the need to engage communities in health behavior change and about the processes required to involve communities (Abrams et al., 1986; Carlaw et al., 1984; Elder et al., 1986; Farquhar et al., 1985; Puska et al., 1985). Widespread agreement about the benefits of using community organizations as primary delivery systems in large-scale health behavior change programs (Green and Raeburn, 1990; McAlister et al., 1982; Tarlov et al., 1987) has been supported by theoretical arguments that durable changes in lifestyles of whole populations require changes in the community environment to support the behavior changes by individuals (Egger et al., 1983; Fortmann et al., 1990; Puska et al., 1983; Tarlov et al., 1987). Several community studies have been conducted in recent years, primarily on cardiovascular risk reduction; initial results from those studies and large-scale smoking cessation trials indicate that behavior change is possible (Carlaw et al., 1984; Egger et al., 1983; Elder et al., 1986; Puska et al., 1985; Fortmann et al., 1990). Most such studies have been carried out with some collaboration by investigators and the communities.

Collaboration between community and researchers, although seen as essential to the research project, varies widely in both the form it takes and the way it is developed. Collaboration can vary from little community involvement, such as community permission to target a particular place for intervention activities by an external agent, to total community control, such as giving a community funds to develop its own solutions to a specific problem. However, for the majority of external funding agencies, a more moderate approach is followed in which the community becomes a partner in the change activity. Increasingly, a strategy called "community organization" is being used, whereby community members become active participants in addressing a problem that affects the entire community (Thompson et al., 1990-91). Theoretically, there are three assumptions that underlie the need to involve local citizenry in a change effort. The first is that behavior occurs in a social context rather than in a vacuum or on an individual basis; the second is that large-scale behavior change requires that the social context be changed; and the third is that change is more likely when the people affected by a problem are involved in defining and solving it (Abrams et al., 1986; Kuriji et al., 1988; Florin and Wandersman, 1990; Thompson and Kinne, 1990). Funding agents and studies that now are attempting to reduce chronic disease risk factors at the community level almost uniformly foster relationships with the community receiving interventions so that local citizens participate in the projects (Chavis et al., 1983; Crosby et al., 1986; Englund, 1986; Millar and Naegle, 1987).

Gaining citizen participation in communities generally requires mobilization of at least some portions of the community. Community, in this context, is a group of people sharing a locality, being interdependent, having interpersonal relationships, and having a sense of belonging to the larger entity (Thompson and Kinne, 1990; Warren, 1958).

Mobilization is the process whereby the community or some of its parts become aware of a condition that has negative implications for the

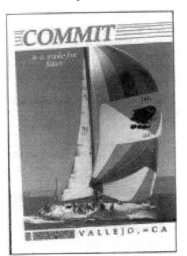

community, identify the condition as a priority for community action, and institute steps to change the condition (Thompson and Pertschuk, 1992). Mobilization is a complex process often idiosyncratic to a community and a project. Partially as a result, few data have been systematically gathered or published about mobilization activities in diverse community studies; rather, an occasional description of the mobilization process may be included in a progress report on research development. A few researchers have examined the process more concretely (Burghardt, 1982; Hunkeler et al., 1990; Stunkard et al., 1985; Thompson et al., 1993), thereby yielding some information on the processes of initially interesting and involving communities in health behavior change.

Although any kind of external funding agency is likely to constrain community efforts to address a problem, research in communitywide projects addressing health promotion poses special problems for involving communities. In a "pure" community approach, community members take the initiative by defining a problem; however, in externally funded projects, the original impetus for the community to accept the existence of a problem comes from external sources that have their own plans for defining and addressing the problem. In addition, the need for integrity of the research and the constraints of funding by government agencies generally put strict limits on the extent to which individual communities can be part of the decisionmaking processes in health promotion projects. Although community members may have their own ideas for addressing a problem, there is likely to be little researcher support for innovation or deviation from a research plan. For example, the Community Intervention Trial for Smoking Cessation (COMMIT) project required communities that were to receive funds to define smoking as a major public health problem. In addition, it utilized a standardized protocol that required the community to implement certain activities before turning to activities that came up from the community.

In spite of the departure from a pure community organization model, the COMMIT project attempted to build a partnership with the

11 intervention communities; it followed a standardized mobilization protocol to build community infrastructures that could address the smoking problems. In this chapter, the mobilization experiences of the 11 communities that participated in COMMIT are described. Because the communities followed a standardized mobilization protocol to organize themselves to address tobacco control, this experience offered a unique opportunity to examine several questions about mobilization and the use of a common strategy for mobilizing communities.

Specific questions of interest included the following: What are the important factors in developing a common mobilization process? Can a single mobilization protocol be implemented across 11 communities? Can mobilization protocol objectives and timelines be met consistently in the various communities? Are the experiences of these communities generalizable to other community health initiatives? What happened in the field as the communities followed the protocol? The lessons learned from the initial mobilization process in the 11 COMMIT intervention communities are presented in this chapter.

ADAPTATIONS FOR RESEARCH PURPOSES   COMMIT builds on a community organization perspective (Blackburn, 1983; Green, 1986; Farquhar, 1978; Kelly, 1979; Labonte, 1989). The partnership arrangement initially planned was one that would reflect "community ownership," important both in theory and in practice. Essentially, the outside experts—the researchers—would be facilitators to guide change, not to control and define it. The general principles of partnership and community ownership were adopted by COMMIT investigators; however, early in the trial, investigators recognized that the design features of COMMIT introduced many potential problems for establishing partnerships with the communities.

After much debate about the shape of the trial (see Chapters 3 and 4), the research direction adopted for COMMIT treated the project as a single study with the equivalence of 22 "subjects": 11 intervention and 11 control communities. With the community as the unit of randomization, it became necessary to define a basic intervention to be tested, with a decision to provide basic commonality in the intervention to permit comparisons across communities (see Chapters 3 and 4). Investigators decided that total local ownership of the project might result in significantly different organizational structures and foci of interventions; indeed, there was a concern that the project might produce 11 different

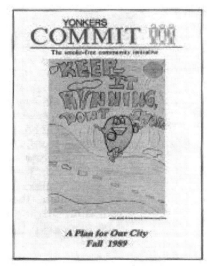

demonstrations rather than a single trial. Researchers also were aware of the danger of too much mandated structure and the threat it might present to local involvement and participation. A compromise approach was developed to maintain trial integrity and provide enough flexibility to accommodate local variations.

Trial integrity was achieved through a protocol that defined a general mobilization process for organizing the intervention communities, establishing a basic structure for organizing local projects, implementing a set of required intervention activities consistent with community customs, and carefully documenting the process (Thompson et al., 1990-91). The general mobilization process and the requirements for establishing the organizational structure are described in this chapter.

The approach used for COMMIT does not meet all the criteria for an equal partnership with the community: As in other community research projects (Chavis et al., 1983; Goodman and Steckler, 1989), scientific goals are a higher priority than the community development goals (Rothman, 1979). Although COMMIT sought to promote partnership whenever possible, it was an unequal process, and the community had less power than either the funding agency (National Cancer Institute [NCI]) or the research institutions receiving funds to administer local projects.

STEPS IN MOBILIZING COMMUNITIES
Significant effort was devoted to defining both the community mobilization process and the resulting structure. The "leadership board" model served as the basic organizational structure. In this structure, a community Board of influential and informed people, often leaders representing key organizations in the community, was formed. The process required an understanding of the community through an examination of secondary sources, conversations with key informants, and involvement of local people with influence in their community to identify and nominate members to serve on a community Board. The approach encourages the inclusion of other community members, especially through task forces, but the focus is on identification and recruitment of known community leaders who have access to, or control over, resources and policy decisions. The model emphasizes participation by members of key community sectors (Thompson and Kinne, 1990) so that the majority of the community is represented.

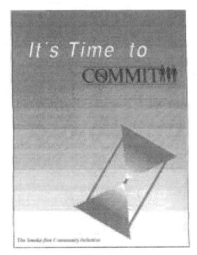

The COMMIT research team established 12 activities (Table 1) that each site was expected to do in support of its mobilization efforts. Most were undertaken during the initial planning phase of the trial before implementation of the intervention. Both the activities and the percent of communities completing each activity are given below:

COMMUNITY ANALYSIS An old Chinese proverb advises: "Go in search of people. Begin with what they know. Build on what they have." This is the challenge facing health promotion advocates as they attempt to design and implement community interventions. The first step in meeting this challenge is to systematically gather information about the strengths, resources, opportunities, and needs in a community. This process has been labeled variously as community diagnosis, community needs assessment, health education planning, and community mapping (Haglund et al., 1990). Ideally, health promotion advocates undertake such a process *with* rather than *to* the community and create opportunities to increase awareness and ownership of any health interventions that result.

The community analysis is designed to provide an indepth, comprehensive look at the community. For lasting change to occur, attention must be paid to the underlying factors that influence behavior, including the factors that might facilitate or inhibit a proposed change within a community as well as the factors that are likely to make a given approach a "good fit" with its host environment. Drawing on the experiences of other community-based health programs, the COMMIT project undertook a series of information-gathering steps in the 11 pairs of communities targeted for study.

Table 1
Mobilization activities and process objectives

Activities To Be Conducted by Each Community	Communities Completing Activities (%)
Establishment of Community Planning Group	100
Planning for Program Office and Staff	100
First Community Board Meeting	100
Creation of Task Force Member List and Recruitment	100
Writing of By-Laws	100
Field Site Management Plan	91
Smoking Control Plan	100
First Annual Action Plan	100
Second Annual Action Plan	100
Third Annual Action Plan	100
Fourth Annual Action Plan	100
Transition Plan	100

Prerandomization   In the first step, researchers prepared a community profile for each of the 22 communities in the trial. Each document blended quantitative information, such as demographic indicators and lists of programs and services, with qualitative information on the community's history and image of itself. The analysis required the collection of extensive information about the communities, including identification of media outlets, health care providers and settings, worksites and business groups, local organizations, available smoking cessation services, and schools and other youth-serving agencies. The analysis also contained a crude assessment of potential intervention channels and resources.

To avoid activation of any of the communities prior to randomization, the report drew primarily on secondary and archival sources (e.g., census data, chamber of commerce publications, local business and trade lists, local media). In addition, a few key informants (people who are knowledgeable about the community) were identified. Discussions with these individuals provided additional information about community structures, key players, influence networks, and previous examples of collaborative effort that focused on public issues.

Postrandomization   For each of the 11 randomly selected intervention communities, a more detailed community analysis was conducted. The postrandomization community analysis assessed the major factors likely to facilitate or inhibit the accomplishment of project goals and the tobacco control activities required for each intervention area. The analysis identified additional key players and stakeholders, provided an assessment of community programs and resources that might be relevant to future tobacco control efforts, and more closely examined the intervention channels. Methods the COMMIT project could use to build on established community organizations were closely explored because a key tenet of the project was to avoid competing with, duplicating, or replacing existing program services. Information gained from the analysis helped staff members work with local organizations.

As part of the postrandomization analysis, investigators developed a description of the community sectors whose participation was considered essential for the project to succeed. Building on the prerandomization analysis, a Community Planning group, consisting of community members representing a variety of sectors and agencies, was convened. The planning group had several responsibilities, including providing input to and refinement of the community analysis. The analysis ended with a community-specific blueprint for forming the community Board, including the sectors to be represented and a list of candidate Board members.

The community analysis is the cornerstone of any community intervention. Across communities, it appears the community analysis is an important tool for both researchers and field staffs as they engage in the initial activation of the community to address tobacco control. In most cases, the community analysis process identified community leaders and other influentials, and it informed participants which groups had been involved in prior health promotion efforts or had a current stake in the tobacco control issue. It laid out a plan for establishing a Board and task forces with a list of possible participants from all fundamental sectors of the community. Community representatives consistently commented that all groups and agencies that became involved in COMMIT were appropriate participants. Yet even after 4 years of effort, all communities could point to one or more groups that did not participate in the project.

What the analysis did not provide in some instances was sufficient insight about the priorities and concerns of key groups that had not been involved previously in tobacco control. This information had to be gathered as the intervention progressed, and many communities were less successful than expected at involving groups that might have provided access to the heavy smoker target group, whether they were unions, blue-collar worksites, racial or ethnic minority organizations, low-income residents, or less educated people. Somehow the analysis failed to provide some communities with the necessary "hooks and handles" to reach into those heavy-smoker enclaves.

Even when such information was available, staff members sometimes did not produce the expected results. In Utica, NY, for example, representatives

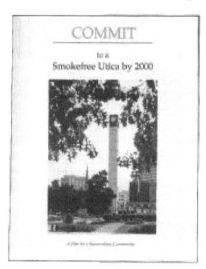

of the minority community were invited to participate in project planning and management via the COMMIT Board and task forces. Later meetings focused on finding ways to tailor COMMIT activities to fit the needs and culture of minority residents. However, despite repeated contacts with appropriate community leaders, other problems, such as drug abuse, crime, and unemployment, continued to receive a higher priority than tobacco use.

Having members of key target groups as volunteers or project employees did pay off in some cases. In Bellingham, WA, the initial Board included both minorities and representatives from blue-collar worksites, and this was seen as important in helping oil refineries become smoke-free. The Vallejo, CA, site attributes much of its success in reaching out to religious organizations to the fact that the staff person doing the outreach was active in the religious community prior to the beginning of the project.

The community analysis was a useful tool for the initial phases of mobilization. Its utility during subsequent years of the trial is more difficult to assess. About half the communities continued to find it useful; however, others complained that it was not user-friendly, seemed redundant, and required the reader to "jump around" the document to find information. Because the community analysis was almost completed before the field staff members and volunteers were deeply involved in the project, many felt little ownership of the document. As a result, some communites reviewed and ratified the community analysis, as required by the protocol, and set it aside and did not consult it again.

Community
Activation
Community activation is the process of familiarizing community members with the issue under investigation—in this case, smoking— and involving them in activities to address the problem. The community analysis provided the basic plan for activating the community. The information gathered in that analysis gave the Community Planning Group the basis for nominating and recruiting Board members and for selling the project to other community members. The short timeframe led many communities to involve research institution staff members in the recruitment process. The haste needed for the initial Board formation reflects yet again the contradiction between the community needs and the research constraints.

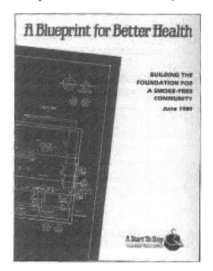

The planning group also had the responsibility for hiring a local field director to run the project. The limited period, the hiring regulations of the research institutions, and the position of the field director vis-a-vis the community Board and the research institution made this task difficult for some communities. The short time allotted to recruiting a field director sometimes made it a process conducted largely by the research institution because the planning group was busy recruiting Board members. Research institutions had their own regulations concerning employees (field directors were the institutions' employees), and this sometimes interfered with the process.

The mobilization protocol acknowledged that the field director would be required to serve two masters: the research institution and the community. For many communities, this duality became an immediate issue in the hiring decision. In some communities, the selection of the field director became a researcher decision, with little or no input by the community Board. In Cedar Rapids/Marion, IA, the Board complained about the research institution's choice but was overruled. (Fortunately, the person hired soon won over the Board members.) In another community (Bellingham), the research institution's first choice of candidates was different from those of the planning group, but the planning group's choice was accepted when members argued that it was their community and they knew best who would be a good fit. (Fortunately, the person selected soon won over the research institution staff.)

The hiring of the field director and the formation of the community Board occurred simultaneously. The basic organizational structure for the communities is shown in Figure 1. The community Board was to be broad based. It would identify and nominate members to serve on four task forces corresponding to the four channels of intervention (public education, health care, worksites and organizations, and cessation resources). Flexibility was allowed in the basic structure: Some Boards added executive committees to make decisions for the Board; two groups added broader community coalitions to meet annually and review project progress; and some Boards added task forces to focus on specific activities.

The process of forming the Board and hiring the field director meant that most communities were prepared to begin in terms of other organizational requirements (e.g., establishing bylaws, recruiting task force members, producing a smoking control plan), and this had implications for the local project. The examples of three communities may be illustrative.

The Board recruitment experience in Brantford, Ontario, Canada, was typical of many communities. The research institution checked the "pulse" of the community through the community analysis and identified influential and interested people in Brantford to participate in the project. The Medical Officer of Health identified individuals who would best represent the

Figure 1
Standardized organizational structure

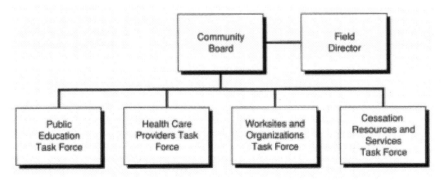

community. The principal investigator of the research institution then contacted those people and requested their involvement. The group that joined (the Community Planning Group) was responsible for planning the Board formation. They also were invited to become Board members; only a few refused. The initial Board had some conspicuous gaps, most notably representatives of local voluntary agencies. However, once the field director was hired, the executive committee of the community Board and the field director developed think-tank sessions to identify people from various sectors to become involved in the project. This approach seemed to work well, and the Board that emerged stayed strong and committed throughout the project.

In Raleigh, NC, the planning group expedited the hiring of a field director so she could assist with the formation of the community Board. Once the field director was on staff, the planning group met with her, identified community sectors that were critical for involvement, and suggested individuals who were good choices to serve on the Board. The planning group members contacted the nominees first; if nominees were willing to serve, the field director followed up. The next step was a letter outlining the project and the expectations held for the volunteers. The personal contact was emphasized as the key to recruiting Board members. This approach was followed throughout the mobilization process in this community. Task forces and replacement members to the Board also were recruited this way as the project continued. Another fruitful recruitment method was inviting the prospective member to serve on an ad hoc committee with a time-limited commitment for a specific event or campaign. Regular meetings of the ad hoc committee with the field director allowed the necessary facilitation without taking the process and product away from the subcommittee.

The research institution in Bellingham selected the small Community Planning Group of seven people. The group worked closely with research institution staff members to identify the important community sectors and potential community Board members from those sectors. They also agreed to recruit specific individuals for the local project. Through their efforts, a Board of 18 members was nominated and recruited within a week after the field director assumed her position. Although the entire group knew a little about the project, the normal complexities of setting up new projects were evident. In an early meeting, the Board members heard a presentation about the project along with a description of their roles and responsibilities. Nevertheless, there were many unanswered questions, including questions about budget and the paperwork required to set up an office. Researchers were honest in their responses; they did not know all the answers at that stage. Group members kept their good humor by telling themselves that the protocol was their "friend"

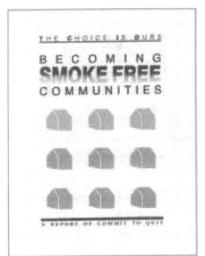

and following it would help them in the organization and implementation process.

The field director's first priorities were orienting the new Board members to the project, explaining their relationship with the research institution, and familiarizing them with the "joys and sorrows" of the protocol. This orientation led to some initial cohesion among the group, which took seriously the task of writing bylaws and recruiting task force members. During the process, some issues emerged that further helped the group come together. Early conflicts among Board members actually facilitated and expedited unity. The issues involved conflicts of interest of Board members who wished to take personal advantage of the project's resources. When the issues came to light, the research institution offered to deal with the problem, but the response from the Board was unanimous: "This is our community; we are responsible for the project; and we will take care of this problem."

Community Buy-In   A major hope in the COMMIT project was that communities would become partners with the research institutions. Because the agenda imposed on the community was artificial—tobacco control was the problem to be addressed, regardless of other problems in the community—effort was needed to promote partnership and ownership. After establishment of the Board and task forces, their first activity was the creation of a comprehensive smoking control plan that would be the framework for intervention activities for the entire project. The plan document was to be produced locally and tied to local facts, figures, and plans. Some communities found the process of producing the plan an important part of the partnership-building process. Other activities, described below, were reported by the field directors as important parts of the buy-in process. There is little doubt that the time required to build feelings of partnership varied among communities; however, representatives from all communities reported that they felt a strong partnership by about the middle of the trial. A few examples follow.

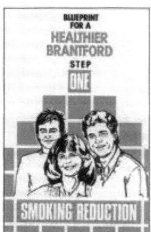

For Brantford, buy-in occurred in small steps. The production of bylaws and the smoking control plan joined people together in understanding the project. The big step occurred with the purchase of office furniture. The frustration of not getting furniture in the field office when it was needed led to a confrontation between the Board members and the staff from the research institution. The research institution responded by changing the process so the community Board could be more active.

For Brantford, as for most communities, a large boost for ownership came when the community Board chairpersons for all the intervention communities were invited to a national COMMIT meeting to see how different groups operated. Other communities also were energized by this meeting. Many Board chairpersons or representatives renewed their energy and gained a common understanding of what it was possible to ask from research institutions.

Some communities relied on specific activities to foster buy-in. For Raleigh, several specific activities pulled the Board and task forces closer together. A COMMIT To Quit contest required much planning that involved many sectors of the community. Board and task force members distributed brochures in health care provider offices, worksites, churches, grocery stores, and malls. They also recruited people and organizations from the larger community to get involvement; that is, they solicited prizes, time, or energy from local radio disk jockeys, a basketball coach, and a drugstore chain. The final tally of more than 1,000 smokers who joined the contest astounded the Board members and made them proud.

A less successful example of buy-in in the same community involved protesting the Philip Morris-sponsored Bill of Rights tour. Despite preparations of Board and task force members to protest the tour under the sponsorship of another tobacco control agency, the research institution stepped in at the last minute to cancel the protest.

Several key activities marked the early buy-in of the project in Bellingham. The initial activity was a daylong retreat of the Board members and task force chairpersons to produce the smoking control plan for the community. After examining the protocol requirements, the group decided to transform the plan into something useful and applicable to their own community. Their plan focused on health, used local people as models and local data, and used a logo created by graphics students at the local college. The group's pride in the way they adapted a protocol requirement to a unique plan for their community contributed quietly to a strong sense of ownership. Other activities also led to ownership in this community. Early formation of a finance committee ensured that the Board knew as much as the research institution about the financial status of the trial. From the beginning, the Board members and task force chairpersons had a friendly relationship with the protocol, viewing it as a roadmap rather than a roadblock. The group also donated space, reduced-cost products, prizes for contests, in-kind resources, and countless volunteer hours, which led to strong feelings of ownership.

Maintaining Community Involvement   Mobilization does not end when the organizational structure is formed. It is an ongoing process that requires attention to volunteers, adaptations of the initial structure, careful attention to allocation of tasks, and rewards, such as information about the outcome of the interventions. Any organization that relies on volunteers may expect attrition as individuals' lives change, their interest wanes, and other activities compete. Recognizing the likelihood of such attrition means that project staff members need to establish processes to bring on new members. As the COMMIT project continued, it was often obvious that the existing organization had to adapt to make the work flow more smoothly. Some groups added a finance committee, a transition committee to begin thinking about what would happen after the project ended, and ad hoc committees focused on specific events and activities. These activities allowed a more directed approach to some of the issues and problems facing the Board. Another common problem that faced some Boards was that apathy developed among their members as the task forces and field staff members did most of the work. This apathy among their members was probably perpetuated by the trial rules about data disclosure; aside from process data, no data were available, to either the communities or the research institutions, about whether the intervention was leading to smoking cessation.

Communities dealt with those ongoing mobilization problems in different ways. Brantford volunteers for the Board were asked for a 4-year commitment up front; this kept their attrition low. The Board continued to be active, especially in the face of controversy. When a proposed task force activity was rejected by officials in the community, the Board responded, "Let's go for it . . . ."

The Brantford group dealt with the above-mentioned data problem by requesting a monthly status report from the research institution that summarized activities and groups reached (e.g., health care providers, worksites). Although the report could not discuss success in outcome, it did reassure the Board that progress was being made in the intervention.

The Raleigh Board recognized that attrition was likely and, 2 years into the project, conducted another recruitment of Board and task force members.

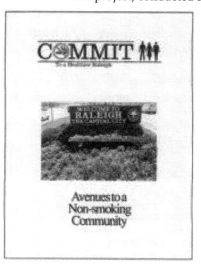

Avenues to a
Non-smoking
Community

As previously mentioned, the Board used ad hoc committees for specific events. Because the bursts of intensive and dedicated activity necessary to a big event are almost impossible to sustain with the same people over a long period, the ad hoc committee approach was ideal for maintaining enthusiasm and interest. A side benefit was that it brought into the COMMIT project other organizations and individuals who continued their interest in tobacco control. The field staff members in this community also divided groups into subgroups for discussion and brought them back together for decisionmaking. This process, requiring that everyone be involved at some level, prevented the tedium of sitting through countless meetings merely listening to reports. The field director also emphasized that lively, timely, and productive meetings were essential to maintaining interest.

The Raleigh community used the process-objective information as a way to document progress. The members were cognizant of the process objectives and took pride in meeting or exceeding them. The baseline data were used by the director of the health department in Raleigh in initiating a policy, and later an ordinance, that restricted smoking in public buildings. Board members saw that event as evidence that things were working.

More than one community (e.g., Bellingham, Cedar Rapids/Marion) suffered from a case of the "middles": The Board was active initially and toward the end of the project but became apathetic in the middle period as work and activities were distributed to task forces and field staff. Some Board members left during this time; however, their leaving provided opportunities to recruit new members who had enthusiasm and different views about tobacco control. In Bellingham the Board became energized when it discovered that it would have a small amount of discretionary funding to give to individuals or groups that proposed ideas for tobacco control. The projects proposed had to be consistent with the overall goals of the protocol but were considered optional activities. This action led to funding activities directed to low-income pregnant women through the county health department. Another activity funded was through the D.A.R.E. (Drug Abuse Resistance Education) program; tobacco control was incorporated as part of the D.A.R.E. curriculum and activities. The Board took pride in reviewing the proposals and deciding about the use of discretionary funds.

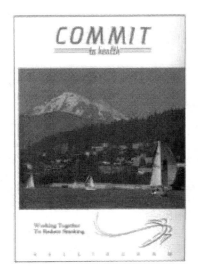

From the beginning, Bellingham used the process data to assess achievements and progress. Quarterly reports of process objectives attained were supplemented with large wall charts that showed the timeline for activities for a year, by task force, with lines colored in as activities were completed. The charts provided an immediate overview of accomplishments.

MOBILIZATION EXPERIENCES ACROSS COMMUNITIES   Although the protocol provided a general mobilization process, there were different experiences among the 11 intervention communities. Both field staff and Board members across the 11 communities cited factors that they found critical in the mobilization process.

One positive feature of the trial was that it provided funds for the communities. This was seen as a great asset by many community members because it meant they could focus on the intervention and not on fundraising activities. Another positive factor mentioned was the approach taken by the trial; it focused on helping smokers to quit rather than portraying them in a negative light.

Many obstacles to mobilization also were seen by project staff and Board members. The short time allocated for initial mobilization was cited by many respondents as a barrier to effective mobilization. As the Bellingham field director noted, "We had to move so quickly, learn what was required of us, and produce accurate and complete plans, that at times we literally felt we were singing in a foreign language." Community Boards and staff members were further frustrated by the time it took to obtain space and set up offices, because such processes had to be approved by NCI (the sponsoring agency) and often by the research institution as well.

Another constraint on mobilization was the approach taken by research institution. Research institutions had different levels of experience with community work, and this led to differing degrees of control. Similarly, research institutions had different types of connections with the intervention communities; where they were not well connected, it was more difficult to mobilize the community. Proximity of the research institutions and intervention communities also had an effect; more distance between the two made it more difficult for research institution staff members to assist with mobilization. The reputation of the research institution within the community was also important. It was easier to approach a community if the research institution working with COMMIT had high credibility and visibility than if the community was unfamiliar with the research institution or had negative experiences with it.

Three intervention communities were dual communities (Cedar Rapids, IA, Fitchburg/Leominster, MA, Medford/Ashland, OR); these resulted from the inclusion of two cities as the target for intervention. In two cases, two communities were combined to make populations sufficiently large to meet research guidelines. In the third case, geographic proximity led to the decision to include both communities. The process of mobilizing them was slowed by the need to contact two sets of city officials, civic organizations, school districts, and so forth. This also complicated hiring, meeting arrangements, and the logistics of some intervention activities. In addition, it was difficult to determine which community should house the field office so that both communities could participate easily in the project.

There was substantial initial confusion over ownership and partnership. In some instances, Board members became frustrated or demoralized when they realized some of the limitations of the protocol because they had developed expectations about the level of control they would have over the intervention. However, other Board members commented that the protocol was a great help to them in both mobilization and implementation because it allowed them to get to work immediately without needlessly repeating earlier efforts. Others commented that it was a broad blueprint that allowed the community to determine strategic details.

In general, the organizational structure required by the protocol was seen as good, and few staff members found it unduly cumbersome. A problem that emerged was the composition of the Board and task forces. The protocol suggested that community leaders be recruited for the Board because of their ability to open doors and lend credibility to the project. Although many communities opted for this approach, some established a Board of people who had reputations for getting things done. There were problems with both approaches. The Boards comprising community leaders soon found it convenient to delegate all the tasks to either field staff or task force members, which somewhat removed the Board from the project. The other approach suffered from a lack of credibility, which slowed down some activities. Many communities combined the two approaches by having a leadership Board with task force members who were more likely to do the work required. However, there was almost unanimous agreement that all Boards and task forces delegated more work to the field staff than had been expected.

As the mobilization process continued, the relationship between research institutions and field staff members became increasingly important. In communities where both understood and accepted the constraints of the protocol and were able to develop a relationship based on trust and mutual respect, mobilization seemed to proceed more smoothly. This tone was passed on to Board members and enhanced the process. In communities where the lines of authority were unclear or information was withheld (e.g., about the budget), the process was delayed. However, it also was noted that in some cases Board cohesion increased when the funding agent or the research institution was seen by the Board as the "common enemy."

A related issue was the transition of activities from the research institution staff to the community and subsequent role clarification. As the field director was hired and began taking responsibility for project activities, the project director at the research institution had to step back gracefully and play a behind-the-scenes role. As the Board became more familiar with the protocol and wanted to take charge of certain activities, the field director had to give way to task force members, other field staff members, and volunteers. In communities where adaptation to changing roles was poor, conflict often was the result.

WHAT COULD HAVE BEEN DONE DIFFERENTLY? In the interest of providing information for other groups and projects contemplating a community intervention in the future, the field staff and Board members were asked to comment on what could be done differently to make the mobilization process run more smoothly. Some responses apply not only to a randomized trial but to any community project.

The most common response was that a more realistic, longer timeframe must be allowed for the initial mobilization. Ideally, field staff members should be hired and Board and task force members thoroughly familiar with the project, their roles, and any constraints before intervention activities begin. Staff members need time to get to know people, to find common ground, and to develop reciprocity. More time would allow the entire group to know whether it had found the appropriate people for the Board and task forces. This is especially important when the agenda is an artificial one to which the community has not given a high priority; momentum must build slowly as people are educated about the problem.

Individuals involved in the COMMIT project also were frustrated by the shortness of the intervention period. Mobilizing an entire community requires much time. Volunteers noted that the project had just begun to develop good community recognition when the project ended.

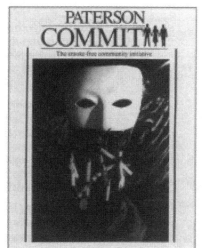

Field directors recommended beginning community projects with small tasks so that immediate success can be seen. For achieving this, a suggestion was made to capitalize more effectively on the development of the smoking control plan as an early mobilization activity. In communities where developing the plan was identified as an objective, a sense of partnership emerged sooner than in those where the community Board had little input into the plan.

Almost all the communities acknowledged that they did not have enough representation from minorities and heavy smokers on their Boards and task forces. Again, more time to explore these populations and engage them in the project was seen as potentially having a large payoff. One person recognized that attention to the protocol shifted priorities away from organizing hard-to-reach groups such as blue-collar and ethnic minority groups. Involving such groups would have enhanced the likelihood of reaching heavy smokers. Putting minority recruitment directly into the protocol would have accomplished the inclusion of hard-to-reach groups and thereby reached heavy smokers more easily.

Many respondents noted that training should have been more specifically focused; for example, training should be more culturally relevant, deal with conflicts, and use the project materials more.

The early products of the trial, such as the prerandomization and postrandomization analyses, were not seen as user-friendly by many communities. This seemed to be partly because the communities' involvement in producing the documents was limited; most groups ratified the documents but never used them as resources for ongoing mobilization activities. It was suggested that the Community Planning Group prepare the analysis so that the community would have some ownership of the report.

CONCLUSIONS The COMMIT mobilization protocol attempted to integrate the best known principles of community organization into an approach that required standardization. Several key principles of community organization were reinforced. Several community studies have noted the need for good community analysis prior to intervening with a community (Bracht, 1988; Haglund et al., 1990). This chapter recognizes that need and suggests that such an analysis include community input as well as comment because understanding the community is a critical step in successful mobilization. Analysis identifies key leaders and actors whose participation is required.

Unfortunately, the trial completely locked communities out of early involvement in trial design and planning. Also, contrary to the basic premises of community organization, it limited their involvement in the community analysis that is the groundwork for later intervention. As a result, there was substantial early confusion over roles and responsibilities.

Community ownership, control, and maintenance are concepts based on the traditions of local autonomy and general community development. In practice, the realization of the overall ownership goal was slow, was not always well understood, and required continuing clarification. Some factors helped: sharing as much information as possible, recognizing the need for joint decisionmaking, and acknowledging that conflict and tension are inevitable in work with large, diverse groups.

Would the COMMIT mobilization status have been different if a standardized protocol had not been used? Would the communities have come to the same place in the same time? Would they have felt more ownership of the project or less? The lessons from the field may not answer these questions, but they do provide insights and suggestions for other groups contemplating community organization strategies for research projects.

REFERENCES

Abrams, D.B., Elder, J.P., Carleton, R.A., Lasater, T.M., Artz, L.M. Social learning principles for organizational health promotion: An integrated approach. In: *Health and Industry: A Behavioral Medicine Perspective*, M.F. Cataldo and T.J. Coates (Editors). New York: Wiley-Interscience Publications, 1986, pp. 28-51.

Blackburn, H. Research and demonstration projects in community cardiovascular disease prevention. *Journal of Public Health Policy* 4: 398-421, 1983.

Bracht, N. Community analysis precedes community organization for cardiovascular disease prevention. *Scandinavian Journal of Primary Health Care* August (Suppl): 23-30, 1988.

Burghardt, S. *Organizing for Community Action*. Sage Human Service Guide, No. 27. Newbury Park, CA: Sage, 1982, pp. 19-20.

Carlaw, R.W., Mittelmark, M.B., Bracht, N., Luepker, R. Organization for a community cardiovascular health program: Experiences from the Minnesota Heart Health Program. *Health Education Quarterly* 11: 243-252, 1984.

Chavis, D., Stucky, P., Wandersman, A. Returning basic research to the community: A relationship between scientist and citizen. *American Psychologist* 36(4): 424-434, 1983.

Crosby, N., Kelly, J., Schaefer, P. Citizen panels: A new approach to citizen participation. *Public Administration Review* 46(2): 170-178, 1986.

Egger, G., Fitzgerald, W., Frape, G., Monaem, A., Rubenstein, P., Tyler, C., McKay, B. Result of large scale media antismoking campaign in Australia: North Coast "Quit for Life" Programme. *British Medical Journal* 286: 1125-1128, 1983.

Elder, J.P., McGraw, S.A., Abrams, D.B., Ferreira, A., Lasater, T.M., Longpre, H., Peterson, G.S., Schwertfeger, R., Carleton, R.A. Organizational and community approaches to community-wide prevention of heart disease: The first two years of the Pawtucket Heart Health Program. *Preventive Medicine* 15: 107-117, 1986.

Englund, A. Strategies for prevention: Role of voluntary and community organizations in implementation. *Cancer Detection and Prevention* 9: 413-415, 1986.

Farquhar, J. The community-based model of lifestyle interventions. *American Journal of Epidemiology* 108: 103-111, 1978.

Farquhar, J.W., Fortmann, S.P., Maccoby, N., Haskell, W.L., Williams, P.T., Flora, J.A., Taylor, C.B., Brown, B.W., Solomon, D.S., Hulley, S.B. The Stanford Five-City Project: Design and methods. *American Journal of Epidemiology* 122: 323-334, 1985.

Florin, P., Wandersman, A. An introduction to citizen participation, voluntary organizations, and community development: Insights for empowerment through research. *American Journal of Community Psychology* 18: 41-54, 1990.

Fortmann, S.P., Winkleby, M.A., Flora, J.A., Haskell, W.L., Taylor, C.B. Effect of long-term community health education on blood pressure and hypertension control: The Stanford Five-City Project. *American Journal of Epidemiology* 132: 629-646, 1990.

Goodman, R.M., Steckler, A. A model for the institutionalization of health promotion programs. *Community Health* 11: 63-78, 1989.

Green, L.W. The theory of participation: A qualitative analysis of its expression in national and international health politics. *Advances in Health Education and Promotion* 1(A): 211-236, 1986.

Green, L.W., Raeburn, J. Contemporary developments in health promotion. In: *Health Promotion at the Community Level*, N. Bracht (Editor). Newbury Park, CA: Sage, 1990, pp. 29-44.

Haglund, B., Weisbrod, R., Bracht, N. Assessing the community: Its services, needs, leadership, and readiness. In: *Health Promotion at the Community Level*, N. Bracht (Editor). Newbury Park, CA: Sage, 1990, pp. 91-108.

Hunkeler, E., Davis, E., Bessanderson, M., Powell, J., Polen, M. Richmond quits smoking: A minority community fights for health. In: *Health Promotion at the Community Level*, N. Bracht (Editor). Newbury Park, CA: Sage, 1990, pp. 278-303.

Kelly, J.G. T'ain't what you do, it's the way you do it. *American Journal of Community Psychology* 7: 239-261, 1979.

Kuriji, K., Ostbye, T., Bhatti, T. Initiating community self-help: A model for public health workers. *Canadian Journal of Public Health* 79: 208-209, 1988.

Labonte, R. Community empowerment: The need for political analysis. *Canadian Journal of Public Health* 80: 87-91, 1989.

McAlister, A., Puska, P., Salonen, J.T., Toumilehto, J., Koskela, K. Theory and action for health promotion: Illustrations from the North Karelia Project. *American Journal of Public Health* 72: 43-50, 1982.

Millar, W., Naegle, B. Time to quit: Community involvement in smoking cessation. *Canadian Journal of Public Health* 78: 109-114, 1987.

Puska, P., Nissinen, A., Salonen, J.T., Tuomilehto, J. Ten years of the North Karelia Project. Results with community-based prevention of coronary heart disease. *Scandinavian Journal of Social Medicine* 11(3): 65-68, 1983.

Puska, P., Nissinen, A., Tuomilehto, J., Salonen, J.T., Koskela, K., McAlister, A., Kottke, T.E., Maccoby, N., Farquhar, J.W. The community-based strategy to prevent coronary heart disease: Conclusions from the ten years of the North Karelia Project. *Annual Review of Public Health* 6: 147-193, 1985.

Rothman, J. Three models of community organization practice. In: *Strategies of Community Organization*, F.M. Cox, J.L. Erlich, J. Rothman, and R.E. Tropman (Editors). Itasca, IL: Peacock, 1979, pp. 86-102.

Stunkard, A.J., Felix, M., Cohen, R. Mobilizing a community to promote health: The Pennsylvania County Health Improvement Program (CHIP). In: *Prevention in Health Psychology*, J.C. Rosen and L.J. Solomon (Editors). Hanover, NH: University Press of New England, 1985, pp. 143-189.

Tarlov, A.R., Kehrer, B.H., Hall, D.P., Samuels, S.E., Brown, G.S., Felix, M.R., Ross, J.A. Foundation work: The health promotion program of the Henry J. Kaiser Family Foundation. *American Journal of Health Promotion* Fall: 74-80, 1987.

Thompson, B., Corbett, K., Bracht, N., Pechacek, T. Lessons learned from the mobilization of communities in the Community Intervention Trial for Smoking Cessation (COMMIT). *Health Promotion International* 8(2): 69-83, 1993.

Thompson, B., Kinne, S. Social change theory: Applications to community health. In: *Health Promotion at the Community Level*, N. Bracht (Editor). Newbury Park, CA: Sage, 1990, pp. 45-65.

Thompson, B., Pertschuk, M. Community intervention and advocacy. In: *Prevention of Coronary Heart Disease*, I.S. Ockene and A.K. Ockene (Editors). Boston: Little, Brown, 1992, pp. 493-515.

Thompson, B., Wallack, L., Lichtenstein, E., Pechacek, T. Principles of community organization and partnership for smoking cessation in the Community Intervention Trial for Smoking Cessation (COMMIT). *International Quarterly of Community Health Education* 11(3): 187-203, 1990-91.

Warren, R. Toward a reformulation of community theory. *Community Development Review* 9: 41-48, 1958.

AUTHORS

Beti Thompson, Ph.D.
Associate Professor
University of Washington School of Public
    Health and Community Medicine
Associate Member
Fred Hutchinson Cancer Research Center,
    MP-702
1124 Columbia Street
Seattle, WA 98104

Linda Nettekoven, M.A.
Project Coordinator
Oregon Research Institute
1715 Franklin Boulevard
Eugene, OR 97403

Dianne Ferster
Executive Director
COMMIT to a Healthier Brant
Suite 403
233 Colborne Street
Brantford, Ontario N3T 2H4
CANADA

Len C. Stanley, M.P.H.
Program Director
Tobacco Control Training Center
Department of Family Medicine
University of North Carolina
Aycock Building, CB-7595
Manning Drive
Chapel Hill, NC 27599

Juliet Thompson
Field Director
Bellingham COMMIT Site
4407 Wilkin Street
Bellingham, WA 98226

Kitty K. Corbett, Ph.D., M.P.H.
Adjunct Investigator
Division of Research
Kaiser Permanente Medical Care Program
3505 Broadway
Oakland, CA 94611
and
Assistant Professor
Health and Behavioral Sciences, CB-103
Department of Anthropology
University of Colorado at Denver
P.O. Box 173364
Denver, CO 80217

Activities To Involve the Smoking Public in Tobacco Control in COMMIT

Russell C. Sciandra, Lawrence Wallack, Carolyn L. Johnson, Janine Sadlik, and Juliet Thompson

INTRODUCTION   Public education is a necessary tool to facilitate smoking control efforts. For many years, the tobacco industry has used public education in the form of advertising to promote the use of its products in such a way that exposure to tobacco cues is virtually impossible to ignore (Johnston et al., 1987; Centers for Disease Control, 1990). The information presented by the tobacco industry regarding the consequences of tobacco use is often fallacious. For example, cigarette advertisements link smoking with images of fitness, health, beauty, and social acceptance (Warner, 1986). There is increasing evidence linking such false advertising to an increase in consumption (Seldon and Doroodian, 1989; Tye et al., 1987). Furthermore, the clout exerted by the advertisers often results in limited coverage in the media of the ill effects associated with tobacco use (Weis and Burke, 1986; Minkler et al., 1987). An excellent example of this occurred when lung cancer became the primary cancer killer of women, exceeding breast cancer, and the issue was largely ignored by women's magazines, which are also primary recipients of tobacco advertising revenues (Kessler, 1989).

Although public education in the interest of reducing public health problems has few resources at its disposal relative to the tobacco industry, some important efforts have been made to use this channel to reduce tobacco use. Flay (1987), in a review of 56 evaluated media tobacco control programs, came to the following conclusions:

- Such programs inform people.

- People are motivated to attempt to quit.

- Potential quitters can be encouraged to take some kind of action (e.g., calling a hotline).

- Smokers can quit for extended periods.

Smoking reductions in mediated quit programs also have been reported by Cummings and colleagues (1987 and 1989), Pierce and coworkers (1990), and Thompson and Curry (1994). Although the cessation rates associated with such programs are low, their public health effect is significant because they reach many people. However, the majority of the tobacco control interventions have been directed at individual smokers in an attempt to encourage them to quit.

In the past few years, new efforts have been added to the general use of public education and the media for tobacco control. Rather than relying only on activities designed to assist smokers in quitting or preventing youth from beginning smoking, tobacco control advocates are taking an aggressive approach to the use of mass media. This approach has been called "media advocacy," and its central approach is to reframe public debate so that more support is generated for effective policy change around a public health issue (U.S. Department of Health and Human Services, 1989). Media advocacy is not targeted to the individual and does not focus on changing individual risk behavior; rather, it focuses on the larger, structural factors that might make a problem a public health issue (Advocacy Institute, 1987). For example, in the tobacco control arena the emphasis is placed on the ethical and legal liability of the tobacco companies, which make a product responsible for much premature morbidity and mortality. An example of effective media advocacy was apparent in the negative framing of the attempt to introduce a new brand of cigarettes, "Uptown," to urban minorities. Antitobacco advocates were successful in convincing the public and opinion leaders that this targeting was a deliberate effort to exploit the minority group. Demonstrations and protests ultimately led R.J.Reynolds to withdraw the product (Freedman, 1990).

RATIONALE AND PROCESS OBJECTIVES
Communitywide public education efforts were central to the Community Intervention Trial for Smoking Cessation (COMMIT). The public education channel was seen as a way to coordinate and promote the activities of the other channels by providing media campaigns to promote smoking as a public health problem, to promote smoking cessation, and to encourage the prevention of smoking.

The overall strategy for the public education channel was to increase community activities that would stimulate public debate about smoking. Of key concern was that such a debate help create a social environment where support for nonsmoking was increased and support for continued smoking decreased.

Three overall goals were developed for the public education channel:

- promote social norms and actions toward a smoke-free community;

- promote the importance of smoking as a public health issue; and

- enhance the effectiveness of smoking control in other program areas.

The process objectives shown in Table 1 were developed to meet these goals.

The activities can be categorized into three major types: (1) activities designed to change the community climate for smoking through media campaigns, (2) activities designed to change the community climate through media advocacy, and (3) activities to enlist smokers in quit attempts.

Changing the Community Climate Through Media Campaigns
To introduce the project to the community, activities in this area began with a kickoff event, the major element of which was a news conference involving as many media outlets as possible. Annually, another major news conference was held to describe the achievements of the past year and plans for the next intervention year. A few months after the announcement of the project, the communities

Table 1
Activities and process objectives for involving the public

Activities for Each Community	Cumulative Objectives (1988-1992)	Number Completed	Process Objectives Achieved[a] (%)
Nationally, Train One Person (e.g., field director) in Media Advocacy	11 people trained	11	100
Train Minimum of Eight Community Members in Advocacy	88 people trained	80	91
Hold News Conference for Smoking Control Plan	11 conferences	11	100
Hold Annual News Conference for Annual Action Plan	44 conferences	44	100
Annually Provide Eight Local News Releases on Tobacco Issues	352 news releases	345	98
Develop Campaigns To Publicize Availability of Cessation Resources Guide and Other Aspects of Smoking Cessation	All communities	11	100
Annually (from 1989) Design and Implement Two Magnet Events	66 magnet events	95	144

[a] *Average for combined communities.*

released their own locally developed smoking control plans. This plan summarized the framework for the entire 4-year intervention period. It used local data and local individuals to present the smoking problem. Another key charge in this area was to publicize smoking control activities in other task force areas. Community campaigns were to be developed to fit with other activities. Each community was required to conduct a campaign to publicize the availability of a Cessation Resources Guide (CRG) (see Chapter 8), a campaign to publicize the Smokers' Network (see Chapter 10), and a campaign to encourage heavy smokers to ask their health care providers for advice about smoking cessation (see Chapter 9). At least two other campaigns, of the community's choosing, also were required.

Media Advocacy   Media advocacy also was an important part of changing the community climate. Within each community, a staff person was trained in media advocacy. The training, conducted during a half-day session by qualified trainers, sought to convey the skills needed to put smoking control on media agendas. The trained staff person was then responsible for organizing media advocacy training sessions in the community. As part of an ongoing effort to find appropriate information for media advocacy, each field office was connected to a communication network that provided regular information on national or regional events that could contribute to public awareness if a local "spin" was put on the story.

Enlisting Smokers in Quit Attempts   The public education channel also had the goal of enlisting smokers in quit attempts. Each community was responsible for designing and implementing two "magnet events" annually. A magnet event is a well-publicized, communitywide activity that stimulates smokers to quit. Examples of magnet events include the American Cancer Society's The Great American Smokeout (GASO), in which a week's worth of activities precede a day when smokers quit for the day, and communitywide "Quit and Win" contests, in which incentives are used to get smokers to quit for a certain period (usually 30 days). Quit and Win contests provide a communitywide outreach that involves not only smokers but also nonsmokers in assisting smokers in quitting. They have been used successfully in several communities (Elder et al., 1991; Lando et al., 1990; Cummings et al., 1990).

CAMPAIGNS   The resources available to COMMIT communities exceeded what is usually available for smoking interventions; however, they were not adequate to mount fully developed media campaigns, especially compared with the media assets commanded by the tobacco industry for promoting cigarettes. Therefore, it was necessary to leverage what was available from the funding agency to maximize its impact. This was done in a variety of ways that are more fully discussed below but can be briefly summarized as drawing on community resources not previously involved in tobacco control.

There was significant variability in how communities implemented media activities. Although most sites were able to initiate the minimum number of activities required by the protocol, there was considerable variety in the quality of the interventions. Moreover, some sites substantially exceeded protocol requirements, whereas others devoted more effort to other intervention channels. This disparity arose from differences among communities (some had limited free-standing media; some had media that overlapped with the comparison community) and from variations in the interests and skills of community staff and volunteers.

Medford/Ashland, OR   The experience of the Medford/Ashland, OR, site was typical of many in the trial. The Medford/Ashland intervention community, one of the smallest in the trial, had a relatively large number of media outlets at its disposal. These included 2 well-read daily newspapers; 3 local, commercial television stations; 1 public broadcast system; 1 public access television channel; and 11 radio stations. Based on previous experience in the community, COMMIT staff members had contacts with several media personalities and spent considerable time and effort maintaining these relationships throughout the trial.

Early in the intervention phase, "COMMIT To Quit," as the program was named in Medford/Ashland, used media advocacy techniques to seize the news media's attention. For example, it held news conferences complete with visual aids comparing cyanide levels in cigarettes to cyanide levels in tainted Chilean grapes declared unfit for consumption. Following this event, COMMIT To Quit became recognized as the "local expert" when reporters were working on tobacco-related stories.

During the first intervention year, the Public Education Task Force relied almost solely on voluntary press coverage of COMMIT events. A few paid print advertisements were run to promote a Worksite Smoking Policy Workshop and a Win a (Cold) Turkey contest as part of the GASO. The task force was disappointed at the numbers of participants generated and decided that the poor reponse was the result of a heavy reliance on public service advertising. Despite cautions from the representatives of voluntary agencies, which use no paid advertising, the task force decided to set funds aside to buy air time. COMMIT To Quit was viewed by media outlets as a voluntary organization and given the nonprofit, column-inch rate in the newspapers and the two-for-one rate in radio and television commercials.

In the second intervention year (1990), the task force contacted a marketing instructor at a local 4-year college and asked whether he would make the design of a 3-month campaign to reach heavy smokers a class project. When he agreed, the class was divided into three groups. Each group had to research the target audience; select a slogan; generate artwork, scripts, and storyboards for television and radio commercials; and propose the media placements. The winning group developed the concept of maximizing the small budget by partnering with a local minor league baseball team. The campaign included a billboard for the ballpark, a full-page advertisement in the program, busboards for the Rapid Transit District buses, and radio commercials. The campaign culminated in participants signing up for a stop-smoking contest, with free admission to the ballpark and a barbeque celebration for those that did so. The winning theme was "Time To Quit!" A request for proposal was sent to all advertising agencies in the county, and an agency contracted to produce a jingle, a 60-second radio commercial, and a 30-second television commercial. (Seven other COMMIT sites later bought copies of the television commercial.) The task force decided to use the agency to create print advertisements and to negotiate advertising purchases throughout the remainder of the project.

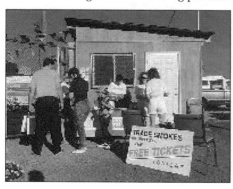

The advertising agency proved a wonderful asset in leveraging advertising dollars. Despite the fact that COMMIT tripled its paid advertising, it continued to receive public service advertising.

During the last year of the intervention (1992), the Public Health Task Force produced a four-page newspaper insert titled "A Resolution You Can Live With." A student poster replaced the Time To Quit artwork on the busboards, and COMMIT donated billboards at the ballparks to a local drug prevention group in exchange for its pledge to address tobacco and nicotine in its programs. The highlight of this year of the project was the production of a 30-minute documentary about COMMIT's 4 years in the community. The documentary was premiered at COMMIT's gala farewell celebration before an audience of dignitaries and volunteers and was later aired in prime time to promote participation in that year's GASO.

In summary, the Medford/Ashland experience demonstrates how the creative use of community resources (college classes, student art, songwriter and composer, filmmaker) and the use of leveraged media buying (partnerships, piggybacking, multiple cosponsors, professional agency) can maximize the reach and frequency of health promotion messages on a shoestring budget.

Utica, NY   The Utica, NY, program devoted more resources to media-related activities than any other site. At the beginning of the project, the volunteer Board suggested that an advertising agency be retained to produce a consistent theme for the project's antismoking messages. The agency that was selected developed a slogan, "Yes, You Can," which was integrated into all the project's messages over the next 4 years. The advertising campaign consisted of radio and television advertisements, bus cards, billboards, and point-of-purchase displays. Some advertising was developed locally, but for the most part, advertisements produced elsewhere were borrowed and tagged with the project's slogan. As in Medford/ Ashland, the program received two- or three-for-one advertising rates in broadcasting. There were several campaigns over the 4 years, all tied together by the "Yes, You Can" theme. The repetition of this theme helped build public awareness of the program.

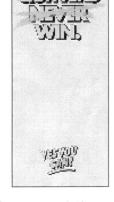

As in other communities, the COMMIT office soon became the recognized source of information and comment for media stories on tobacco. The computerized communication network provided by the trial gave advance notice that news was breaking nationally; this allowed staff members and volunteers to contact local media to alert them and provide local comment and statistics. Being in the news so frequently built credibility and awareness of the program. Sometimes this had unforeseen benefits.

The Utica field director stopped in a pharmacy to pick up a prescription, and the pharmacist recognized her from television as the COMMIT spokesperson. As a professional pharmacist, he was interested in doing something about smoking. This chance encounter led to activities involving a major pharmacy chain in a series of smoking cessation activities.

Bellingham, WA   The Bellingham, WA, site had to cope with several media problems. None of the major television outlets viewed by residents had local offices. One cable station existed, and it provided some local access but little else.

The local newspaper was read widely but was part of a chain, which placed constraints on local practices. Nevertheless, COMMIT staff members and the Public Education Task Force took on the challenge of providing the information to the community.

The task force did not elect to use one theme for the entire intervention period of the project. It tied campaigns to specific community activities and events that would capitalize on local values and characteristics. The first media campaign developed by volunteers and staff took place during the 1989 holiday season (November 1989 through January 1990). This holiday gift campaign was based on the theme that "The best gift you can give yourself and your loved ones is the gift of your own good health." Several radio commercials were developed with the collaboration of a local disc jockey who donated his time. The commercials urged listeners who were interested in giving themselves good health by stopping smoking to call the COMMIT office number to receive a free "holiday quit kit." The commercials began playing on four local radio stations just after Thanskgiving and continued until the first part of January. The radio stations were selected to reach diverse audiences and included a local popular news station, a country-western music station, a rock music station, and another station that had a variety of programming. Good coverage was obtained by varying the time of day when the commercials were aired. Costs were kept reasonable by obtaining two or three advertisements for every one that was purchased.

Individuals who responded to the radio commercials were given a gift package that included a quit kit (containing quit tips, items to keep their hands busy while quitting smoking, cartoons, sugarless mints and gum, and various other aids intended to make cessation easier), a gift card to present to a friend or family member stating the respondent was giving the person the gift of his or her health, and self-help materials on smoking cessation. The response was overwhelming. From the first day the messages aired, telephone calls and visits were received from people who heard the messages and wanted to quit. In 6 weeks more than 400 gift packages were distributed.

The Bellingham group also developed the "Be a Winner" campaign that commenced in fall 1990. The COMMIT staff members and volunteers worked with a local television production company to develop a message that winners were people who tried, often many times, to achieve a goal. Football players provided the basic image, and they were shown running down the field many times and finally scoring a touchdown. This theme was used in the hope of reaching blue-collar smokers and convincing them that repeated attempts to win (i.e., quit) were normal in many aspects of life. In this way, perhaps they could be motivated to try to quit more than once. The football and winner theme was chosen to coincide with the National Football League season, and especially the playoffs, so that interest in a Quit and Win contest that was scheduled to begin in January would be high.

The response to the campaign was good. Although no quantitative data were collected on the campaign, anecdotal data indicated that people saw the commercials (they were mentioned when people signed up for the contest) and liked them. The connection with the football theme was seen as positive, and no negative comments were received.

Raleigh, NC The project in Raleigh, NC, began with a large kickoff event that was well received; however, staff members soon discovered that it was difficult to convince the daily newspaper to cover issues considered by COMMIT volunteers to be important. Their strategy became one of presenting unique analyses of tobacco issues and staging visually interesting events by members of the community.

The kickoff event coincided with Raleigh's Downtown Beautification Project. After learning of the attention that would be paid to the project, the COMMIT project donated 100 oak tree saplings to the city, a symbol of Raleigh's "turning over a new leaf." During the presentation, COMMIT volunteers tied to the saplings construction-paper leaves with the names of recent quitters on them. This activity received much media attention.

The Raleigh group had great success in publicizing the 1990 Surgeon General's report as well as several local youth-buying operations. The media response to the first part of their COMMIT To Quit program, a Quit and Win contest, was outstanding. However, as the project continued, it was apparent that gaining media attention was not always easy. For example, the 1991 COMMIT To Quit occurred at the same time as the Persian Gulf War, and it was difficult to keep the media's interest. Furthermore, staff members discovered that it was hard to sustain enthusiasm in a yearly event; the media prefer new angles.

The Raleigh group, being in the heart of tobacco country, faced particular hardships. The newspapers often overlooked them. Any competing events seemed to draw the media away from COMMIT activities. Even the introduction of "big name" speakers did not generate media coverage. The biggest, consistent media success for this community was the coverage generated by underage teen-buying operations.

MAGNET EVENTS All COMMIT communities had numerous magnet events. Every community had at least one Quit and Win contest, with a total of 26 such contests held throughout the trial. The contests varied in length and awards but had some commonalities. First, efforts were made to extensively promote the contest in the community. In addition to the usual media outlets, small media also were used to advertise the event. For example, contest organizers convinced grocery stores to print information on grocery bags; leaflets were distributed in specific neighborhoods; posters with attached entry forms were distributed to retail stores, doctors' offices, public buildings, and worksites; and brochures were distributed. Second, some biochemical verification of smoking status (usually expired carbon monoxide) at the end of the contest was required. Third, there was a period for registration before the big "quit day," which was usually tied to a date that is noteworthy for smoking cessation (e.g., New Year's Day, the GASO). Fourth, many prizes were distributed, with a major grand prize of $1,000 in almost every contest. Fifth, the event ended with a celebration for all participants and their families. The examples that follow give a flavor of the activities involved in conducting Quit and Win contests.

Fitchburg/ Leominster, MA   Fitchburg/Leominster, MA, initiated the first of their three Quit and Win contests in 1990. Planning for the activity, called Time To Quit, began 2 1/2 months before the contest. Most preparation work was done by field staff. COMMIT paid for advertising, which included radio commercials, newspaper advertisements, discussions on local talk radio, and a videotape that was aired on the local cable television channel. Posters and registration cards were sent to community worksites and health care providers. Entry forms also were included in the COMMIT newsletter. A local supermarket printed 200,000 grocery bags with registration forms that could be cut out and mailed.

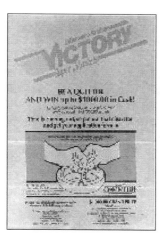

One hundred and five smokers registered for the contest; of those, approximately 40 quit for a month. Most registrations came from the COMMIT newsletter. Every week during the contest, COMMIT staff members sent postcards containing support messages and quit tips to the participants. These were reported to be helpful in reinforcing quit attempts. The end of the contest, which coincided with the American Lung Association's (ALA) Non-Dependence Day, was celebrated in the parking lot of the local mall. A local radio station donated 3 hours to broadcast the events, including the drawing of winners, and to interview contest participants and volunteers.

The contest was considered a success; however, volunteers also learned from this first activity. COMMIT staff members and volunteers believed a longer planning period was necessary. There also was a feeling that promotion of the event was too narrowly focused and began too close to the start date; thus, fewer people enrolled than might have. For example, the grocery bags appeared only 1 week before the start date. The following year (1991), planning began much earlier, and promotion was more extensive. In addition, entrants received a "scratch" lottery ticket just for entering. Other venues were targeted for recruitment, including bingo halls, bowling alleys, and Lamaze classes. Worksites were enrolled, and a between-worksites competition of four platoons of firefighters brought more entrants. Approximately 200 smokers participated in this second effort.

Paterson, NJ Paterson, NJ, has a high proportion of ethnic minorities; thus, involvement in a Quit and Win contest had to appeal to several different groups. The COMMIT Board and task forces planned a long-term,

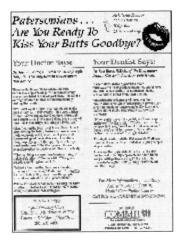

comprehensive contest that focused on recruiting the heavy smokers in the community. The contest began on January 24, 1991, and ended June 30, 1991. The basic format of the contest involved an ongoing recruitment effort, with drawings made monthly for a prize ($250) to be given to a quitter at the end of the contest (provided he or she remained in the quit category), followed by a final cash award of $1,000 given to a quitter whose name was drawn from all quitters at the end of the contest.

The recruitment effort dominated the activity. The group began with the usual methods of information dissemination: media promotion, use of a graphic artist to design a contest theme, distribution of promotional items, and mailings of entry forms. The contest also was promoted in Spanish-language media. As time went on, volunteers became more active in getting registrants; they went to barbershops, beauty shops, day-care centers, family centers, supermarkets, shopping malls, and other areas to sign up smokers to participate. Additional promotion efforts included giving economic incentives to youth to sign up smokers, and even police departments were contacted to invite area convicts to participate. The Worksites and Organizations Task Force contacted all local workplaces to sign up smokers; 7,000 flyers were sent home with children in the Paterson school system, and 9,000 payroll stuffers were distributed to all area hospital and city employees. By the end of June, 501 smokers had participated in the contest. A grand finale was held during a local festival, with the overall winner's name drawn by the mayor of Paterson.

This ambitious effort required significant time and resources, and the COMMIT staff members and volunteers learned from the event. First, they learned that recruiting smokers was more difficult and tedious than anticipated. Ultimately, door-to-door recruitment was seen as the most effective method of getting smokers involved in the contest. This group also experienced problems with late promotion of the event, largely as a result of initial difficulties with the graphics firm that was to design and conduct the publicity. Although these problems eventually were resolved, time was lost in promoting the event. Logistics problems also emerged in this community; there were some incomplete entries that led to the inability to find entrants. Overall, however, this contest was considered successful. It reached the targeted smokers as evidenced by the demographic characteristics of the participants (which closely matched the community demographics); it increased the number of smokers who signed up for the Smokers' Network; and it greatly increased the visibility of COMMIT.

Santa Fe, NM Santa Fe, NM, held a 3-month Quit and Win contest in 1991 that culminated on the ALA's Non-Dependence Day. Participants were eligible for interim awards. Relapsers in the first month of the contest were encouraged to sign up again for the remainder of the contest. A total of 377 people initially joined the contest, with an additional 46 April relapsers joining in May or June. Contest participants were encouraged to find people to support them in their quit efforts. At the grand finale, quitters (verified by expired carbon monoxide) were eligible for first-, second-, or third-prize drawings, based on the amount of time they had been tobacco-free. Followup

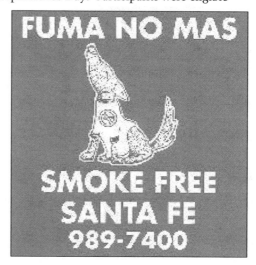

telephone calls were made to entrants every week to ascertain whether they needed materials or support in quitting or remaining abstinent. A grand finale was held on the Santa Fe Plaza on July 5, 1991. Music was provided by a local group; a puppet show was held for children that included content on smoking; a city council member read a proclamation declaring July 5 Non-Dependence Day; and the awards were given.

This event ran smoothly, and recruitment of participants exceeded expectations. All task forces were involved in the recruitment process and in promotion of the event. The Public Education Task Force worked with a public relations firm to plan the promotion of the activity and helped to plan all aspects of the promotion. Schools were involved in spreading the word about the contest. Puppet shows presented to children were designed to get the message to parents. Peer educators helped with mailings and other logistics. Cessation Resources Task Force members assembled materials and delivered them to health care facilities and provider offices. They also convinced local cessation resources to provide discounts during the contest. The Health Care Provider Task Force ensured that materials were available in all provider offices. They also set up five "minicontests" between

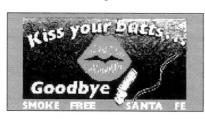

individual offices and clinics. The Worksites and Organizations Task Force contacted local businesses and organizations to inform them of the contest and to recruit from the employees or membership. Few problems were encountered in this community. One disappointment was the inability to find a celebrity to hand out the awards. This was attributed to the event occurring on the holiday weekend. Another problem was that the ALA changed Non-Dependence Day from July 5 to July 3; nevertheless, the Smoke-Free Santa Fe group continued with July 5 as the date of the finale.

Yonkers, NY   Yonkers, NY, ran its second contest, called "A Thousand Good Reasons To Quit Smoking," from January to February 1992. The activity focused on the effects of smoking on children; thus, each entrant in the contest was required to designate a youth supporter between the ages of 5 and 18. The grand prize for the contest was a $1,000 U.S. savings bond for the child's education and a $250 gift certificate for the quitter. Only residents of Yonkers were eligible. All quitters had to undergo cotinine testing to verify their smoking status. Many community sectors participated. The school system sent home 12,000 newsletters advertising the contest with elementary school students. Several worksites permitted staff members to personally register smokers. Media promotion was used, and many articles about the contest appeared in the local newspaper. Prizes were donated by several local businesses; these included monetary donations, a weekend for two at a local inn, dinner for two at a theater club, movie tickets, and gift certificates. A total of 164 smokers entered the contest.

Staff members and volunteers felt the contest was successful but had hoped for a larger enrollment. Staff members felt that there were several constraints on the enrollment. First, the prize that went to the winner was not large because the youth supporter received most of the benefits. Second, a number of smokers did not enroll with youth and had to be contacted to provide the name of a youth supporter. This suggested that many smokers may have declined to enroll because of that stipulation. Third, the cotinine testing presented a problem because it required 2 weeks to obtain laboratory results. Participants found it annoying to come in to provide a saliva sample. Fourth, a staff suggestion to initiate a contest between schools and worksites to sign up smokers was vetoed by the Board. Fifth, the grand finale was not well attended, probably because it was held in a relatively obscure location in a local mall.

Cedar Rapids/   Cedar Rapids/Marion, IA, took advantage of the newly imposed ban
Marion, IA   on smoking on commercial air flights to institute a magnet event. Working with a representative of the ALA Iowa affiliate, COMMIT staff members and volunteers planned an event at which materials would be distributed at the Cedar Rapids airport on the day the ban started. Permission was readily given by the airport administration, and "panic packs" were assembled. These were packages that contained tips for surviving the flight, a CRG, balloons, hard candy, buttons, wrist snappers, and headless matches. The event was held in late afternoon on the day of the ban and was well covered by the media. The event served the additional purpose of providing an energy boost for COMMIT staff members and volunteers who saw that, with a little extra effort, it was possible to "seize the moment" and get substantial media attention.

Medford/ The third intervention year (1991) in this community began with
Ashland, OR a locally produced and televised "Freedom From Smoking" cessation program cosponsored by a television station, the local power company, and the county library system. A small group of smokers was recruited to meet daily for a week and share experiences in following each activity in the cessation guide. Five thousand guides were distributed throughout southern Oregon. Each night during the news, the anchor showed a segment of the discussion among the smokers and directed viewers to the next day's assignment in the guide. Print advertisements and other promotional features directed smokers to pick up guides at several prominent locations. The program continued to use a combination of press releases and print, radio, and television commercials to promote activities, and participation rates increased each year.

Medford/Ashland, OR, These two areas conducted a "friendly" competitive
and Bellingham, WA magnet event. Because each community has a minor league baseball team, COMMIT staff members collaborated on a joint activity. The impetus came from Medford (the ballpark is located in Medford, not both communities), where a promotional campaign was designed to link with the local baseball team, the Southern Oregon Athletics (minor league team for the Oakland Athletics). Conditions of the competition were that both communities would have a smoke-free family night at the baseball game and sign up smokers for the Smokers' Network. Dates were set for when the teams would be playing against each other. The Southern Oregon Athletics challenged the Bellingham Mariners (minor league team for the Seattle Mariners) to go smoke-free for the night, and the challenge was reversed when the Medford team came to Bellingham. In both communities, COMMIT purchased (or received donated) tickets to the game. Also, smokers or chewers received a free ticket in exchange for a packet of cigarettes or a can of snuff. Arrangements were made for the announcer to mention frequently the COMMIT To Quit message.

In Medford, the teams backed out of their commitment to go tobacco-free for the night for fear that playing would be affected. Fifty smokers signed up to participate and received free tickets to the game. The smoke-free family section censured an individual who tried to light up a cigarette in that section of the ballpark, and many smokers in the smoking section were cajoled by family and friends into going to the COMMIT booth for testing. Although participation was less than expected, the clown hired by COMMIT, the favors passed out, and a bright, sunny day made it an enjoyable event. One of the COMMIT volunteers noted that the event was charming because it recruited smokers and rewarded nonsmokers.

Bellingham COMMIT needed to beat the number of participants recruited by Medford/Ashland COMMIT. The group was successful in convincing the Bellingham Mariners players to go tobacco-free for the night. Media coverage of the event included interviews with players who stated that youth should not start chewing because it is a difficult habit to break. Thirty participants gave a package of cigarettes or chew in exchange for a free ticket; however, the game was repeatedly delayed by bad weather. By the time the game began, there were virtually no spectators. Determining that Medford/Ashland had won, the Bellingham field director had a plaque made for the Oregon site and presented it to the COMMIT Board representatives at an annual meeting in February 1991.

The between-community competition generated a great deal of interest and fun. Media coverage was excellent in both communities. Interestingly, the between-community competition portion of the event was not much added effort because the events were already scheduled in each community. It is surprising that more events like this did not occur throughout the various intervention communities. There was much sharing of material and promotional campaigns, but it may have been threatening to various staff members to feel that they had to compete with each other.

Other Magnet Events

Quit and Win contests were not the only magnet events devised to draw smokers into quit attempts. Every community conducted numerous activities around the GASO or, in the case of the Canadian communities, "Weedless Wednesday." Activities focused on this annual event included providing cold turkey sandwiches, setting up a "survival camp" for smokers who pledged to quit for the day, providing smokers' quit kits to interested smokers, having someone dress as a 7-foot turkey to symbolize "quitting cold turkey," organizing competitions to see which worksites could have the most quitters and supporters during the GASO, and providing the community with messages about tobacco control.

Numerous other magnet events were held in the intervention communities. In Medford/Ashland, staff members and volunteers designed, constructed, and staffed a float for an Independence Day parade. Brantford, Ontario, Canada, held a community forum to gain community input on tobacco control. Brantford also held a "Butt Out" party to encourage quitters to keep their New Year's resolutions. Bellingham COMMIT sponsored a team for an annual fitness race from Mount Baker to Puget Sound. Paterson organized a rally against cigarette advertisements on billboards. Other events also were held.

MEDIA ADVOCACY

Media advocacy is the strategic use of mass media to advance a public policy initiative. Media advocacy involves capitalizing on news events (or creating news events) to stimulate broad-based coverage and reframe public debate, in contrast to the tendency of the news media to present health problems as a function of personal choice or circumstances. Media advocates focus on factors shaping the environment in which individuals' decisions about health behavior are made. By exploiting the news media's appetite for conflict, controversy, irony, innovation, and the "local angle," advocates can redefine the issue as a social problem and promote a public policy solution.

The ability of COMMIT to openly advocate for legislative and regulatory change was limited by restrictions on the use of Federal funds. Therefore, communities used the media to advocate for the view that tobacco is a communitywide problem and for certain general principles, such as the right to a smoke-free environment. A consistent theme was to shift attention (and blame for the problem) from tobacco users to tobacco-product manufacturers and marketers. This enabled smokers and nonsmokers to identify a common enemy—the tobacco industry.

Utica, NY   The Utica site conducted a series of media advocacy events throughout the intervention. Many of these events were intended to focus public attention on the predatory nature of the tobacco industry and to portray it as an intruder from outside the community (as opposed to the community-based COMMIT program). Among the media advocacy events staged by Utica COMMIT were:

- picketing and leaflet distribution at a dance performance sponsored by Philip Morris;

- an appearance by members of the national boomerang team, which had refused tobacco industry sponsorship;

- a news conference with alcohol and other substance abuse agencies calling on the proposed director of national drug policy to break his nicotine addiction;

- a news conference announcing the results of a survey checking merchant compliance with the law against selling tobacco to minors; and

- a youth antitobacco rally in the hotel room next to an RJR Nabisco, Inc., "smokers' rights" meeting.

Media advocacy, which is based on opposition and conflict, makes many community health professionals and volunteers uncomfortable. Advocacy challenges traditional notions of public health based on education and consensus building, and COMMIT sites encountered some resistance from community members unwilling to engage in confrontation. However, as the program continued to repeat advocacy events, members of the coalition became more comfortable with the concept. By the 3rd year, it was community members who, learning of the smokers' rights meeting described below, organized the counterdemonstration and contacted the media. The event was a watershed in Utica, marking the advent of a new level of activism by grassroots tobacco control advocates.

Several volunteers in Utica had signed up to receive regular information from smokers' rights groups, and in early March 1991, they were notified of a smokers' rights meeting to be held in Utica. A coalition member contacted the field director, who also had received a notice, and both agreed to talk to as many coalition members as possible about the upcoming meeting. Fortuitously, all the task forces were meeting at about that time, and they all were informed of the upcoming event. Volunteers were outraged that the tobacco industry was bringing its extensive lobbying into their community, and they agreed that something had to be done, although there was no immediate agreement on what that would be.

After much discussion, the group decided there should be some physical presence at the meeting but that it was important not to be too confrontational and not to do anything illegal. COMMIT staff members noted that it was important to frame the smokers' rights meeting as part of an industry lobbying campaign, in this case, directed at proposed State legislation to further restrict youth access to cigarettes. The group decided this meant that youth and children should be involved. The field director and COMMIT volunteers mobilized a local advocacy agent for low-income, at-risk youth to participate. A local physician, who was also a COMMIT volunteer, was recruited to attend, along with her daughter. Another volunteer, whose father had died of lung cancer earlier that year, agreed to come. While participants were being recruited, the media were alerted about the event. News releases were prepared, and spokespersons were briefed on the areas they should cover.

The COMMIT group had rented a room in the same hotel as the smokers' rights group. Forty-two COMMIT volunteers, staff members, and young people arrived 30 minutes before the smokers' rights meeting and were briefed on the counterdemonstration agenda. They were told they could observe the smokers' rights meeting as long as they did not disturb the proceedings. Teens handed out antitobacco flyers to people who came to the smokers' rights meeting. The tobacco company employee was surprised by the countermeeting. He asked a radio reporter who had contacted the media. Without asking their ages, he also gave written materials about cigarettes and lighters to the teens who entered the smokers' rights meeting.

Broadcast and print news coverage of the dual event surpassed all expectations. The field director, the physician, and a local teen were interviewed by media at the event. Four radio stations covered the activity, and two asked the field director to appear on half-hour talk shows. The television station gave the event coverage on the nightly news. The newspaper ran a story and a photograph, which generated an editorial and seven letters to the editor, only two of which were for smokers' rights.

Board members were enthusiastic about the event and the publicity it generated. A few who had initially expressed reservations about possible negative publicity were especially pleased and expressed hope that other, similar opportunities would appear. The Utica physician used an excellent reframing strategy in her letter to the editor. She said, "Utica smokers don't need political consultants from R.J. Reynolds telling them what to do. They need the support and concern of their families, friends, and neighbors. We will be here next week, next month, next year. R.J. Reynolds' political consultant left town the same night" (McCall, 1991).

Brantford, Ontario, Canada   The Brantford community had a difficult time involving volunteers in media advocacy; indeed, the Public Education Task Force was initially reluctant to become involved in this area at all. Volunteers were not comfortable with the type of confrontation and conflict displayed in Utica and were inclined to move more slowly. It was not until an individual was hired to deal specifically with the media that things began to happen with the community media.

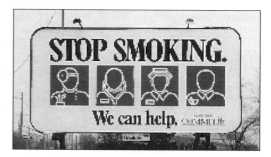

The media staff member designated a spokesperson for each news conference, and she fully briefed that spokesperson ahead of time. Other staff members and community volunteers were recruited to assist with the conference as required. She also ensured that press kits were available ahead of time, and she was willing to reorganize her time to be responsive to the changing needs of the media.

The majority of the staff person's time was spent in building relationships with the media. Because of the patience and prompting she provided, the media now turn to COMMIT for information. However, the form of media advocacy taken in Brantford is largely confined to writing letters to the editor and writing op-ed pieces.

Bellingham, WA   From the beginning, media advocacy was a problem in Bellingham. In the first year of intervention, a large media advocacy workshop was held. It was well attended by COMMIT volunteers and other community members. The workshop was thorough and covered issues besides the confrontation methods. At a subsequent COMMIT Board meeting, there was significant discomfort about the workshop and the methods of media advocacy that had been portrayed. Board members had no problem with trying to increase media coverage and shifting blame for the tobacco problem from smokers to the tobacco industry but found it difficult to advocate by using conflict and confrontation. From the outset, Board members wanted the project to be encouraging and reinforcing and, indeed, would not even allow the universal nonsmoking emblem to be used on the COMMIT letterhead.

Over time, the Board members relaxed their stance somewhat. They, like their Brantford counterparts, began writing letters to the editor of the local newspaper. Some volunteers were especially good at writing pieces about the effects of smoking relative to other risks. They wrote effective pieces about the cyanide in Chilean grapes compared with the cyanide in cigarettes and about the benzene in Perrier compared with the benzene in cigarettes. They began leaving stickers in restaurants complimenting owners for a smoke-free environment or stating that their dining experience would have been enhanced by a smoke-free environment. They encouraged youth-buying operations and urged media coverage of the results. However, the kind of media advocacy that occurred in Utica never really got a foothold in this community.

WHAT COULD HAVE BEEN DONE DIFFERENTLY?

This public education channel was a source of both frustration and pride for most of the communities. Initial reaction to changing the community environment through media campaigns was positive. The media seemed pleased to hear about COMMIT, wrote stories about COMMIT, and provided cut rates for advertising. However, it soon became clear that the media would tire of writing and covering the same themes over and over. Their focus is on items that are new and newsworthy. Few COMMIT staff members had the skills and resources to constantly attract the media.

In retrospect, more attention should have been paid to training field staff members to deal with the media. Training sessions where staff members produced news bites and news releases would have been good practice for the implementation of the activities in this channel. Training also should have been given in adding gimmicks to the press conferences about the annual action plans so that media representatives had a reason to continually attend.

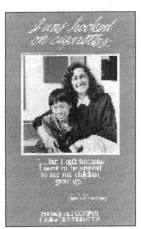

It might have been wise to build in an activity and resources for establishing a relationship with a public relations or advertising firm from the beginning of the project. Such groups are experts in gaining access to media and in designing campaigns to meet the needs and desires of specified target groups. Communities that used such groups seemed to do better than those that relied on volunteers or field staff members to conduct those activities. For example, the "Yes, You Can" campaign designed for Utica lasted the length of the project and provided a foundation for many media promotions. The "Kiss Your Butts Good-bye" campaign in Paterson also provided a visible identification with the COMMIT project. The "Hooked" campaign in Cedar Rapids/Marion was an eye-catching symbol of the addictive nature of tobacco. All these campaigns could be shaped by the advertising firms into the more specifically required campaigns such as "Ask a Doc" or promotion of the CRG or Quit and Win contests.

COMMIT staff members and volunteers were comfortable with the idea of using paid media. Many had previously worked with other volunteer groups and were accustomed to relying on public service announcements to promote projects. The COMMIT projects saw real advantages in having control of the content of messages and the times those messages were aired. This advantage, when combined with the ability to leverage more air time than was paid for, was seen as beneficial for the trial. In addition, staff members and volunteers liked the ability to target media outlets that were most likely to reach the target population. However, the amount of money allowed for media campaigns was still relatively modest, and many staff members thought that more resources should have been allocated for media campaigns.

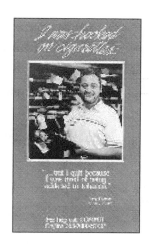

Most communities were frustrated by media advocacy expectations. As previously noted, media advocacy is not an easy thing to do, and many staff members and volunteers elt uncomfortable with it. Even more indepth training did not seem to provide many people with the skills needed to do good media advocacy. The reluctance to get involved in this cannot be attributed to the lack of information. A computerized system regularly provided each community with relevant national news items, along with sound bites and brief statements that could be used in news conferences, op-ed pieces, and so forth. The constant competition for getting on the media's agenda was frustrating to many COMMIT staff and volunteers. Careful preparation of news releases and planned press conferences that were ignored because of some other breaking story wore down many people involved in the project.

Probably the main reasons media advocacy was not used more were the fear of confrontation and the reluctance to engage in open, conflict-filled debate. To be comfortable in this process requires more training than COMMIT staff members or volunteers received. In addition, most Boards did not want to alienate other community members by publicly proclaiming their stance on specific issues. The one exception was in the area of youth. Without exception, Boards, staff members, and other volunteers were willing to take a stand when youth were involved. Thus, communities were willing to openly advocate for restrictions on youth access, even if it meant conducting undercover merchant compliance checks and presenting the results to the media. Similarly, Boards were willing to support the banning of billboards that advertised products considered harmful to youth or exploitive of youth, women, and minorities (i.e., alcohol and tobacco products).

It may not be possible to expect everyone to be a media advocate and confront a tobacco company employee as was done in Utica. It may not be possible for community members to boycott stores that sell tobacco products. Communities that have received support from the tobacco industry for cultural sports events may be reluctant to give up that support in the absence of other sponsors. As Wallack and Sciandra (1990-91) noted, much more work and research are needed on this issue.

This channel also provided some of the best experiences in the various communities. The magnet events were universally well received. For the staff, it was gratifying to see some real progress in terms of people who actually quit smoking. Staff members were working "blind" when it came to knowing whether their activities had any effect on smokers. This was because of the design of the trial that blinded investigators and the staff to trial outcomes throughout the intervention period. The appeal of the Quit and Win contest is understandable in that context. Staff members and volunteers alike could document how many smokers joined and how many quit smoking at least for a certain period. In addition, these events were usually fun and interesting. Many artifacts could be distributed, many volunteers could become involved, and a celebration at the end gave the event some closure.

One thing that is clear about the contests is that many resources—human and otherwise—go into them. A recent study of the COMMIT Quit and Win contests noted that for the 26 trial contests, the mean cost per participant, including staff and contributed community resources, was $78.57 (Shipley et al., submitted for publication). Estimating a 16 percent, 8-month continuous abstinence rate, the authors determined that the mean cost per quitter was $428. Interestingly, a high correlation (> .70) was seen between resources expended and participation. Finally, the most highly correlated measure (.82 on a per smoker basis) was between participation and the total value of nonprize resources. These findings suggest that such contests are a good way to draw smokers into quit attempts.

In summary, the public education channel, as most of the others, had good and bad points. Whether the communities achieved the channel goals of promoting social norms and actions toward a smoke-free community, increasing the perception of smoking as an important public health issue, and enhancing the effectiveness of smoking control in other program areas remain to be determined as the data are analyzed. The major positive point of this channel was the gratification of working with smokers and seeing them quit. The main downside was trying to understand how to deal with media, keep them interested, and deal with the new strategy of media advocacy.

REFERENCES

Advocacy Institute. "Smoke Signals: The Smoking Control Handbook." Prepared for the American Cancer Society, 1987.

Centers for Disease Control. Cigarette advertising—United States, 1988. *MMWR. Morbidity and Mortality Weekly Report* 39(16): 261-265, 1990.

Cummings, K.M., Kelly, J., Sciandra, R., DeLoughry, T., Francois, F. Impact of a community-wide stop smoking contest. *American Journal of Health Promotion* 4(6): 429-434, 1990.

Cummings, K.M., Sciandra, R., Davis, S., Rimer, B. Response to an anti-smoking campaign aimed at mothers with young children. *Health Education Research* 4: 429-437, 1989.

Cummings, K.M., Sciandra, R., Markello, S. Impact of a newspaper-mediated quit smoking program. *American Journal of Public Health* 77: 1452-1453, 1987.

Elder, J.P., Campbell, N.R., Mielchen, S.D., Hovell, M.F., Litrownik, A.J. Implementation and evaluation of a community-sponsored smoking cessation contest. *American Journal of Health Promotion* 5: 200-207, 1991.

Flay, B. *Selling the Smokeless Society: Fifty-Six Evaluated Mass Media Programs and Campaigns Worldwide.* Washington, DC: American Public Health Association, 1987.

Freedman, A. New smoke from RJR under fire. *Wall Street Journal*, February 20, 1990. p. B1.

Johnston, L.D., O'Malley, P.M., Bachman, J.G. *National Trends in Drug Use and Related Factors Among American High School Students and Young Adults, 1975-1986.* DHHS Publication No. (ADM) 87-1535. Rockville, MD: U.S. Department of Health and Human Services, Public Health Service, Alcohol, Drug Abuse, and Mental Health Administration, National Institute on Drug Abuse, 1987.

Kessler, L. Women's magazines' coverage of smoking related hazards. *Journalism Quarterly* 66: 316-323, 1989.

Lando, H.A., Loken, B., Howard-Pitney, B., Pechacek, T.F. Community impact of a localized smoking cessation contest. *American Journal of Public Health* 80: 601-603, 1990.

McCall, M. Letter to the Editor. Utica, NY: *Observer-Dispatch*, April 10, 1991.

Minkler, M., Wallack, L., Madden, P. Alcohol and cigarette advertising in Ms. magazine. *Journal of Public Health Policy* 8: 164-179, 1987.

Pierce, J.P., Macaskill, P., Hill, D. Long-term effectiveness of mass media led antismoking campaign in Australia. *American Journal of Public Health* 80: 565-569, 1990.

Seldon, B., Doroodian, K. A simultaneous model of cigarette advertising: Effects on demand and industry response to public policy. *Review of Economics and Statistics* LXXI: 673-677, 1989.

Shipley, R., Hartwell, T., Austin, W., Clayton, C., Stanley, L. (for the COMMIT Research Group). Community-wide stop-smoking contests in the COMMIT trial: Resource inputs, contest participation percentages, and the association between the two. *American Journal of Public Health*, submitted for publication.

Thompson, B., Curry, S. Characteristics and predictors of participation and success in a televised smoking cessation activity. *American Journal of Health Promotion* 8: 175-177, 1994.

Tye, J., Warner, K., Glantz, S. Tobacco advertising and consumption: Evidence of a causal relationship. *Journal of Public Health Policy* 8: 164-179, 1987.

U.S. Department of Health and Human Services. *Media Strategies for Smoking Control Guidelines.* DHHS Publication No. (PHS) 89-3013. Rockville, MD: U.S. Department of Health and Human Services, Public Health Service, National Institutes of Health, 1989.

Wallack, L., Sciandra, R. (for the COMMIT Research Group). Media advocacy and public education in the Community Intervention Trial to reduce heavy smoking (COMMIT). *International Quarterly of Community Health Education* 11(3): 205-222, 1990-91.

Warner, K. *Selling Smoke: Cigarette Advertising and Public Health.* Washington, DC: American Public Health Association, 1986.

Weis, W., Burke, C. Media content and tobacco advertising: An unhealthy addiction. *Journal of Communication* 36: 59-69, 1986.

AUTHORS

Russell C. Sciandra
Director
Tobacco Control Program
New York State Department of Health
Empire State Plaza
Corning Tower, Room 515
Albany, NY 12237

Lawrence Wallack, Dr.P.H.
Principal Investigator
University of California, Berkeley School
   of Public Health
516 Warren Hall
Berkeley, CA 94720

Carolyn L. Johnson, R.N.
Program Manager
Healthy Start Program
Jackson County Department of Health and
   Human Services
Building A
1005 East Main Street
Medford, OR 97504

Janine Sadlik
Executive Director
Court Street Diagnostic and Treatment
   Center
430 Court Street
Utica, NY 13502

Juliet Thompson
Field Director
Bellingham COMMIT Site
4407 Wilkin Street
Bellingham, WA 98226

Changing Public Policy Around Tobacco Control in the COMMIT Communities

David S. Carrell, Carolyn L. Johnson, Len C. Stanley, Juliet Thompson, and Sandy Tosti

INTRODUCTION   Public policy is a potentially powerful tool for changing individual and group behaviors (Jason et al., 1991). Through ordinances, regulations, and other policies, local governments can influence a wide variety of behaviors concerning the promotion, sale, and consumption of tobacco products (Bierer and Rigotti, 1992; Thompson et al., 1990-91; U.S. Department of Health and Human Services, 1991). Creating smoke-free indoor air spaces, preventing illegal sales of tobacco to minors, and prohibiting the distribution of free cigarette samples are policy actions that can influence individual behavior and community norms regarding health-related behaviors. Over the past decade local governments have become the primary innovators in the use of public policy as an instrument for preventing or controlling tobacco use (Samuels and Glantz, 1991; U.S. Department of Health and Human Services, 1993).

This chapter describes the contributions of the Community Intervention Trial for Smoking Cessation (COMMIT) intervention activities to tobacco control policy changes in selected communities and distills lessons from these experiences that may be useful to others engaged in or considering similar undertakings. Although every attempt to bring about policy change is unique, some themes, challenges, and strategies are common. Familiarity with the experiences of others can be valuable.

Intervention designers anticipated that many COMMIT activities were likely to translate into demands for more aggressive and better enforced tobacco control policy (COMMIT Research Group, 1991). Media campaigns were designed in part to raise public awareness of tobacco hazards and foster community ownership of the problem. COMMIT Board and task force membership often included local government officials, other influential members of the community, and advocates for improving the health of the community. As these individuals became more fully informed about the hazards of tobacco use, their commitment to intervention opportunities (including policy change) was expected to increase. Invigorated grassroots advocacy groups helped to keep these issues on local government agendas and in the public eye. The COMMIT field office acted as a clearinghouse for technical information (e.g., how to conduct compliance checks, provide model language for proposed clean indoor air policy) and a center of communication among various local groups and influential leaders. Recognition and ownership of tangible local problems, public support for government action, committed leaders, coalition building, and technical know-how are among the important factors affecting the political climate for local policy change (Reich, 1988; Kingdon, 1984; Weiss and Tschirhart, 1993).

Although policy change was recognized as an important avenue of community change, it was not a primary objective of COMMIT. Federal regulations prohibited use of COMMIT monetary contributions for lobbying in State and local political arenas. However, there were no such restrictions on indirect activities, such as provision of information and coalition building. In addition, project staff and Board and task force members were allowed to advocate for policy change as long as they did so on their own behalf, not as representatives of COMMIT. During the intervention, important policy changes occurred in many intervention communities.

Tobacco control policy is defined here as any ordinance, regulation, or directive issued by a *governmental* body intended to alter individual behavior regarding the promotion, sale, or consumption of tobacco products. Some governmental policies affect the general public, such as smoking restrictions in city- or county-owned facilities. Others may affect only city or county employees, such as office no-smoking policies or city personnel policies requiring newly hired police officers and firefighters to be nonsmokers. It is important to remember that "policy" includes both the scope and content of the policy "on paper" as well as related efforts by official agencies to monitor and enforce its provisions. Other entities, such as employers, retailers, and restaurants, also set policy that may influence the public. Such regulations are sometimes referred to as "informal" public policy. When shopping malls, public schools, or individual restaurants decide to become smoke-free, a limited but potentially significant portion of the community is affected. Smokers encounter domains in which they cannot smoke, and nonsmokers enjoy and become accustomed to smoke-free air. (For a discussion of informal, nongovernmental policies, see Chapters 10, 12, and 13.)

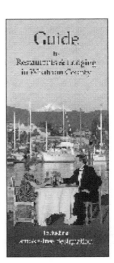

RATIONALE   The rationale for promoting tobacco control policy change in community-based health promotion interventions is compelling. First and foremost, public policy is believed to have a powerful influence on the broad social environment or context within which health-related individual behavior occurs (U.S. Department of Health and Human Services, 1989; Glynn, 1991; Bracht, 1990; Frankel, 1988; Wynder, 1988). Regulating or preventing the promotion and use of tobacco products may significantly affect social norms and practices concerning tobacco use. Over time, as the public presence of smoking, environmental tobacco smoke (ETS), and tobacco product promotion is reduced within a community, members of that community may grow increasingly accustomed to tobacco-free environments. Whereas it was once normal for people to smoke in enclosed public places, for cigarettes to be advertised on television, and for merchants to sell tobacco to underage youth (despite laws to the contrary), public attitudes toward these activities have begun to change. Many communities now consider smoke-free public environments to be the norm and have come to believe that youth should be protected from the hazards of tobacco use by putting a stop to illegal sales and youth-oriented promotion of tobacco products. Public policy can be an effective tool for promoting and reinforcing norm changes by giving official, communitywide sanction to the regulation of tobacco-related behaviors.

Policy is also an important health promotion tool because it is capable of reaching people who are difficult to reach through other intervention channels, such as cessation counseling or public education campaigns. Some members of minority populations, blue-collar workers, and youth are included in this category (Escobedo et al., 1990). Many of those who do not receive public health education messages or health care provider-based cessation interventions will be employed at worksites or will patronize public places where smoking is restricted or banned for health protection reasons. Protecting youth from the health hazards of both firsthand and secondhand tobacco exposure continues to be a powerful argument for policies restricting smoking in public places and preventing tobacco sales to minors.

Finally, substantial experience from Project COMMIT indicates that there is a potential for synergy between local policy efforts and other intervention activities, such as youth education, workplace policy, cessation campaigns, and media advocacy efforts (see also U.S. Department of Health and Human Services, 1991). Messages conveyed through public school curricula, the media, or health care providers can be bolstered and reinforced by the messages implicit in smoking restrictions at the workplace, in restaurants, or in public buildings. Once smoke-free office policies are demonstrated to be feasible and desirable in local city or county offices, private sector offices may be encouraged to follow suit. Thus, policy can be an important component of a community's multifaceted approach to reducing tobacco-related morbidity and mortality.

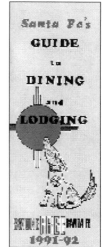

Over the past two decades the tobacco control policy movement in the United States has moved its focus away from Federal and State policy arenas and is now aggressively and effectively pursuing means within local jurisdictions (U.S. Department of Health and Human Services, 1993). As policy activity within cities and counties continues to build momentum, excellent opportunities to improve public health through tobacco control policy will continue to present themselves.

CHANGING POLICIES   This section illustrates the challenges, strategies, and themes—some common and others unique—encountered in local policy change efforts. Vending machine bans, clean indoor air ordinances, smoke-free school policies, and a billboard ban are described. Many of the policy activities focused on youth. This was because policy changes directed at restricting youth access are generally not controversial; thus, such activities could be used to gain the participation of many community members.

Vending Machine Bans   Communitywide policy change was not a focus of COMMIT intervention activities. However, some of the COMMIT intervention communities' efforts to reduce youth access to tobacco resulted in policy actions to restrict or ban cigarette vending machines. Children can easily purchase cigarettes from unattended vending machines with little fear of being detected. Vending machine ordinances are particularly popular among tobacco control advocates because vending machines are one of the most common sources of illegal sales to underage youth, particularly the very young (U.S. Department of Health and Human Services, 1990). As a result, local youth and community groups are often eager to assume ownership of and work toward addressing this problem, and the case for banning machines can be effectively communicated to local policymakers. As of 1992, 161 communities throughout the United States were known to have ordinances restricting or banning the use of tobacco vending machines (U.S. Department of Health and Human Services, 1993). In this section, experiences with vending machine ordinances in the North Carolina, California, and Oregon intervention communities are described.

Raleigh, NC   In 1991, COMMIT sponsored a 14-month initiative, the Tobacco-Free Youth Project, designed to reduce illegal tobacco sales to youth through merchant education. This initiative continued beyond COMMIT and was a major factor in the successful passage of a Raleigh, NC, city ordinance restricting placement of cigarette vending machines. Although banning vending machines was not one of COMMIT's intended goals, the ordinance came about as a direct result of the activities and actions of people involved in the initiative. Strategic framing of the issue, effective use of locally collected information, and a readiness to seize the moment were key ingredients in the passage of this ordinance.

Compliance in Raleigh with an existing State law prohibiting tobacco sales to persons younger than 18 years of age was poor, as is the case in many communities throughout the United States. Because the local community was generally unaware of the extent of illegal sales (or even the existence of the State law), it was decided that an awareness-raising effort was needed.

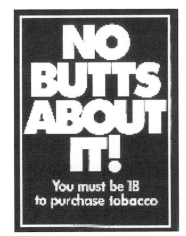

Project personnel believed that city authorities were unlikely to improve enforcement efforts unless they perceived the community to be informed of and concerned about the problem. Therefore, the Tobacco-Free Youth Project initiative began with an undercover compliance check (see Chapter 13 for a complete description of such operations) to document the ease with which underage youth could purchase cigarettes, both over the counter and from vending machines. The procedure involved underage youth going out with an adult superior to buy cigarettes, which they are not legally allowed to do. Two-thirds of over-the-counter and more than 90 percent of vending machine purchase attempts were successful.

To communicate this information to the general public, a youth-led press conference was orchestrated that received excellent media coverage and followup through editorials, feature stories, and a local radio talk show. Two months later, in an attempt to keep the issue in the public eye, the same youths presented their compliance check results to the Raleigh City Council. They also presented national data showing that vending machines are a primary source of cigarettes for very young (11- to 12-year-old) adolescents. Their presentation concluded with a plea to ban vending machines by a city ordinance. The youths reminded the council that, although it may be feasible to achieve compliance with tobacco sales laws by educating merchants, "You can't educate a vending machine" (unpublished quotation). The Raleigh City Council had voted down a similar proposal several months earlier; however, this time they referred the vending machine proposal to their newly created Substance Abuse Commission, to whom the youths again presented their compliance check results.

Subsequent negotiations between the Raleigh city attorney, tobacco industry representatives, and local vending machine owners yielded a compromise proposal allowing machines only in establishments licensed by the State to serve liquor, which mollified the vending machine owners. Although the Tobacco-Free Youth Project went back to the city council with data showing that most liquor-licensed establishments were family restaurants or local motels where youngsters gathered, by that time the compromise proposal had been drafted into a policy statement that the city council was reluctant to alter. The city council soon passed a precedent-setting municipal tobacco vending machine restriction in the capital city of the largest tobacco-producing State in the Nation. The Tobacco-Free Youth Project claimed victory.

Vallejo, CA   Before the COMMIT intervention began in Vallejo, CA, the North Bay Health Resources Center launched a 5-year project called the Solano County Cancer Prevention Program to address the problem of illegal access to tobacco by youth.

The cancer prevention program laid thorough groundwork in Vallejo in 1988 and 1989 by conducting undercover compliance checks to assess the ease with which over-the-counter and vending machine sales could be made to minors. This activity was followed by a merchant education campaign, another compliance check, more merchant education, and a third compliance check in May 1990. By this time the COMMIT intervention was under way with 1 year of community organizing and intervention behind it.

COMMIT was a resource to the Solano County Cancer Prevention Program during this first year by providing background data from the COMMIT baseline survey regarding local public opinion in support of tobacco control efforts. In addition, the coalition network built by COMMIT provided a natural clearinghouse for information sharing and cooperation among the various related agencies in Vallejo.

In June 1990, COMMIT cosponsored a dinner meeting with the cancer prevention program to bring together community leaders and interest groups to discuss ways to deal with illegal sales to youths and the lack of consistency in civil fines levied on merchants for illegal sales. The primary outcome of discussion among the 30 community representatives attending the dinner was a proposal to ban vending machines and prohibit free distribution of tobacco products in Vallejo.

A key advantage in the passing of the proposal was a political one: The chair of the Solano County Cancer Prevention Program was also a member of the Vallejo City Council.

Members of the cancer prevention program joined forces with the Minority Coalition for Cancer Prevention, a Vallejo organization that targeted African-Americans, to expand their own networks and mobilize a newly formed ad hoc coalition to propose the legislation to the Vallejo City Council.

COMMIT served as a resource here also, with staff members providing supporting survey data as background information. Because many members of this new coalition were also COMMIT Board and task force members, COMMIT meetings provided an avenue for information sharing. In fact, individual COMMIT volunteers were directly involved in testifying at the city council hearings and orchestrating the passage of the vending machine ordinance. Those individuals, representing their own organizations, included the administrator of the local private hospital (and COMMIT Board chair), the executive director of the local American Lung Association (ALA) (and COMMIT Board member), and the project directors of the Solano County Cancer Prevention Program and the Minority Coalition for Cancer Prevention (and COMMIT Board members).

The most important factor contributing to the successful passage of the vending machine ordinance was the role of three Vallejo youth groups: the Students Against Cancer (a subgroup of the minority coalition), the city-sponsored Youth Activities Commission (whose two adult advisers were another city council member and a COMMIT task force member), and the Vallejo chapter of Friday Night Live.

Ironically, these three youth groups were pulled together earlier in the year by a North Bay Health Resources Center staff member on contract with

COMMIT to involve community teens in an activity that would monitor youth access to tobacco. As the teens organized themselves around this activity, became educated about youth access problems, and began to develop ways to educate the public about the problem, the coalition was mobilizing and planning its strategy for proposing a vending machine ordinance.

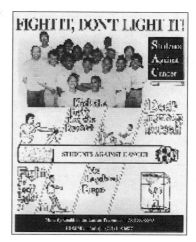

For their COMMIT activity, the three youth groups launched a media campaign called "Fight It, Don't Light It." One of the teens sketched a poster drawing, which was enlarged, duplicated, and placed inside Vallejo transit buses in June 1990. This was the first time the transit company allowed anyone to place "advertisements" in the interior of its buses.

The contribution of this COMMIT youth group was significant for two reasons. First, the youth coalition was organized and in place at the time of the city council's public hearings on the proposed ordinance. Now knowledgeable about the issues of youth access, the teens were invited to speak at the public hearings. The passion of the teens' testimony and the public evidence of their ability to buy cigarettes just prior to the council meeting swayed at least one council member from a "no" to a "yes" vote.

Second, the posters indicated their design was the work of Vallejo teens. Although the posters appeared in city buses after the ordinance was passed, they added impetus to the fact that local youth demanded that their community protect their health.

One source of embarrassment in the vending machine ordinance campaign was the lone vote in opposition to the ban. That council member was a member of the COMMIT Board of Directors!

After the ordinance passed, the COMMIT Board chair wrote a letter to the editor of the Vallejo Times Herald praising the work and wisdom of the city council.

Medford/ Ashland, OR
Community-based youth groups also played a central role in efforts to obtain vending machine bans in Medford/Ashland, OR. In preparation for these efforts, a COMMIT task force reviewed the community analysis report (see Chapter 5) to identify existing youth groups that could be asked to participate. It was felt that local youth would be most effective in pressuring law enforcement agencies to regulate access to tobacco products by minors.

COMMIT staff members approached the Medford Mayor's Youth Commission, a group of 15 high school students representing 5 high schools.

The group was looking for a project and was willing to put youth access to tobacco on their agenda. With organizational assistance from COMMIT, they conducted a compliance check in which 95 percent of over-the-counter purchase attempts were successful. The group presented these findings at a press conference and to the Medford City Council. The presentations concluded with a plea for police cooperation in enforcing the existing State law.

The following day the chief of police called a press conference to pledge support for an educational campaign to increase voluntary compliance among area merchants. In conjunction with this announcement, the Youth Commission sent a letter asking store managers to provide in-service training for their clerks. A cash register sign reminding clerks and patrons of the State law also was included in the mailing.

In 1990 the Mayor's Youth Commission repeated the compliance check, this time including vending machine purchases. The success rate for over-the-counter purchase attempts dropped to 72 percent, but 100 percent of vending machine attempts were successful.

With evidence that illegal sales were persisting and with other background information provided by the COMMIT staff, the students met with the city attorney who helped them draft a vending machine ordinance proposal. The proposal would restrict tobacco vending machines to premises not accessible to persons younger than age 18, private workplaces, or retail locations where the machine would be within direct view of an employee who could see the facial features of machine users at all times. Failure to comply would result in a $250 fine.

The students testified at a public hearing to consider the proposal. Only one vending machine distributor testified against the ordinance. Another tobacco distributor was quoted in the newspaper as being supportive of the goal to help prevent youth from smoking. He complained that the only reason he had cigarette machines is that some local employers requested them. The council adopted the ordinance by a unanimous vote.

Realizing that youth access to vending machines remained unabated in the county's 10 other cities and unincorporated areas, the following year COMMIT staff members and task force volunteers approached the youth group of a countywide drug prevention organization. The group was readily mobilized and eager to conduct its own compliance check.

With evidence of successful purchases in 75 percent of over-the-counter and 100 percent of vending machine purchase attempts, the students presented their findings to the district attorney and asked that an ordinance similar to that in Medford be drafted. Representatives of the youth group also made a presentation to the county commissioners, who subsequently ratified the ordinance.

COMMIT then focused attention on the city of Ashland. High school students associated with Students Against Drunk Driving (SADD) and Responsible Educated Adolescents Can Help (REACH) were recruited to conduct compliance checks, draft an ordinance, and make a presentation to the city council. The night of the public hearing, because of final exams, only one student was available to testify. Despite this, the city council adopted an even stricter ordinance limiting tobacco vending machines to places not accessible to minors.

Both ordinance campaigns in Oregon took about 3 months to plan, execute, and complete. It was very labor intensive for COMMIT staff members to plot the locations of businesses on maps, set up routes for each team, obtain subjects' permission as required by the research institute, obtain parental permission as required by local law enforcement agencies, recruit volunteer drivers, perform fundraising for the money used in purchase attempts and a pizza party following the compliance checks, draft ordinances, rehearse their testimony before appearing in front of government bodies, and make presentations. Such efforts are essential to the success of these campaigns.

The presence of several municipal or county jurisdictions within a single geographical area can complicate policy change efforts and multiply the amount of work required. In the campaign for a county vending machine ban, the Oregon COMMIT staff members had to gather data and present arguments in each separate city within the county and in the unincorporated areas. The result was three different ordinances, each with different provisions.

After COMMIT staff members worked for 3 years of effort to work within the many jurisdictions, the State of Oregon passed a law prohibiting tobacco vending machines from places accessible to minors but exempted hotels, motels, industrial plants, and restaurants with liquor licenses. This excludes, for example, many pizza parlors. Not only was this a much weaker law, but it also included a preemption provision, requested by the tobacco industry, that prevented local governments from having more stringent ordinances. This law undermined many of the provisions of the ordinances enacted in Medford/Ashland and continues to prevent other communities from aggressively controlling illegal cigarette sales to youth.

Initial sponsorship of State laws by the "right" organizations does not eliminate the preemption threat. The Oregon law was originally promoted by a coalition composed of the American Heart Association, American Cancer Society, State Department of Health, and ALA. However, once a proposed law enters the State legislative arena, the tobacco industry lobbyists can be counted on to do everything within their power to alter, minimize, or undermine the proposal's original intent. Often, what tobacco lobbyists convince legislators is a "fair compromise" is a relatively weak State bill that is difficult to enforce or incorporates preemptive language forbidding cities and counties from adopting more stringent local ordinances (Pertschuk and Shopland, 1989).

Clean Indoor   The enactment of new or strengthened clean indoor air ordinances
Air Ordinances   was a policy change strategy pursued in many COMMIT
communities. During the trial, policy changes restricted smoking in a
variety of public places, including government buildings and vehicles,
restaurants, office buildings, schools, retail shops, sporting venues, and
public transportation facilities. This section describes the events leading
up to the adoption of three such ordinances, one in Medford and two in
Raleigh.

Medford, OR   When the COMMIT intervention began, Oregon had a State law
requiring designated smoking areas in public buildings, and Ashland had
already adopted a smoke-free policy for city employees. The COMMIT staff
members thus focused their attention on Medford. A consultation with the
city personnel director was arranged to provide information on the benefits
of clean indoor air policies and to discuss effective strategies for developing
and implementing a policy that was acceptable to employees. Medford was
advised to conduct an in-house survey of its employees to determine their
attitudes toward an office smoking ban. The survey indicated strong support,
even among smokers. Three months later Medford adopted a smoke-free
workplace policy for its employees.

Jackson County, within which Medford and Ashland are located,
decided to take a more radical step. Following informational consultations
with COMMIT staff members, county officials announced in July 1990
that all county-owned buildings would become smoke-free within 30 days.
Designated smoking areas were to be eliminated entirely. The ruling exempted
the baseball park, the fairgrounds, an outdoor music arena, and the airport.
The policy banned smoking in the county jail (by employees and the
190 inmates) and in all county vehicles. The policy was supported by the
public employees union and the sheriff's employees union, both of which
had been notified beforehand of the county's intentions.

The media reported that the county adopted the policy in response to
rising health costs. The county, which underwrites its own insurance, had
an active wellness program and expressed concerns about the health effects
of ETS.

Despite the lack of forewarning, the ban was implemented with little
fanfare or controversy. Six months later a group of inmates staged a brief
hunger strike to protest conditions in the jail and included the smoking ban
along with other complaints. Jailers reported that cigarettes replaced other
drugs as the primary contraband smuggled into the jail and that inmates were
observed drying lettuce leaves, wrapping them in paper, and short-circuiting
the television cord to get a light.

Raleigh, NC, Wake   The first clean indoor air ordinance passed in Raleigh during the
County Ordinance   COMMIT project was a Wake County ordinance banning smoking
in all county buildings, including offices housing county employees. The
campaign to pass this ordinance was led by the director of the county health

department, a dynamic dentist who worked closely with COMMIT staff and volunteers throughout the effort.

The power to adopt the proposed ordinance ultimately rested with the Wake County Board of Commissioners. Through an informal polling of commissioners, the health department chief learned that support for the ordinance existed but that an influential tobacco grower on the board was likely to challenge the policy change.

COMMIT personnel recommended that the county conduct an in-house survey of employee attitudes regarding the proposed no-smoking policy. Such surveys can provide powerful evidence to challenge unsubstantiated claims of those opposed to such policies (tobacco farmers in this case). Previous surveys in other communities (outside North Carolina) indicated that between two-thirds and three-fourths of employees favored workplace restrictions on smoking. However, without tangible evidence of *local* opinions, some feared that the views of the silent majority would be overshadowed by the impressions created by a small but vehement minority opposing the ordinance. Furthermore, to the extent that a survey would involve those affected by the ordinance in the decisionmaking process, a sense of ownership can be promoted that can, in turn, fortify support. COMMIT staff members and county officials felt that employees would be more inclined to support a policy they helped develop than one mandated from "on high."

When the commissioner opposed to the ordinance learned that the county was preparing to conduct an employee survey, he attempted to influence its content. For example, he suggested that, in addition to questions about ETS, the survey should ask employees whether breathing perfume, aftershave, or another person's body odors was bothersome. Such questions were perceived by those conducting the survey as an attempt to trivialize the survey and the public health issue it addressed. The commissioner's questions were not included.

Results of the employee survey were presented at a public hearing attended by more than 100 tobacco farmers and their families. Emotional pleas by farmers about the eventual hardships the ordinance would cause them and their families were answered by survey evidence that 77 percent of employees—including many smokers—supported the proposed restrictions. By doggedly insisting that the issue be positively framed in terms of *protecting employee health* and by giving the commissioners survey evidence justifying a yes vote, backers of the ordinance successfully guided it through local political channels with a 7-to-2 vote, despite vocal and well-orchestrated opposition.

Prior to its formal implementation, a single exception to the ban was granted to one section within the county courthouse. Although the exception was presented as a compassionate provision for smokers under the stress of the legal system, the widely acknowledged truth was that a prominent judge was a smoker and was furious about the ban. The often-repeated maxim "all politics is local" applies to local politics as well.

Raleigh, NC,   In 1991 Raleigh passed citywide restrictions on smoking in public
City Ordinance   places. Again, the campaign was spearheaded by the director of the
Wake County Department of Health working in conjunction with COMMIT advisers, members of the Raleigh City Council, lawyers, and personnel from the Wake County Department of Health and the North Carolina State Division of Health.

This is a case in which a legacy of State-level tobacco policy efforts placed limitations on what was politically feasible at the local level. Some historical background is thus in order.

Raleigh is the capital of North Carolina and home to numerous State office buildings. In 1989 the director of the North Carolina Division of Health, a physician, imposed a smoking ban in all State health department offices under the division's jurisdiction. Within 24 hours the Governor held a press conference in which he publicly rescinded the ban. Such policies, the Governor maintained, were unfair to the tobacco industry and would not be tolerated. Two years later when the Raleigh city ordinance was proposed, it was clear that any attempt to regulate smoking in State buildings would be opposed.

Public opinion in Raleigh was far ahead of the Governor on this issue. As two previous COMMIT surveys confirmed, high percentages of Raleigh residents favored restrictions on smoking in a variety of public places. These survey results provided the impetus for proposing a comprehensive no-smoking ordinance for the city. The State policy legacy meant that careful political maneuvering would be required to secure its passage.

The proposed city ordinance was among the most stringent in the country at the time. It banned smoking in enclosed entertainment venues, sports arenas, educational facilities, shopping malls, elevators, health care facilities, pharmacies, and publicly accessible restrooms and on public transportation. The ordinance also required employers to provide "reasonable provisions" for smoke-free workplaces, and restaurants were required to reserve at least one-third of their tables for nonsmokers.

Ironically, this ordinance was passed by the Raleigh City Council with virtually no public opposition by the tobacco industry. Several factors accounted for the absence of opposition.

Perhaps the single most important factor was a strategic decision, made early in the process, to exclude all State government buildings from the provisions of the ordinance. The stated rationale for this was that State buildings are under separate jurisdiction. In reality, the decision was motivated almost entirely by political considerations. In North Carolina, as in many States, the tobacco industry can exert considerable political influence within the State legislature. If the Raleigh ordinance had included State buildings, the tobacco industry would have had an opportunity to redefine the issue as a State issue and unleash its lobbying machinery against the ordinance, perhaps defeating it entirely. By conceding State buildings from the outset, this controversy and the involvement of the tobacco lobby were avoided entirely.

Another factor accounting for the relative absence of tobacco industry opposition during this campaign was the leadership provided by the health department chief. There is no substitute for the careful planning, political aptitude, thoroughness, and diligence she exhibited in spearheading this effort. The value of such leadership cannot be overstated.

Another notable development during this campaign involved the use of survey data to counter the opposition's attempts to spread misinformation. Prior to the city council vote, the Restaurant Owners' Association and the chamber of commerce suggested to the news media that there was considerable public opposition to the proposed ordinance. These claims were reported in the local newspaper. Supporters of the ordinance responded immediately by providing the newspaper with results from COMMIT's 1989 Evaluation Cohort Survey (COMMIT Design and Evaluation Working Group, 1989) refuting the unsubstantiated claims. Ordinance supporters felt that publication of these survey results served to contain the opposition.

Another interesting phenomenon observed during the city ordinance campaign was the reluctance of many local businesses to publicly reveal their support for the proposed policy. Fear of alienating other members of the business community appeared to be the motivation behind this behavior. Representatives of these businesses were willing to recount their own experiences with workplace smoking policies at COMMIT-sponsored workshops and for use in a COMMIT-produced policy handbook. When they were asked to testify at public hearings, their enthusiasm waned. Of more than a dozen major companies in Raleigh that could have helped the cause of the campaign by describing their own positive experiences with smoking policies, only two would testify at public hearings. Both of these had strong connections with health care—the North Carolina Medical Society and Duke University.

Several contacts within the business community indicated that the decision not to participate was made at the highest levels within some organizations and was motivated out of fear of alienating the tobacco industry, whose representatives sit on the boards of some of these corporations. For other businesses, the reluctance to testify seemed to be an attempt to avoid open conflict with the chamber of commerce, which openly opposed the ordinance. In either case, the experiences in Raleigh suggest that unwillingness to publicly endorse a city ordinance does not necessarily indicate opposition within the business community.

Indeed, once the ordinance went into effect, some businesses used the mandate as an excuse for implementing more stringent workplace policies than required. That is, they banned smoking entirely when "reasonable accommodation" of nonsmokers was all the ordinance required. Apparently, these businesses were taking advantage of an opportunity to pursue their own more aggressive agendas while channeling any criticisms thereby generated toward the city.

Smoke-Free School Ordinances

In 1991 the school districts of Medford and Ashland adopted regulations that virtually banned smoking from public school facilities but only after successfully overcoming several political and operational barriers.

At the start of the COMMIT intervention there was some awareness within the Medford and Ashland School Districts of smoking as a public health issue. Both districts had established wellness committees focusing on school health issues and had participated in local health fairs and The Great American Smokeout events. Still, smoking was allowed in designated teachers' lounges, and there were designated smoking areas for students on high school campuses. Student smoking areas had been established to accommodate neighbors bordering the school who complained about students smoking in their front yards.

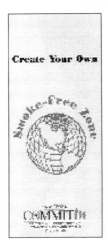

In 1990 both the Medford and Ashland School Districts' wellness committees began to spearhead efforts to achieve smoke-free school buildings, although efforts were slowed by union negotiations. Custodians wanted a policy that would allow them to drive off campus to smoke during their breaks. Initially, there was no plan to eliminate designated outdoor smoking areas on school grounds. However, in June 1991 the State legislature passed a law making possession of tobacco by minors illegal. This legislation also required schools to adopt policies regarding smoking and the use of other drugs on public school grounds.

Concerned that previous State laws regarding youth access to tobacco products had been poorly and inconsistently enforced, COMMIT staff members arranged two meetings to discuss the new State law and the need for coordination of policies across the county's seven school districts. In attendance were representatives from COMMIT, the school districts, law enforcement, and the juvenile justice system. Frustration with the poor enforcement of minor-in-possession laws by local police was expressed.

Ultimately, school officials decided to take an active approach to enforcement and handle most violations in-house; they would not simply notify local police when violations occurred. Each school district adopted its own multistage disciplinary policy. Generally, these policies began with confiscation of the tobacco (or other drug) for a first offense and ended with suspension from school in the case of frequent repeated offenses.

With respect to smoking policies for teachers and staff, COMMIT personnel presented the argument that adults, and especially teachers, should act as role models for healthy lifestyle behaviors for children. They argued that teachers and students should be subject to the same smoking policy; smoking should be banned entirely, for everyone, on all school grounds.

Heeding this appeal, the Ashland School District adopted a tobacco-free campus policy that stipulated no tobacco use by anyone at anytime on any school grounds, including the football stadium. The Medford School District adopted a similar policy but allowed teachers to smoke in their cars in the faculty parking lot.

Billboard Ban   In spring 1990 the city of Bellingham, WA, passed an ordinance phasing out all billboards within the city limits. By 1996 this ordinance will have eliminated what in most communities is a pervasive form of tobacco advertising. Passage of the billboard ban was the result of cooperation by several different community groups. Although motivations for supporting the ban differed, the groups' collective efforts produced an outcome that was beneficial to all.

Two years before the question of a billboard ban caught the attention of local policymakers, a COMMIT project staff member sought and obtained information from Scenic America, a national organization advocating removal of billboards as a means of beautifying the environment. Her interest in Scenic America was less associated with its goal than its means; elimination of billboards was one way to reduce the promotion of tobacco products because a large percentage of Bellingham's billboards regularly displayed cigarette advertisements.

In an attempt to initiate local action on this issue, the Scenic America materials were sent to a Bellingham City Council member who chaired the council's Public Works Committee and who was a personal friend of the COMMIT field director. In a followup contact, the council member was polite but indicated no interest in the matter.

About a year later Bellingham was in the throes of a transition. In summer 1987, a large regional shopping mall had opened north of the downtown area, an event that divided both the business community and the general public. The result was a relocation of businesses from the downtown area to the mall, leaving one city building after another vacant.

At this same time Bellingham was receiving numerous requests for permits to erect billboards on newly vacated downtown properties, a development that alarmed several members of the city council. The council swiftly imposed a moratorium on all new billboards until it could study the issue.

At this point the council member who had been given the Scenic America materials reconnected with the COMMIT field director and asked whether she would be willing to testify at a Public Works Committee hearing on the billboard issue. Support was building within that committee for addressing the billboard problem by proposing a full ban on all billboards to the city council.

Several billboards at that time displayed liquor advertisements featuring a reclining blond model in a revealing black gown. These advertisements played an important role in the outcome of the proposal because they angered and activated other local groups, including alcohol abuse treatment professionals, parents, and women's groups.

The hearing was attended by an attorney representing the community's largest billboard owner, another local billboard owner, and numerous local advocates and concerned citizens. Most of the people in the latter group favored the ban. Much of the testimony focused on the liquor advertisements. The COMMIT representative detailed the enormous amounts of advertising revenues spent by both tobacco and alcohol companies each year, how the advertising affects youth who are captive viewers, and how the advertising gives youth the impression that alcohol and tobacco are socially acceptable.

One argument that played well in the discussion was that, because it was impossible to selectively ban "bad" advertising messages, the only recourse was to eliminate the vehicle for these messages.

Many, including the billboard owner's attorney, were surprised and moved by the power of the COMMIT field director's testimony. When it was the attorney's turn to speak, he looked sheepish and confessed in an apologetic tone that he did not even let his own youth wear T-shirts with beer logos on them.

To enhance the effectiveness of her presentation, the field director had invited a retired Washington State senator who was a highly respected member of the community to accompany her in the hearing. The retired senator briefly reiterated and endorsed the field director's remarks.

The proposed ordinance was approved by the Public Works Committee and shortly thereafter passed by a majority vote of the city council. A 6-year phase-in period was provided to give billboard owners time to absorb and adjust to the economic impact of the ordinance.

Several months later COMMIT was asked to provide the same testimony to the Whatcom County Council as it reviewed its outdoor advertising policies. This time the billboard owners were more organized and presented more effective counterarguments. Instead of instituting a ban, the county council voted to forbid construction of any new billboards and specified that when existing structures were removed, they could not be replaced. Ultimately, the billboards will go, but it will be a more gradual process.

When attempts are made to change policy, the importance of laying foundations early on to ensure that some of those changes take place in the future cannot be overemphasized. Providing a council member with the billboard abatement materials long before the issue was on the local political agenda illustrates this point. That the mayor was a member of the COMMIT community Board also was not accidental. The COMMIT project wisely chose to hire a field director who was well known in the community and who knew how to "work the community" to ensure some success. The initial informational contact with the chair of the council's Public Works Committee was facilitated by a previously established relationship. The willingness of a highly regarded community influential (the retired senator) to advocate for this policy provided additional credibility and stature to the effort.

Another critically important strategy is to be poised and ready to "seize the moment" whenever it may arise. The success of the billboard bans turned largely on the fact that when an opportunity presented itself, tobacco control advocates were able to assemble their resources swiftly and strike with a certain element of surprise. Surprise was not an element in the hearings for the *county* ordinance, and the results were less impressive.

It is also essential to consider how issues are framed. From beginning to end, the supporters of the billboard ban focused exclusively on the issue of youth exposure to unhealthy images and messages. Because they did not deviate from that posture, the hazards of being portrayed as antibusiness or as infringing on first amendment rights were avoided. Opponents' attempts to reframe the issue must be assiduously resisted.

Diligence is essential in all efforts to change local policy, the process of which is often long and arduous. Even after ordinances are adopted, opponents may later attempt to have them overturned. As this volume goes to press, the billboard ban in Bellingham (which is not yet fully phased in) is under attack by a small but vocal group of local entrepreneurs who view the policy as an infringement of their business opportunities.

CHALLENGES TO POLICY CHANGES It is often the case that more is learned from failures and mistakes than from successes. This section examines two unsuccessful attempts at policy change. The first involved a county ordinance to address youth access problems; the second was an attempt to pass a local clean indoor air ordinance that was preempted by a tobacco industry-sponsored State law.

Unsuccessful Youth Access Ordinance Early in the intervention (1989), the Public Education Task Force in Bellingham identified the need for a policy initiative restricting youth access to tobacco products. Task force members arranged a joint meeting of the mayor of Bellingham, the chief of police, two city council members, and a task force member who was a highly respected and influential member of the community. Everyone at the meeting agreed that this was a great idea, but there was no commitment by anyone to spearhead the initiative. Vague promises were made that something would happen, but nothing was forthcoming.

Several months later the county health officer contacted the COMMIT offices and discussed the possibility of putting forth some sort of effort toward restricting youth access to tobacco. His idea was to cast this effort as a health department initiative promoting the health and well-being of youth rather than as an effort to beef up law enforcement or a program that could be construed as blaming the business community (retailers) for the problem. The effort would include the entire county.

The proposal called for licensing all tobacco vendors in the county and collecting a licensing fee. The fees would be earmarked for health department-sponsored educational and enforcement activities. The proposal also prohibited the sale of single cigarettes.

One surprising twist in this venture was the rapid response of the tobacco industry. The proposal was first presented to the county executive and chief of police in a closed-door meeting with the health officer and county counsel on a Friday afternoon. The following Monday morning the health officer received a telephone call from a representative of the tobacco industry asking about the proposed health department activity and requesting that the industry be kept informed of any further progress in this area. All involved became understandably paranoid. Nevertheless, there appeared to be no further involvement on the part of the tobacco industry.

Prior to the presentation of the proposal to the county council, COMMIT conducted two compliance checks to document the ease with which underage youth could purchase tobacco products in the county (for a discussion of compliance checks, see Chapter 13). Additional political groundwork was completed by the health officer, who made several informational presentations to various sectors of the community (such as a meeting of small retailers). At the health officer's request, COMMIT made a presentation to the county health advisory board. It was the health officer's belief that all stakeholders should have input into the initiative.

The presentation was made, and the proposed ordinance was forwarded to the county council for action. This was the last anyone heard of it. Apparently, the council simply did not put the proposal on its agenda for discussion. The reasons for this are unknown.

There are a multitude of potential barriers and challenges that must be successfully negotiated to pass an ordinance of this type. It is thus difficult to say with certainty why the effort failed. That there were seven separate municipal jurisdictions within the county that had to sign off on the policy undoubtedly complicated matters. In addition, the local political climate during the time the ordinance was under consideration was unfavorable for any significant policy change: Budgetary anxieties were high, and relationships between the county executive, the county council, and the health officer were strained.

There was a sense among some people close to the effort that key players involved were not able to respond swiftly enough—to seize the moment—at critical junctures during the process. Leadership plays a central role in determining the tone and course of such endeavors. In the opinions of some, the deliberate and at times overly cautious style of the health officer leading this effort did little to mitigate what was already a slow and inherently cumbersome process that called for exceptional political sophistication. The best of motives do not mitigate such shortcomings.

Ultimately, the passage of a State-level youth access bill made all attempts to reactivate the county ordinance moot because the State bill preempted similar local policies.

State Preemption of a Clean Indoor Air Ordinance

In 1992 an attempt was made to pass a county ordinance in Wake County, NC, restricting smoking in public places. Although this ordinance was almost identical to a successful city ordinance passed a year earlier (described above), the controversy surrounding it was much larger.

The successful city ordinance had been proposed by the county board of health but was actually voted on by the city council. In the case of the attempted county ordinance, when the county commissioners succumbed to tobacco industry pressure and would not consider the proposal, the Wake County Board of Health decided to conduct hearings and exert its authority to protect the public health. Citing the recently released U.S. Environmental Protection Agency report (U.S. Environmental Protection Agency, 1992) as a justification for action, the board of health passed a countywide policy (as a health board directive) in early 1993.

The opponents to this action consisted of tobacco farmers, the tobacco industry, and restaurant owners. The industry's primary strategy was to challenge the board of health's authority to regulate smoking in public, arguing that the board was not an elected lawmaking body.

Meanwhile, the industry sponsored a preemption bill at the State level that was passed in June 1993 and took effect in October. It purported to be a clean indoor air bill. It required that allowing smoking (or nonsmoking—many say the wording is deliberately unclear) be guaranteed in 25 percent of seating sections in public places across the State. A "small print" clause at the end of this bill stated that no municipalities could pass more stringent regulations. A "grandfather" clause permitted more stringent ordinances only if they were in place before October 1993.

Most preemption laws are extremely damaging to local policy efforts. However, in this case the process had a surprise ending. Local tobacco control proponents joined forces with the League of Municipalities (which was furious at this transgression of local ordinance-making authority) and other allies across the State to urge local governments to quickly enact smoking control policies under the grandfather clause. Some counties went to their county commissioners or city councils for ordinances, but many proposed ordinances through the more sympathetic and less industry-influenced county boards of health.

In the ensuing flurry of local policy action, more than 40 counties in North Carolina passed or strengthened no-smoking ordinances, rendering the industry's preemption bill much less effective than it otherwise would have been. A local newspaper story describing the tobacco industry's attempt to preempt local actions of this sort ran under the headline "Snatching Defeat From the Jaws of Victory" (Williams, 1993).

In retaliation, the tobacco industry targeted one "weak" county with lawsuits challenging the authority of every North Carolina county board of health to pass smoking control regulations. It will take years to resolve, and counties do not have the resources for protracted legal battles, so the outlook is not optimistic. The industry (through a 15-restaurant front group) had already sued the Wake County Board of Health for its ordinance on similar grounds.

As this experience illustrates, the strength that tobacco control proponents have at the local level can be offset by the strength of the tobacco industry in State legislative and legal arenas.

WHAT COULD HAVE BEEN DONE DIFFERENTLY? How could the design of the COMMIT intervention be altered to improve opportunities for and the outcomes of policy change efforts? The major design feature that significantly impeded progress in these efforts was the prohibition on the use of COMMIT resources, especially money, to engage in political lobbying efforts (such as advocating an improved clean indoor air ordinance). Virtually everyone

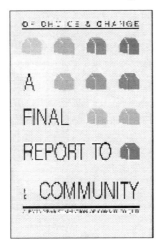

involved in the project's policy-related activities felt frustrated by this restriction. It was unavoidable in that COMMIT's funding came from the Federal Government, and Federal law prohibits use of Federal funds for State or local lobbying activities in deference to principles of jurisdictional separation.

Identifying funding for political lobbying is an ever-present challenge. The Federal Government is not the only entity that limits use of its funds. Even independent, nonprofit organizations that are otherwise free to engage in lobbying efforts may have self-imposed limits of this nature, often to avoid being seen as overly "political" by the public or to avoid the appearance of conflict with elected officials.

There is no simple solution to this problem. In some cases it may be possible to forge an alliance with another local group supportive of the policy change that is able and willing to fund a particular lobbying activity. In Paterson, NJ, the National Council of Negro Women (NCNW) initiated a campaign to petition State legislators and citizens to support a bill prohibiting cigarette advertisements on billboards in low-income and minority neighborhoods. Although this was not a COMMIT-sponsored activity, COMMIT played an important role in the effort. The NCNW member who organized the campaign was also a member of the COMMIT Board. Once NCNW decided to pursue the campaign, it turned to COMMIT for advice and assistance, illustrating the importance of being open to creative approaches to dealing with restrictions on use of funds.

GENERIC LESSONS The experiences recounted above and numerous others not mentioned here suggest certain generic lessons or rules of thumb useful in planning and carrying out tobacco control policy change campaigns. This section summarizes some of these lessons.

First, framing tobacco control policy issues in terms of health promotion, such as the protection of young people from unhealthy influences, is usually the best strategy. Opponents will often attempt to reframe the issues as antibusiness or in terms of infringements of individual rights. Anticipate this and be prepared to respond without delay.

As illustrated in several examples above, attempting to pass ordinances in geographical areas where political jurisdiction is shared by several entities can be especially challenging. Sometimes this is unavoidable, as is the case when a county ordinance is needed and the county encompasses several municipalities. Whenever possible, work within one jurisdiction at a time. Be prepared to devote considerable attention to consensus building when working with more than one jurisdiction.

Be poised to seize opportunities as they arise. Unanticipated developments often occur in the political arena. As some of the examples discussed above indicate, such developments can often be used to advance the tobacco control policy agenda.

When policies are being considered, do not let momentum and attention wane while a governing body "sits" on the issue. Keep your issue in the news to build public pressure. High public visibility creates pressure for political figures to act.

Strategies for maintaining visibility include announcing new endorsements or resolutions of support for the initiative by locally influential groups such as medical societies, parent and teacher associations, and health promotion organizations; writing opinion editorials and letters to the editor; conducting and reporting followup data-gathering efforts (such as compliance checks for sales of chewing tobacco after having done the same for cigarettes); requesting time in the policymaking body's meeting agenda to present new findings or arguments; and linking your issue to media coverage of related events or activities (such as a quit-smoking contest) by highlighting the connections between the issues.

Attentiveness to stages of change is essential in policy change efforts. For example, in youth access policies many communities may feel tough enforcement is the only way to make an ordinance work. However, raising a strong cry for more aggressive police action may only alienate the community, particularly when law enforcement is preoccupied with other problems. When there is little awareness of the legal buying age for tobacco (let alone awareness of how easily underage youth can purchase tobacco), educating the community as well as policymakers must be the first order of business.

Once awareness of a problem exists, fostering ownership of the problem and, ultimately, promoting community involvement in the solution are important second and third steps. When the community becomes involved in a policy change effort, it is much more difficult for opponents to claim that the need for policy action is merely a false perception created by a few zealots.

A corollary to this kind of community ownership is to involve a broad, diverse group of advocates in the effort. In addition to building clout and momentum, this also helps protect against being labeled and dismissed as "those zealots" or "those health people." A coalition of advocates from multiple sectors of the community tells the public and policymakers that this issue is important to many people and that something needs to be done about it.

Recruit "victims" or others directly affected by an issue to be public spokespersons. Even if they are not the most articulate, they tend to be the most powerful proponents. Sometimes this is *because* they lack the polished style of a professional or "expert." Youth can be particularly powerful. They can say things to elected officials that adults could never say, and they can give the issue a reality that can impress even the most cynical media representatives.

Locally collected data, such as opinion surveys and compliance check results, can be powerful tools, especially when opponents are trying to deny the magnitude or relevance of the issue in the local community. Such surveys, conducted by major employers and city and county agencies, were used to great advantage several times during the COMMIT project.

The enactment of an ordinance is not a guarantee of success from a health promotion perspective. Getting a law on the books does not mean that it will be enforced. Nor does it mean that the underlying health promotion objective—changing community norms concerning health-related behaviors—has been accomplished, especially if increasing community awareness and involvement did not contribute to the law's passage. Remember that forging strong community alliances, fostering leadership opportunities for youth and other members of the community, and involving citizens in the public health policymaking process are worthy ends in themselves.

Know your opponents and understand their strategies. Exchanging information with advocates undertaking similar efforts in other communities can be invaluable. National information networks can facilitate this.

Count on the tobacco industry to use State preemptive legislation to foil local tobacco control efforts whenever they can. To combat this, be watchful of all State laws related to tobacco control, even if they appear to be uncontroversial. Seemingly minor 11th-hour changes in the wording of proposed laws have been used by the tobacco industry to cripple otherwise sound legislation. A dismal example of this occurred in Washington State in 1993, when a bill originally intended to strengthen the law against illegal sales of tobacco to youth was ultimately passed with language preempting many local ordinances that were stronger than the new State policy. The bill also incorporated weakened enforcement provisions.

Finally, be bold and persistent. In the examples cited, many times the "gatekeepers" were acting on the basis of assumed or feared reactions by industry, businesses, influential officials, or even their allies. Politicians are especially prone to see certain issues as "sacred cows" and are loath to take stands perceived to be politically risky. However, with diligence, community-based advocates armed with locally relevant data and forming a united front with other community groups and supporters can challenge the status quo and bring about effective change.

REFERENCES

Bierer, M.F., Rigotti, N.A. Public policy for the control of tobacco-related disease. *Medical Clinics of North America* 76: 515-539, 1992.

Bracht, N. (Editor). *Health Promotion at the Community Level.* Newbury Park, CA: Sage, 1990.

COMMIT Design and Evaluation Working Group. "1989 Evaluation Cohort Survey." (5/26/89 version.) Unpublished document, 1989.

COMMIT Research Group. Community Intervention Trial for Smoking Cessation (COMMIT): Summary of design and intervention. *Journal of the National Cancer Institute* 83(22): 1620-1628, 1991.

Escobedo, L.G., Anda, R.F., Smith, P.F., Remington, P.L., Mast, E.E. Sociodemographic characteristics of cigarette smoking initiation in the United States: Implications for smoking prevention policy. *Journal of the American Medical Association* 264(12): 1550-1555, 1990.

Frankel, B.G. Reducing tobacco consumption: Public policy alternatives for Canada. *Canadian Medical Association Journal* 138: 419-423, 1988.

Glynn, T. Comprehensive approaches to tobacco use control. *British Journal of Addictions* 86: 631-635, 1991.

Jason, L.A., Ji, P.Y., Anes, M.D., Birkhead, S.H. Active enforcement of cigarette control laws in the prevention of cigarette sales to minors. *Journal of the American Medical Association* 266(22): 3159-3161, 1991.

Kingdon, J. *Agendas, Alternatives, and Public Policy.* Boston: Little, Brown, 1984.

Pertschuk, M., Shopland, D.R. (Editors). *Major Local Smoking Ordinances in the United States: A Detailed Matrix of the Provisions of Workplace, Restaurant, and Public Places Smoking Ordinances.* NIH Publication No. 90-479. Rockville, MD: U.S. Department of Health and Human Services, Public Health Service, National Institutes of Health, National Cancer Institute, 1989.

Reich, R.B. Policy making in a democracy. In: *The Power of Public Ideas*, R.B. Reich (Editor). Cambridge, MA: Harvard University Press, 1988. pp. 123-156.

Samuels, B., Glantz, S.A. The politics of local tobacco control. *Journal of the American Medical Association* 266: 2110-2117, 1991.

Thompson, B., Wallack, L., Lichtenstein, E., Pechacek, T. (for the COMMIT Research Group). Principles of community organization and partnership for smoking cessation in the Community Intervention Trial for Smoking Cessation (COMMIT). *International Quarterly of Community Health Education* 11(3): 187-203, 1990-91.

U.S. Department of Health and Human Services. *Reducing the Health Consequences of Smoking: 25 Years of Progress. A Report of the Surgeon General.* DHHS Publication No. (CDC) 89-8411. Rockville, MD: U.S. Department of Health and Human Services, Public Health Service, Centers for Disease Control, Center for Chronic Disease Prevention and Health Promotion, Office on Smoking and Health, 1989.

U.S. Department of Health and Human Services. *Youth Access to Cigarettes.* DHHS Publication No. OEI-02-90-02310. Rockville, MD: U.S. Department of Health and Human Services, Office of Inspector General, Office of Evaluations and Inspections, 1990.

U.S. Department of Health and Human Services. *Strategies To Control Tobacco Use in the United States: A Blueprint for Public Health Action in the 1990's.* Smoking and Tobacco Control Monographs–1. NIH Publication No. 92-3316. Rockville, MD: U.S. Department of Health and Human Services, Public Health Service, National Institutes of Health, National Cancer Institute, 1991.

U.S. Department of Health and Human Services. *Major Local Tobacco Control Ordinances in the United States.* Smoking and Tobacco Control Monograph No. 3. NIH Publication No. 93-3532. Rockville, MD: U.S. Department of Health and Human Services, Public Health Service, National Institutes of Health, National Cancer Institute, 1993.

U.S. Environmental Protection Agency. *Respiratory Health Effects of Passive Smoking: Lung Cancer and Other Disorders.* EPA600/6-90/006F. Washington, DC: Office of Research and Development, Office of Health and Environmental Assessment, 1992.

Weiss, J.A., Tschirhart, M. Public information campaigns as policy instruments. *Journal of Policy Analysis and Management* 13(1): 82-138, 1993.

Williams, B. Snatching defeat from the jaws of victory. *Raleigh News and Observer*, September 19, 1993. pp. F1, F7.

Wynder, E.L. Tobacco and health: A review of the history and suggestions for public health policy. *Public Health Reports* 103: 8-18, 1988.

AUTHORS

David S. Carrell, Ph.D.
Research Assistant Professor
Community Health Care Systems, SM-24
University of Washington
Seattle, WA 98195

Carolyn L. Johnson, R.N.
Program Manager
Healthy Start Program
Jackson County Department of Health and
    Human Services
Building A
1005 East Main Street
Medford, OR 97504

Len C. Stanley, M.P.H.
Program Director
Tobacco Control Training Center
Department of Family Medicine
University of North Carolina
Aycock Building, CB-7595
Manning Drive
Chapel Hill, NC 27599

Juliet Thompson
Field Director
Bellingham COMMIT Site
4407 Wilkin Street
Bellingham, WA 98226

Sandy Tosti, M.A.
7335 Franco Lane
Vacaville, CA 95688

Activities To Enhance the Use of Cessation Resources in COMMIT

Edward Lichtenstein, Paul R. Pomrehn, and Russell C. Sciandra

INTRODUCTION   Cessation resources include a wide range of methods and materials aimed at encouraging and assisting people to quit smoking. The range includes educational or self-help materials such as books, pamphlets, and audiotapes or videotapes; support services such as smoking hotlines or information services; and group and individual treatment programs offered by nonprofit agencies or proprietary firms or individual practitioners. The Community Intervention Trial for Smoking Cessation (COMMIT) project made several key assumptions that influenced protocol development and implementation. First, because a wide variety of services and resources are generally available in communities through existing agencies, it was not necessary for COMMIT to develop new cessation services. If other COMMIT programs increased demand for services, local agencies would be responsive.

Second, the individual smoker is probably the best judge of which method meets his or her needs and should be offered a range of options. Third, because 90 percent of smokers quit on their own, providing motivation and improving their access to self-help materials appear to be the most promising intervention strategies (Pomrehn et al., 1990-91).

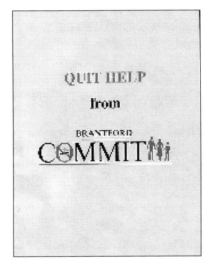

Considerable COMMIT resources were directed toward public education (Wallack and Sciandra, 1990-91), health care settings and providers (Ockene et al., 1990-91), and worksites and other organizations (Sorensen et al., 1990-91), with the expectation that the supply of cessation resources— for example, cessation classes and individual counseling—would expand as need and demand increased. As reflected in the protocol, communities were charged with promoting cessation resources that were available and providing regular notice of opportunities for smokers to quit. Because heavy smokers (≥ 25 cigarettes a day) were the primary target for COMMIT, communities also sought to identify and use avenues for reaching them.

This chapter has a twofold purpose: first, to present the rationale for the three required activities, describe how they were implemented, and offer some practical advice for communities interested in mounting such services with their own resources; and second, to describe how several COMMIT sites used the protocol or conducted optional activities to target heavy smokers and culturally diverse smokers. Both successes and failures are chronicled along with suggestions to guide communities in doing better.

CESSATION RESOURCES ACTIVITIES AND PROCESS OBJECTIVES
Each COMMIT channel had overall goals, a set of impact objectives, and a set of mandated activities designed to meet these objectives if they were successfully implemented (see Chapter 4). The overall goals of the cessation resources and services channel were to:

- increase smokers' awareness of cessation resources in their community;

- assist smokers in identifying cessation assistance; and

- promote participation in community cessation programs and services.

The impact objectives for cessation resources reflect the emphasis on increasing awareness of cessation programs, distributing self-help materials, and reaching out to heavy smokers. This corresponds with the trialwide goal to increase the capacity to modify smoking behavior. In accordance with the focus on self-help or nonassisted quitting, low objectives were set for attending cessation clinics by heavy smokers. The impact objectives were:

- By 1993 80 percent of smokers will be aware of the availability of stop-smoking programs or classes in their community as measured in the evaluation cohort survey.

- By 1993 cessation materials will be distributed to the equivalent of 20 percent of smokers as measured by the cessation resources survey.

- By 1993 cessation clinics will have been attended by the equivalent of 8 percent of smokers as measured by the cessation resources survey.

- By 1993 the Smokers' Network will have enrolled 8 percent of heavy smokers as measured by the COMMIT Program Records System.

The cessation resources channel consisted of five major activities. These activities and their process measures are listed in Table 1.

DEVELOPING AND DISTRIBUTING A CESSATION RESOURCES GUIDE
Smokers are likely to be unaware of all the available resources in their community. Information about timing, location, and expense is important to smokers who are seeking assistance in quitting or who are advised to do so by friends or health care professionals. Many health care professionals—for example, physicians, and dentists—and friends and relatives of smokers would like to be able to provide cessation resource information to smokers as they advise them

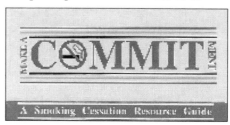

Table 1
Cessation resources activities and process objectives

Activities for Each Community	Cumulative Objectives (1988-1992)	Number/ Percent Completed	Process Objectives Achieved[a] (%)
Produce Cessation Resources Guide	All communities	11	100
Annually Deliver Cessation Resources Guide to:			
Physicians	90%		107
Dentists	90%		104
Targeted worksites	90%		101
Targeted organizations	90%		78
Semiannually Produce and Distribute Newsletters	66 newsletters	92 newsletters	139
Develop Network Recruitment Plan	All communities	11	100
Recruit Heavy Smokers Into a Network	8%	8.4%	105

[a] *Average for combined communities.*

to quit. For these reasons, a community-specific Cessation Resources Guide (CRG) was developed in each COMMIT site.

Resource guides are community-specific, nonevaluative descriptions of local cessation resources. The guides listed organizations or individuals offering smoking cessation programs, sources of self-help materials and cessation aids, and any other resources deemed appropriate by each local task force. A brief description of each service included names and telephone numbers of contact persons and often some information about fees or costs. Decisions about which services to include were made locally and were generally inclusive; those who wished to be listed were. There was virtually no conflict over listings. Most sites included the names of physicians and dentists who had received COMMIT-supported training in cessation counseling (Ockene et al., 1990-91). Several of the guides were formatted as 3×8 pamphlets that easily fitted into a purse or pocket and unfolded into a small poster that could be displayed on a bulletin board. The guides sometimes included motivational material to encourage smokers to quit on their own, such as a self-administered

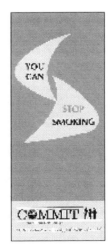

quiz on nicotine addiction or some other attention-getting visual or verbal material. In one site, a Spanish-language edition was prepared and distributed.

The CRG was probably the most popular and successful COMMIT activity across all 11 communities. Table 2 lists the number of CRG's distributed by each community as derived from the COMMIT Program Records System (Corbett et al., 1990-91). Distribution channels were determined partly by the protocol, with some opportunity for local creativity, and typically involved physicians' and dentists' offices, clinics, hospitals, pharmacies, and health fairs. CRG's also were part of self-help packets distributed during community events such as The Great American Smokeout or "Quit and Win" contests (as described in Chapter 11). In Medford/Ashland, OR, one of the smallest COMMIT sites, nearly 35,000 guides were distributed primarily through health care provider offices and worksites. A key distribution tactic developed by the Medford/Ashland site was the use of clear plastic racks for the CRG's; they were seen as useful and convenient by health care offices. Such racks helped make the guides visible for patients and providers, a strategy emulated by many other communities and proven to be popular at those sites.

The cost of the guides included staff time to collect the information, formatting and layout, printing, and distribution. Obviously, startup costs are greatest, and economies of scale will be realized with larger printings. As popular as this service was during COMMIT, it is not surprising that many sites wished to see it maintained after project funding ended.

A CRG could be produced by a county health department; a voluntary organization, such as the American Cancer Society or American Lung Association; or some consortium of these. A small fee (e.g., $25 per listing) could defray expenses, or one of the pharmaceutical companies producing the nicotine patch might be willing to bear some of the cost. In addition,

Table 2
Cessation Resources Guide distribution, by community

Vallejo, California	76,575
Brantford, Ontario, Canada	16,617
Cedar Rapids, Iowa	16,183
Fitchburg/Leominster, Massachusetts	12,323
Paterson, New Jersey	17,445
Santa Fe, New Mexico	3,566
Utica, New York	46,217
Yonkers, New York	42,089
Raleigh, North Carolina	191,830
Medford/Ashland, Oregon	34,990
Bellingham, Washington	8,719

there could be flexibility in how often such a guide needs to be revised and updated; every 3 years could be sufficient. Many of the COMMIT communities printed extra covers and gave a computerized listing of the contents of the CRG to a local health voluntary agency or health department so that the guide could be updated annually or biannually.

RECRUITING HEAVY SMOKERS INTO A NETWORK

Quitting smoking is a process, and smokers typically go through the stages of quitting several times before achieving long-term success (DiClemente et al., 1991). Therefore, it is desirable to maintain communication with those who are contemplating quitting or trying to quit as a way of encouraging quit attempts, preventing relapse, and encouraging relapsers to try again. For this reason, each

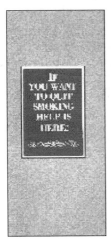

COMMIT community established a computerized registry, called a Smokers' Network, that provided a database of smokers who desired regular communication on cessation opportunities. Smokers joined the COMMIT network voluntarily when participating in community-wide Quit and Win contests (see Chapter 6) or when attending health fairs or other promotional events. Some sites used standing displays or posters with tear-off registration forms that could be mailed to the COMMIT office. Several sites struggled to meet network recruitment goals early in the trial, but most eventually succeeded. By the end of the COMMIT trial, seven sites each had recruited at least 8 percent of their total local population of adult heavy smokers. The range of percentage of heavy smokers in the network was 3.1 to 21.7 percent, and for light-to-moderate smokers 1.8 to 10 percent, with average trial percentages of 8.4 and 3.9, respectively. This indicates that efforts were generally successful in enrolling heavy smokers into the registry; more surprising was that a greater portion of heavy smokers enrolled than light-to-moderate smokers.

There were inherent barriers to entering the network: Smokers had to choose to complete and sign the card and sometimes had to mail it to the COMMIT office. COMMIT's contractual Federal funding required that registration cards contain the following statement, "The information you provide will be kept confidential, and will only be used for the purposes of this mailing list and will only be available to the appropriate staff, or as required by law. You may request removal from this mailing list at any time by contacting (local COMMIT ID) at the phone number and address provided in the newsletter." Although this statement may have inhibited some smokers from registering, many sites minimized this impact by sizing and creative placement on the registration cards. Sites found it neccessary to use incentives (e.g., pens or coffee mugs imprinted with nonsmoking messages) to help with network recruitment. Others distributed promotional items, such as a paper clip holder with a "join the network" message, to physicians' offices or

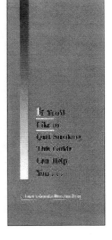

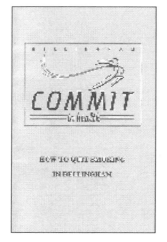

worksites. Many sites creatively developed registration cards for magnet events, such as Quit and Win contests, so that as smokers registered for contests, they concurrently registered for the Smokers' Network.

Perhaps the major lesson learned from COMMIT's network experience is that it is possible to use various cessation and promotional activities to develop a mailing list of smokers. Simple registration cards can be easily filled out and subsequently entered into a database for future contact. Individual agencies conducting smoking control activities could develop their own lists for their own purposes, or such lists could be shared or merged into a centralized resource for a community. Such a network could serve a variety of purposes, including newsletter mailings, supportive mailings or telephone calls to prevent relapse or urge recycling to another quit attempt, or offerings of new cessation programs or services. Such a system also can tell sponsors where in the community people are getting their tobacco information.

For COMMIT, the network was limited to the receipt of periodic newsletters. Enrolling in a network may be a signal that a smoker is considering quitting or is ready to quit (DiClemente et al., 1991). A mechanism that provides a more timely response than that of an infrequently issued newsletter can capitalize on this opportunity.

DISTRIBUTING A SEMIANNUAL NEWSLETTER   The COMMIT newsletters also were aimed at maintaining ongoing communication with smokers to encourage movement along the process-of-change continuum (DiClemente et al., 1991). Although COMMIT newsletters were initially aimed primarily at network-registered smokers, most sites distributed them more broadly, including to physician offices, worksites, organizations, and even locales where smokers were likely to be found. The newsletters attempted to be sensitive to and supportive of smokers and their needs. Content usually included a calendar of local smoking cessation events, tips on quitting, stories or testimonials from local people who had quit, interesting facts about smoking, and often humorous material in the form of cartoons or stories. Most newsletters used testimonials from successful quitters as a way of providing role models for quitting. Forthcoming programs or activities, such as Quit and Win contests, were also routinely featured. The newsletter was produced by COMMIT staff or volunteers using the desktop publishing capabilities of ordinary personal computers. Production sometimes strained the resources of COMMIT personnel who had limited prior experience with such an activity, but by the close of the intervention, the activity had become routine.

During the final 2 years of intervention, COMMIT sites averaged three newsletters a year, and all distributed the required minimum of two. At two sites, newsletters were mailed to all homes in the community, which resulted in many telephone calls to the COMMIT office as well as to other agencies concerned with smoking control. However, such a broad mailing, even with bulk mail rates, can raise cost barriers to programs with limited funding. Most agencies involved in tobacco control already produce newsletters or bulletins for their membership. This technology and capability can be readily adapted to newsletters or to other mailings directed at smokers. Newsletters could be piggybacked onto existing mailings, thereby reducing postage costs, one of the major barriers for this activity. A less desirable but still cheaper option is to include smoking cessation material within a broader health newsletter. Many health maintenance organizations already do so.

In summary, the three mandated cessation resources activities were successfully implemented across the 11 COMMIT sites. The CRG appeared to be the most popular and deserving of attention from communities wishing to enhance their tobacco control capabilities.

SPECIAL RECRUITMENT AND INTERVENTION ACTIVITIES Heavy smokers are less successful in quitting smoking compared with light smokers (Ockene et al., 1991). Less educated and economically disadvantaged populations are likely to have greater proportions of smokers and are also less likely to use or be reached by conventional cessation programs. The goals of increasing awareness of cessation resources and promoting participation in programs apply equally to disadvantaged segments of the community, but special tailoring of approaches and means is required. For these reasons, COMMIT communities were encouraged to develop and implement optional programs to reach the heavy or disadvantaged smoker. All COMMIT sites did so, and this section describes some of the successes and failures and offers some suggestions for future programs.

Paterson, NJ, an urban site with a high proportion of African-American residents, used an existing network of well-attended hypertension screening clinics to reach the black community. CRG's and self-help materials were displayed at these clinics and were well received. Information about smoking, smoking cessation, and COMMIT activities also was distributed at screening sites in Yonkers, NY. Yonkers COMMIT also participated in city-sponsored summer cultural festivals, including the Arab-American Festival and the

African-American Heritage Festival. Network cards and CRG's were distributed, and carbon monoxide testing was offered. Thus, network recruitment and CRG process objectives also were served by this activity.

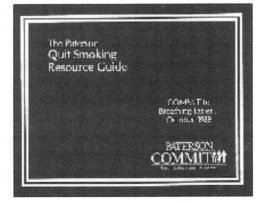

In Utica, NY, COMMIT staff members and volunteers identified 90 distribution locations for CRG's in neighborhoods with expected high concentrations of heavy

smokers. Indicators used to identify these locations included neighborhood socioeconomic status (SES), proximity to large blue-collar worksites, and retail sites known to be popular places for cigarette purchases (e.g., convenience stores, gasoline stations, corner grocery stores). Merchants agreed to cooperate by providing readily visible locations for brochure holders. The holders were restocked monthly by COMMIT and cooperating agencies. The Utica site also provided one-on-one cessation counseling in Women, Infants, and Children (WIC) program clinics, which serve young, disadvantaged women who have high rates of smoking prevalence. WIC nurses were trained in counseling techniques by COMMIT staff. There were Valentine's Day quit smoking challenges for WIC clients, and successful quitters received donated prizes.

The Cedar Rapids/Marion, IA, site used a local telephone information service, CityLine, to provide cessation services using taped messages and a voice mailbox. The telephone service was promoted through the media. During a 9-month period, the service received 2,450 calls, and 972 "Quitpacks" (cessation materials) were requested. The CityLine was particularly useful for promoting cessation events such as The Great American Smokeout and the "Cold Turkey Challenge."

Fitchburg/Leominster, MA, decided to target smokers in what was referred to as the Four B's: barber shops, bars, bowling alleys, and bingo sites. Field staff members began targeting smokers in these locations and eventually other locations where it was determined that high volumes of heavy smokers would congregate. Activities involved visiting locations with bingo nights and bowling leagues to recruit smokers for the network. This activity also was done to recruit participants for annual Quit and Win contests. A great deal of information was gained about the views and opinions of smokers concerning cessation, policies, and general behavior. Staff members succeeded in recruiting more smokers for the network than were recruited through previous efforts. Field staff members also began to set up booths at community blood donor activities sites, food distribution sites for welfare recipients, and functions held in neighborhood centers. Smoking cessation activity was particularly successful at blood donor activities sites because American Red Cross volunteers routinely tell donors not to smoke for half an hour after donating. This afforded COMMIT volunteers an interesting lead-in when many smokers inquired as to why they should wait the half hour. COMMIT volunteers actually served as attendants in the recovery area, which afforded more opportunity to interact with smokers. By volunteering, COMMIT staff members were rewarded with reciprocal volunteerism from American Red Cross members who recruited smokers even when staff members were not present.

The staff at the Medford/Ashland site also had observed that there was much smoking in bowling alleys and that bowlers were often blue-collar workers likely to have high smoking rates. They designed a campaign to appeal to bowlers—"Spare Your Lungs to Quit and Win"— featuring a Medford native who is a nationally known professional bowler. Unfortunately, few smokers signed up for the program at the various bowling alleys where campaign publicity was displayed. A great deal of staff time and energy was expended with minimal return in participation or quitting. Staff members concluded that this was not cost-effective. On the more positive side, Yonkers distributed bowling towels and COMMIT network cards at a Big Brother/Big Sister Bowl-a-thon, thereby bringing awareness of COMMIT to an existing, well-attended bowling event.

The Bellingham, WA, site also targeted one of the Four B's—bars or taverns. "Adopt a Tavern" was the name of a program wherein members of the Cessation Resources Task Force each adopted three to five places that they visited approximately once every 2 months to leave COMMIT brochures and newsletters in public places. All were good locations for reaching smokers. They included three golf courses, the Department of Social and Health Services, pharmacies, a bingo hall, two blue-collar taverns, one laundromat, Norway Hall, a Veterans of Foreign Wars hall, a Dairy Queen, the YWCA (Young Women's Christian Association) and YMCA (Young Men's Christian Association), and three alcohol abuse centers.

These examples illustrate the various ways that COMMIT cities tried to reach heavy smokers and ethnically diverse populations of smokers. These efforts typically required much staff and volunteer time. One lesson learned is that it requires extra resources—time and money—to reach ethnically diverse and disadvantaged segments of the smoking population. Staff members sometimes experienced frustration when outcomes did not seem commensurate with effort.

One general strategy that emerged is to integrate or piggyback smoking cessation messages and materials into existing activities or programs. This was done with hypertensive screening clinics, blood donor clinics, ethnic cultural festivals, and bowling matches. This strategy "captures" ethnic or disadvantaged smokers at events they have chosen to attend. This is efficient and economical and helps to integrate smoking cessation with ongoing health screening and health promotion activities. Relatedly, identifying settings with heavy or ethnically diverse smokers—for example, taverns, low SES food markets—and then bringing cessation materials to such settings also proved useful.

Heavy smokers ($\geq$25 cigarettes a day) may profit from more intensive, pharmacologically assisted programs (e.g., the nicotine patches). COMMIT sites reported that there was great interest in nicotine patches when they came on the market in 1991. Cessation programs providing access to nicotine patches seemed to attract more participants than those that did not. In 1991 there appeared to be a pent-up demand for nicotine patches and, therefore, an opportunity to use them to attract heavy smokers. Several years later, this may be less true. Some COMMIT sites were also successful in nurturing Nicotine Anonymous support groups modeled after the 12-step Alcoholics Anonymous programs.

In summary, COMMIT's cessation resources activities were effectively implemented, and communities displayed much ingenuity in shaping them to particular needs. Efforts to reach ethnically diverse, disadvantaged, and heavy smokers varied widely both in content and in success in reaching the target population. The most promising strategies appear to involve (1) identifying activities (e.g., hypertension clinics) or events (e.g., cultural celebrations) that such smokers already attend and integrating smoking cessation activities into them or (2) bringing cessation materials to the natural enviroment of heavy smokers by identifying locations they are most likely to frequent.

REFERENCES

Corbett, K., Thompson, B., White, N., Taylor, M. (for the COMMIT Research Group). Process evaluation in the Community Intervention Trial for Smoking Cessation (COMMIT). *International Quarterly of Community Health Education* 11(3): 291-309, 1990-91.

DiClemente, C.C., Fairhurst, S.K., Velasquez, M.M., Prochaska, J.O., Velicer, W.F., Rossi, J.S. The process of smoking cessation: An analysis of precontemplation, contemplation, and preparation stages of change. *Journal of Consulting and Clinical Psychology* 59: 295-304, 1991.

Ockene, J.K., Hymowitz, N., Lagus, J., Shaten, J. (for the Multiple Risk Factor Intervention Trial [MRFIT] Research Group). Comparison of smoking behavior change for Special Intervention and Usual Care study groups. *Preventive Medicine* 20: 564-573, 1991.

Ockene, J.K., Lindsay, E., Berger, L., Hymowitz, N. (for the COMMIT Research Group). Health care providers as key change agents in the Community Intervention Trial for Smoking Cessation (COMMIT). *International Quarterly of Community Health Education* 11(3): 223-237, 1990-91.

Pomrehn, P., Sciandra, R., Shipley, R., Lynn, W., Lando, H. (for the COMMIT Research Group). Enhancing resources for smoking cessation through community intervention: COMMIT as a prototype. *International Quarterly of Community Health Education* 11(3): 259-269, 1990-91.

Sorensen, G., Glasgow, R.E., Corbett, K. (for the COMMIT Research Group). Promoting smoking control through worksites in the Community Intervention Trial for Smoking Cessation (COMMIT). *International Quarterly of Community Health Education* 11(3): 239-257, 1990-91.

Wallack, L., Sciandra, R. (for the COMMIT Research Group). Media advocacy and public education in the Community Intervention Trial to reduce heavy smoking (COMMIT). *International Quarterly of Community Health Education* 11(3): 205-222, 1990-91.

AUTHORS

Edward Lichtenstein, Ph.D.
Research Scientist
Oregon Research Institute
1715 Franklin Boulevard
Eugene, OR 97403

Paul R. Pomrehn, Ph.D.
Associate Professor
Department of Preventive Medicine
University of Iowa
2812 Steindler Building
Iowa City, IA 52242

Russell C. Sciandra
Director
Tobacco Control Program
New York State Department of Health
Empire State Plaza
Corning Tower, Room 515
Albany, NY 12237

Activities To Promote Health Care Providers as Participants in Community-Based Tobacco Control

Elizabeth A. Lindsay, Norman Hymowitz, Robert E. Mecklenburg, Linda C. Churchill, and Blake Poland

RATIONALE   The goal of the Community Intervention Trial for Smoking Cessation (COMMIT) was to implement community-based interventions that had been demonstrated to help smokers, especially heavy smokers, achieve and maintain cessation. Building on the extensive experiences of past and ongoing smoking cessation studies supported by the National Cancer Institute (NCI), community-based heart disease prevention efforts, and other groups involved with smoking cessation, COMMIT combined interventions into a comprehensive program designed to have an effect on the smoking patterns of entire communities (COMMIT Research Group, 1991; Lichtenstein et al., 1990-91). Through a community organization approach, citizens from the community, with professional staff member support, assumed the major role in planning, adapting, and implementing the interventions. The COMMIT protocol was a mix of activities designed to create a supportive context for not smoking as well as activities that provided direct education or other services to smokers. To create a context for stopping smoking within this channel of activities, COMMIT promoted nonsmoking policies in all health care facilities. To reach smokers directly, planners considered who had personal access to heavy smokers and who might influence them. Physicians and dentists are among the few direct communication lines (i.e., person-to-person contact) to the majority of heavy smokers. On average, 70 percent of smokers see their physicians each year (Centers for Disease Control and Prevention, 1993), and more than 60 percent visit their dentists (Hayward et al., 1989).

A series of studies with physicians and dentists have demonstrated that, if appropriately trained and motivated, these health care professionals can give cessation advice and support to a large enough number of smokers who respond successfully to justify the time spent (Wilson et al., 1988; Cohen et al., 1987, 1989a, and 1989b; Ockene et al., 1991 and 1990-91; Janz et al., 1987; Gilbert et al., 1992; Ockene, 1987; Gerbert et al., 1989; Jones et al., 1993). Several trials demonstrated that physicians and dentists have an important effect on smokers. Although the success rates varied and often were modest, if this effect were spread across a community of physicians and dentists, the impact would be substantial and greater than any other single strategy (Russell et al., 1979). Although other health care providers also could be important in helping smokers, there is little research on which to base an approach to other health professionals.

Proponents of physician interventions argue that, in addition to having frequent contact with both healthy and ill smokers, physicians are ideally placed to influence smokers to quit because they are respected and trusted (in a way that cajoling friends or family members may not be) and patients see their physicians when perceived vulnerability to health threats is highest. Thus, there is an opportunity for intervention, especially if complaints can be related to patients' smoking.

There were preliminary evidence and a strong rationale that the dental profession also could play an important role in smoking cessation. More than 85 percent of dentists are general practitioners and thus in family practice (U.S. Department of Health and Human Services, 1990). Because of the frequency and continuity of dental care, the relationship between the dentist and the patient, and often the patient's family, is well established. Knowledge about each patient's social background can be useful during the intervention process. Regular dental care provides opportunities for accelerating the prequitting decisionmaking process and for postquitting followup reinforcement. Patients can be shown tobacco effects in their own mouths (e.g., gum disease and buildup of plaque on teeth) effects that are real to them at the moment rather than a more distant threat to their future health. In addition, dental visits often are longer than medical visits and can provide quality, face-to-face interactive time that provides many opportunities to reinforce patients' reasons for wanting to stop and for assisting patients with the process (Mecklenburg et al., 1993). In the early stages of the COMMIT intervention, the major national dental organizations adopted policies urging members to integrate tobacco intervention services into their clinical practices. For example, workshops on smoking cessation were offered at national and State meetings.

Previous studies made it clear that training physicians and dentists in smoking cessation was not sufficient in and of itself for a practice to reach the number of smokers necessary to produce a measurable change in smoking cessation at the 1-year followup (Kottke et al., 1989; Cummings et al., 1989). A comparison of studies that produced significant changes in smoking cessation with those that did not pointed to the importance of the presence of a reminder system in the office routine to cue health care professionals to address the smoking issue with patients. This meant motivating and training office staff members to set up office procedures that would make cessation interventions happen systematically.

There is evidence that the potential for physician and dental professional effect on smokers goes unrealized. Physicians and dentists believe that they should advise patients to stop smoking and have taken steps to eliminate smoking in their offices, but they often feel unprepared to intervene or feel that their intervention is unlikely to make a difference (Secker-Walker et al., 1989). In two random statewide surveys of Michigan adults, Anda and colleagues (1987) reported that fewer than half of smokers indicated that their physicians had ever asked them to quit. Based on surveys of physicians in the United States, Ockene and colleagues (1988) reported that, although physicians feel a responsibility to help smokers, fewer than two-thirds advise all smoking patients to quit. COMMIT baseline surveys of physicians and dentists indicated that 71 percent of physicians and 51 percent of dentists said that they routinely asked patients about smoking (Lindsay et al., 1994; Jones et al., 1993). In comparison, baseline surveys of smokers in the COMMIT communities indicated that only 39 percent of smokers had been told to stop smoking by either their physicians or their dentists (Lindsay et al., 1994). It appears that physicians had intentions to address the smoking issue with patients but perceived that they were intervening more often than they actually were. It is important to note that patients' recall of whether their physicians did raise the issue with them also will include errors, and therefore, it could be concluded that there was little congruence between perceptions of physicians and patients.

CHALLENGES AND BARRIERS Barriers to physicians' efficacy have been explored by several surveys. These barriers include restrictions of the time that can be spent with each patient, remuneration for counseling patients, medical school training that provides little in prevention skills, low success rates that are discouraging, and lack of knowledge about how to be more successful (Anda et al., 1987; Orlandi, 1987; Orleans et al., 1985). There was evidence that few physicians or dentists went beyond offering advice to stop and rarely made referrals, handed out self-help literature, set quit dates, or offered followup (Ockene et al., 1991). Addressing these issues became an important foundation for the protocol activities planned for the health care provider channel.

In summary, medical and dental care teams became the focus of the health care provider channel activities. There was evidence that physician and dentist offices could change with appropriate motivation, education, and followup. There also was evidence that patients would appreciate the advice of these health care professionals and often would respond by trying to stop smoking. It also was clear that an integrated approach should be promoted that involved key roles for office staff members and a smoke-free office environment. It was important to mobilize other health care providers in the community, but at the time of protocol development, there was no systematic approach to recommend because of the lack of research among nurses, pharmacists, and other providers. Therefore, the primary mandate was to involve all health care providers in planning activities but to focus training on medical and dental care teams. COMMIT planners anticipated that activities directed at health care professionals beyond physicians and dentists would evolve as appropriate according to the needs of individual communities, but no resources were allocated specifically for this purpose.

GOALS AND PROCESS OBJECTIVES FOR HEALTH CARE PROVIDERS Based on the understanding of how health care providers can influence smoking cessation, the following overall goals were set to guide activities in this channel:

- Involvement and leadership: Health care providers will be aware of, promote, and play an active role in smoking intervention efforts in the community.

- Changes in clinical procedures: Health care providers will regard smoking cessation advice as the minimal standard of practice; they will ask all patients whether they smoke; and some providers will go beyond providing advice.

- Policy changes: All health care facilities will adopt and effectively implement policies for a smoke-free environment.

- Public response: Smoking patients will more actively seek assistance from the health care system to stop smoking.

The health care provider channel received considerable emphasis in COMMIT, which is clearly evident by the range and number of intervention activities involved (Table 1).

INTERVENTION ACTIVITIES

Activities of "Influentials"

As a community health project, COMMIT needed "buy-in" and leadership from many members of the health care community. Participation took many forms. Each community identified influential health care professionals who were interested in smoking as a community health problem. In addition to their involvement in continuing medical and dental education, these influentials stimulated community change by promoting smoke-free health care facilities; supporting new regulations—and the enforcement of existing regulations—on the sale of tobacco to minors and smoking in public places, schools, and worksites; and serving as spokespersons with the media, schools, and community groups. COMMIT organizers invited known leaders from the physician and dental communities to take on educational roles and to guide activities in a health care provider task force, which involved representatives from many other professions. Most communities involved nurses and pharmacists in these efforts. Chiropractors were active participants in some communities, and in others, occupational and public health nurses played important roles.

Physician and Dentist Training

There were three levels of training activities provided for medical and dental care teams designed to achieve the educational goals and facilitate regular counseling of all smokers following a standard protocol. These activities have been described in detail elsewhere (Lindsay et al., 1994; Ockene et al., 1990-91; Manley et al., 1991); they include a basic program, comprehensive program, and a more advanced program to develop skills to teach others the basic and comprehensive programs.

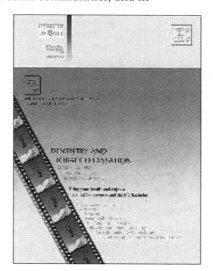

Table 1
Health care provider activities and process objectives

Activities for Each Community	Cumulative Objectives (1988-1992)	Number Completed	Process Objectives Achieved (%)
Three or More Local Influential Medical Care Providers Trained	33 providers	74 providers	224
Three or More Local Influential Dental Care Providers Trained	33 dentists	49 dentists	148
Annually, At Least Three Physicians Will Be Active on Community Board	132 physicians	211 physicians	160
Annually (from 1989) At Least One Dental Care Provider Will Be Active on Community Board	33 dentists	93 dentists	282
Annually (from 1989) At Least Three Dental Care Providers Will Be Active on Community Board	99 providers	124 providers	125
At Least One Physician Attended National Training	11 physicians	23 physicians	209
At Least One Dentist Attended National Training	11 dentists	17 dentists	155
At Least Two Dental Care Providers Attended National or Regional Training	22 providers	25 providers	114
Basic Training of Physicians	80%		101
Basic Training of Dentist/Dental Care Providers	65%		94
Comprehensive Training of Physicians	25%		100
Comprehensive Training of Dentist/Dental Care Providers	20%		95
Physician Office Staff Training	30%		200
Dentist Office Staff Training	30%		147
Resource Materials Sent to Physician Offices	90%		111
Resource Materials Sent to Dentist Offices	90%		111
Promotional Materials Sent to Physician Offices	90%		110
Promotional Materials Sent to Dentist Offices	90%		108
Presentations to Physician Offices Not Smoke-Free	60%		147
Presentations to Dentist Offices Not Smoke-Free	60%		138
Presentations to Health Care Facilities Not Smoke-Free	100%		100

[a] Average for combined communities.

The most advanced level of training was provided centrally for several individuals from each community and was intended to develop leadership and educational skills for medical and dental care teams within the intervention communities. These central training events provided guidelines for how to deliver the NCI-developed programs (basic and comprehensive programs) and how to plan community-level educational programs. *Basic* (approximately 45 minutes, like that of traditional rounds presentations) and *comprehensive* training (a minimum of a 2 1/2-hour workshop) that included didactic presentations, opportunities for discussion, and planning as well as skills-building exercises were then made available to all medical and dental care teams at the community level.

In the 11 COMMIT communities, there were 909 primary care physicians (mean = 83 per community) and 731 general care dentists (mean = 66 per community) in the intervention communities. During the 4 years of the COMMIT intervention, an estimated 80 percent (727) of primary care physicians and 65 percent (475) of general care dentists attended some level of training.

WHAT HAPPENED: SUCCESSFUL COMPONENTS AND CHALLENGES

Goal 1. Involvement and Leadership

Representatives from many health professions spent time as volunteers to provide leadership through the COMMIT Board and task forces. Most of these volunteers took on a 4-year commitment and sustained their involvement with project. The chairs of the health care provider task forces usually were physicians. Participants on this task force provided many different kinds of leadership and support to the COMMIT intervention. The specific contributions were dependent on individual interests and skills and the opportunities afforded by the particular form of activities in each community. The role of the knowledgeable expert

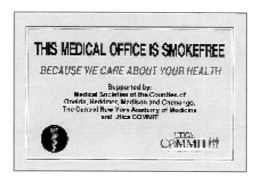

on health was always important for media events. Radio, television, and newspapers often looked to the health care provider leaders for comment on the smoking issue. The experts participated in talk shows, wrote articles for newspapers, and responded to health issues at press conferences. For example, at the time of the release of the 1989 U.S. Surgeon General's report (U.S. Department of Health and Human Services, 1989), there was an opportunity to discuss implications of the report at the community level.

Physicians, dentists, and other health professionals played leadership roles in creating smoke-free hospitals and other medical and dental facilities, submitting articles for the *COMMIT Newsletter*, and encouraging their colleagues to prescribe the nicotine patch when it was first introduced. The importance of this visibility and the sense of local expertise are difficult to measure but are critical in the diffusion process as a context for promoting other activities.

Task Force Issues   The protocol's emphasis on physician and dentist training interfered with smooth functioning of task forces in several communities. Planning of training events was time consuming, and committees spent an inordinate amount of time attempting to deal with physician and dentist reluctance to attend comprehensive training. At the same time, there was concern that, even with training, these health care professionals could have only a minimal effect on patients' smoking behavior.

Representatives of other health care professions could see an important role for their groups in COMMIT but did not see sufficient resources allocated for this purpose. This lack of resources was overcome in many communities by local initiatives, but the group process suffered because of the resentment engendered by this perception of inequality and inappropriate attention to physicians and dentists. At the same time, there was a reluctance among staff members and other members of the task force to address issues because of the (1) traditional independence, rank, and respect for physicians and dentists and (2) possibility of not meeting project objectives.

Some communities reported that the task force lacked a strong, visionary, and powerful leadership committed to the spirit as well as the letter of the protocol. Some groups tended to focus on meeting the minimum requirements of the protocol and did not push their creativity beyond the minimum. This was unfortunate because a community approach, by its nature, should be comprehensive and coordinated. For example, physicians and dentists are in an excellent position to refer smokers to other health professionals for quit-smoking therapy, and they may work jointly by providing a prescription for nicotine replacement therapy. In urban settings, where physicians and dentists often work in combination clinics and free-standing health centers, such cooperation and interaction among physicians, dentists, nurses, and other health professionals may be more readily anticipated than in private office settings that are often more limited in scope.

Although these limitations within the protocol were a problem for many communities, there were many examples of pushing beyond the protocol requirements. For example, the Santa Fe, NM, group developed a videotape that was circulated among a variety of health professionals. In Paterson, NJ, a poor urban community with a large minority population, hypertension nurses and clinicians who conducted onsite high blood pressure screening programs throughout the community were trained to measure the carbon monoxide in the expired air of smokers and to counsel smokers, particularly those with high blood pressure, to quit smoking. In several communities, "grand rounds" presentations and comprehensive symposia and workshops, although targeted to physicians and dentists, were extended to include other professionals. In one instance, a comprehensive training event included presentations (e.g., a lawyer from the Rose Cipollone case in New Jersey [*Cipollone* v. *Liggett Group*], a presentation on environmental tobacco smoke, an update on smoking and health issues) of interest to a diverse audience. By offering Continuing Medical Education (CME) credits for nurses and other health professionals, it was possible to attract a varied concerned audience, boost attendance, and add to the success of the program. Sometimes training was provided specifically for other health care providers. For example, in Fitchburg/Leominster, MA, special training was offered to hospital nurses who wanted to take advantage of the "teachable moment" when smoking patients in a smoke-free hospital must deal with a period of abstinence.

Goal 2. Changes in Procedures

Changes in Procedures Require a Chain of Events

To ensure that medical and dental care teams put state-of-the-art procedures into place, a chain of events appears necessary (Figure 1). This is a complex process, and breakdowns at any stage in the chain will compromise the overall impact on patient outcomes. There were challenges to be met and solutions to be found at every link of this chain.

Link 1. Physicians and Dentists and Their Office Staffs Must Want To Learn About and Be Willing To Attend Training for Smoking Cessation. Most communities were able to provide basic training to more than 80 percent of physicians and 65 percent of dentists. However, physicians and dentists were reluctant to attend comprehensive training. Some communities made an effort to schedule the comprehensive training at "attractive" times, such as in association with the American Cancer Society's The

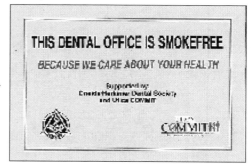

Great American Smokeout (GASO) or in conjunction with a New Year's "Quit and Win" contest. Some communities expanded the training program to enhance its attractiveness to other health professionals and to use the event as an occasion to train and educate members of the COMMIT Board and task forces, local health department staff members, and other key people in the community. This ensured strong attendance and enhanced the ability

Figure 1
Chain of events that enable health professionals to help patients

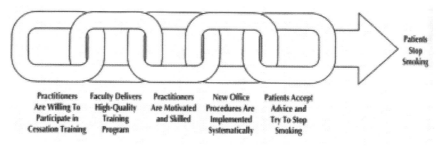

of the entire community to intervene on smoking. However, not all communities followed this procedure.

In many communities, training events were cancelled because of insufficient registration. Most task forces spent many meetings considering how to attract professionals to 2 1/2 hours of training about smoking cessation. A wide range of incentives was offered, such as CME credits, dinners in pleasant locations, and in one community, eligibility for a drawing for a weekend of skiing. Across the COMMIT communities, there were many variations on optimum timing for training events; virtually every possibility was explored. In some communities, experts were imported, local opinion leaders made personal telephone calls, and so forth. In several communities, the organizers took the program to health care providers in their offices. This strategy provided an excellent opportunity to meet with office staff members, help them tailor and "mobilize" the office for intervention on smoking, and provide necessary followup and continued contact.

The nicotine patch became available early in 1992, during the final 9 months of the 4-year intervention period. Some communities saw the patch as an opportunity to make a final push to attract health care providers to training events. Rather than physicians raising the issue of smoking cessation with their patients, many smokers were asking their physicians about the patch. The need to know more about how to prescribe the patch provided a window of opportunity to attract physicians to training. In addition, drug company representatives were willing to work with COMMIT staff members to help promote and stage the training events.

However, in some communities the task force did not respond to this opportunity because it had already reached its objectives and because of the perception that there was not sufficient demand among physicians and dentists for more training on smoking cessation. This reality was borne out in one community that cancelled a workshop as the result of a lack of registration during the height of the nicotine patch campaigns.

Link 2. The Faculty Members for Training Events Need To Have the Knowledge, Skills, and Motivation To Deliver Effective Training to Their Colleagues in the Community. Some communities reported that they felt they needed "an out-of-town expert" to attract physicians and dentists to a training event. Others noted that the individuals trained to lead sessions were not available or tended not to be committed to the need for training or, in some cases, the content of the recommended training. On the other hand, the local physician and dentist leaders were important in many communities because of their role in persuading their colleagues to attend at least one training event. The local professionals also demonstrated that the recommended intervention could be implemented within regular practices and were able to address in a credible manner the practical concerns related to the local situation.

Most often, the organizers were satisfied with the quality of the presentations but not with the level of participation. There are advantages to a mix of outside expertise and inside leadership. In addition, when the audience at the training events included nurses, dental hygienists, or other health care providers, there was not only more satisfaction in terms of levels of participation but also more interest and richness in what the audience brought to the session.

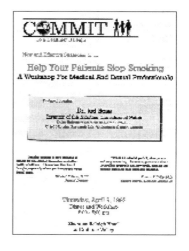

Link 3. The Education Provided Must Be Effective Enough To Motivate Practitioners To Address Smoking More Systematically and To Provide Enough Knowledge and Other Resources To Enable Changes in Procedures. (Note: It was important that the presentations provided through COMMIT have an effect on health professionals' behavior similar to the effect of the educational programs tested in the research that provided the basis for the training program [Wilson et al., 1988; Ockene et al., 1990-91; Gilbert et al., 1992; Kottke et al., 1989; Cummings et al., 1989].) There was a wide range in the quality of the educational programs provided. In many instances, staff and participants reported high-quality presentations. Sometimes the faculty members for these sessions would present what they were comfortable with rather than the NCI training package. There was no centralized evaluation of training sessions; therefore, it is unknown whether specific training events had the effect on practices that was intended in the original training objectives.

Link 4. After Attending These Training Events, Physicians and Dentists and Their Office Staff Members Need To Take Action by Setting Up Their Offices To Facilitate Smoking Control Activities and To Provide Effective Advice and Support to Their Smoking Patients. It takes motivation, knowledge, and support to make changes in procedures. It also is necessary to reduce the barriers to action that exist for health care providers. Health care providers have often listed lack of reimbursement for smoking cessation advice as an important barrier to implementing the procedure, and it was found that in communities where this activity is billable (for example, Bellingham, WA, and Brantford, Ontario, Canada), knowledge about the use of appropriate billing codes appeared to be one of the most powerful elements in the training program. It is not known whether those who attended training changed the way they dealt with smokers because the observation of changes in practices among those who attended training was not part of the evaluation process. Project staff members noted that little change in office systems was evident unless COMMIT staff members personally visited offices. In other words, training of office staff members was essential. Instructing physicians and dentists to make changes in their office systems to help them remember to address smoking often did not lead to these systems being set up. Even with in-office training, many offices resisted setting up a reminder system but welcomed the other office support resources that COMMIT offered.

Link 5. Patients Need To Respond to the Advice and Support Provided by These Health Care Professionals and Successfully Stop Smoking. Even if a health care professional does everything right, a patient's ability to successfully stop smoking depends on many factors. Degree of nicotine dependence; level of motivation beliefs about the determinants of health, self-confidence, perceived self-efficacy and locus of control; and presence of a supportive environment at work, home, and among peers contribute to individuals' willingness and ability to follow through on their physicians' advice (U.S. Department of Health and Human Services, 1989). Previous studies have shown that stopping smoking is a long-term process and that it is often important to help smokers move through stages of change prior to their final successful attempt to stop. For example, helping contented smokers become discontented with their habit, shortening the number of years that individuals think about stopping before making their first attempt, helping relapsers start thinking about quitting again, and supporting ex-smokers are all potentially important effects of the interventions taught to health care providers through the training and materials. Baseline and midpoint surveys of smokers in the COMMIT communities indicated that smokers do take the advice of their physicians seriously and, if advised, do try to stop smoking (Ockene et al., 1991 and 1990-91). Final analysis of the COMMIT surveys of smokers will provide some insight into their responses to these aspects of the intervention. Unfortunately, specific physician intervention cannot be linked with patients' success in stopping smoking.

Goal 3. Policy Changes   Leaders in the health care provider community approached by COMMIT organizers to participate on the Board and task forces often already had played a key role in advocacy and policy issues change within their communities prior to the beginning of COMMIT. This history varied by community, but when these leaders were already in place, it often gave those communities a headstart on this aspect of COMMIT work. However, this history may not be an advantage if these individuals have alienated stakeholders through their previous efforts within the community. The baseline survey demonstrated that most large health care facilities in most communities had some smoking control policies in place. However, the objective to have totally smoke-free hospitals, including their psychiatric and substance abuse wings, was ambitious. Success with enforcing this strict definition varied, but overall progress was made in strengthening the number and comprehensiveness of the policies. Some communities were more successful than others in this area. Factors that appear to have a positive impact on large health care facility changes were the influence of State health department initiatives, leadership provided by State or county medical and dental societies, interest of key influentials, and influence and momentum from the national media and professional journals.

At the end of the 4-year intervention, approximately 96 percent of medical offices and 88 percent of dental offices were totally smoke-free.

In the comparison communities, the rates were approximately 91 and 92 percent, respectively (Poland, 1993). The identification of leadership, staff support for the activities, and the climate created by the overall intervention may have been key factors in explaining the difference in physicians' offices. However, it appears that dentists' offices were not similarly influenced.

Goal 4.
Public Response

The baseline surveys for COMMIT indicated that smokers would welcome their physicians' or dentists' offer to help them stop smoking. Seventy-one percent of heavy smokers and 81 percent of light-to-moderate smokers said that they would try to stop if directed to do so by

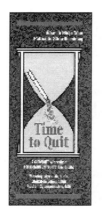

their physicians (Ockene et al., 1990-91). These data contradict what health professionals have expressed as a concern, that is, that their patients are not interested in talking about smoking cessation and may respond in a hostile manner to such overtures. It is important to correct this misconception. However, it is also important to state that some approaches by health care providers are more welcome than others. Poland's interviews (Ockene et al., in preparation) with patients in Brantford revealed diversity among patient responses. Some were immediately defensive when the topic was raised by their physicians; some indicated the need for more empathy from their physicians; and others simply wanted to be told to stop. There was a sense among many patients that physicians had little to offer them to help with smoking cessation. Health care providers need to know that there are standards of practice for cessation intervention developed through consensus that they can learn by attending an appropriate training event. At the same time, they must listen carefully to their patients to understand the individual nature of the help each patient will need.

To encourage patients to become aggressive consumers of stop-smoking advice, most communities sponsored Ask Your Doc campaigns, often in association with cessation events such as the GASO, Quit and Win contests, and making New Year's resolutions. COMMIT posters throughout the town and in health care provider offices and public service announcements on the radio encouraged the public to quit smoking and to ask their health care providers for help. One community purchased advertising space to announce which physicians and dentists were particularly interested in providing smoking cessation counseling. The aggressive marketing of the nicotine patch early in 1992 led many smokers to ask their physicians about the patch and smoking cessation, which was an excellent time for a community to set up an Ask Your Doc campaign as well as to offer additional training events.

Linkages to Other
Activities in the
Intervention

Many COMMIT activities were promoted through medical and dental offices, and this linkage made an important contribution to the comprehensive strategy. In general, office staff members were receptive to requests to distribute cessation resource guides and self-help material and to publicize the Smokers' Network and other magnet events such as Quit and Win contests. These activities did not increase their workload and in some cases provided tools that made their job easier.

Taking advantage of and coordinating with ongoing events in the community enhanced the effect of the physicians' and dentists' interventions. Not only could practitioners encourage patients to quit smoking, they could encourage them to use self-help materials distributed in association with a community Quit and Win contest and use the contest as an occasion to select a quit date. Indeed, one community conducted a competition among physicians' offices, with the prize a color television set for the winner's waiting room. The winning office enrolled 150 smokers in the Quit and Win contest.

In general, a good response can be expected from medical and dental office staff members if the focus is on enhancing what they already feel they need to do and making that easier for them. Organizers can expect a less enthusiastic response when a request involves any extra work or does not fit within the regular office routine. A key factor is how an office is set up to provide resources to patients. An office with mechanisms in place will be much more receptive than one that is disorganized with regard to this aspect of its work. Sometimes providing the rack on which materials can be distributed will persuade some offices to distribute antismoking materials to patients.

The Nicotine Patch— An Opportunity for Linkages The availability of the nicotine patch provided a focal point for linkages among several task forces and activities. Several communities, such as Utica, NY, built a campaign around the availability of the nicotine patch. For example, media attention given to the patch encouraged the public to ask questions of COMMIT offices and health care providers. This, in turn, provided an opportunity to distribute cessation resources and hold training events for health care providers. On the other hand, several communities were reluctant to become involved with the patch promotion, particularly if it meant affiliation with one pharmaceutical company rather than a more generic approach.

THE FUTURE— RECOMMENDATIONS The first and most important recommendation is to approach the health care provider community as a whole and develop a team approach to how they can best be part of a communitywide program. Allow the leadership to emerge from the group without preconceptions about the professional affiliation of the leadership. Physician and dentist trainings are valuable tools and are an important part of the approach, but they should be part of an overall strategy for all health care providers.

Remember that physicians and dentists are members of a community as well as health care professionals. Include them on working groups and task forces responsible for formulating local policy, whether the policy concerns smoke-free hospitals or a communitywide ordinance banning sales of cigarettes to underage youth. Physicians and dentists also are members of special societies that can play leadership roles in the formulation of policy and legislation. Call on the lung association, cancer society, or heart association local affiliates for guidance and tap the resources of the

State or local medical and dental societies. Local boards of health, health departments, and hospital associations also have an interest in promoting sound policy for the control of tobacco. Call on them. The more key people included in the development of the policy in the first place, the more support will be generated for the policy later.

Policies and practices in individual clinics can create a nonsmoking environment that can affect smokers. Creating no-smoking offices with no ashtrays, signs posted, literature available, and support for staff training is part of a comprehensive approach to tobacco control.

To promote changes in practices and policies in physicians' and dentists' offices requires applying everything known about helping people and communities change behavior. Just as smoking cessation is a process, integration of smoking intervention in an office is a long-term process. One strategy is almost never enough to bring about changes. Some professionals will need motivation; some will need information; others will be ready to act but need the skills to implement new procedures (Prochaska and DiClemente, 1983).

Creativity and good marketing strategies are essential. If physicians or dentists will not attend training programs, it is possible to use other means to reach them. Bring pizza for office staff members and show them a videotape during lunch hours on how to help smokers stop smoking, set up a wall rack with self-help quit-smoking material, present the physician or dentist with the "Heart Rx Kit" from the American Heart Association, and review the material on smoking cessation. Revisit the office, bringing more materials and supplies and using each visit as an occasion to encourage intervention on smoking. Involve the office in the GASO activities, Quit and Win contests, and other community events. The physician or dentist may never become as personally involved in the smoking issue as is wished, but small changes in procedures among many health professionals are important outcomes. People do not take action unless they feel that they should and that what they do will make a difference. In addition, practical issues that make the actions feasible also will determine whether change happens.

During the COMMIT intervention, the acceptance by the medical profession regarding smoking as a professional responsibility was different from that by the dental profession. Randomized controlled trials had demonstrated the efficacy of physicians' interventions, and the professional literature urged the medical profession to take action on the smoking issue. Lomas and colleagues (1991), in their studies of the implementation of consensus guidelines, concluded that it takes approximately 7 years for an accepted change in procedure to be integrated by the majority of physicians. Dentistry was many years behind medicine in recognizing the relationship between smoking and oral disease. The connection has been made stronger in the past 5 years with an increase in the number of published research articles and literature reviews as well as the establishment of new standards in dental education curricula. Although substantial action was taken at the national level to promote the role of the dental care team in smoking control, it appears that at the community level the profession was not yet ready to accept this responsibility.

Although the medical profession appeared ready to accept smoking control as part of regular practice, there were many factors that determined whether physicians learned how to implement it effectively and whether they put what they learned into practice. Attracting medical and dental care teams to the COMMIT training events was challenging in most of the COMMIT communities, and in some communities, it was almost impossible. Baseline surveys showed that physicians felt adequately prepared to help their patients stop smoking, yet they were not doing things known to be part of an effective approach (Lindsay et al., 1994). This lack of perceived need to know could have been a block to attending training. Physicians needed to know that there was more that they could do within the confines of their regular practices to help patients stop smoking. Those factors should be considered in promoting training to community health care providers.

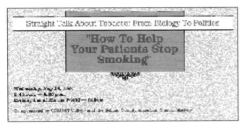

The CME literature shows that information exchange presented in a regular lecture format affects knowledge and attitudes but is rarely sufficient to bring about any change in procedures. More experiential learning strategies, such as discussion and practice with followup in the office and supplemented by techniques to cue or reinforce the procedure, are critical to integrating changes into practice (Davis et al., 1992). Basic training (less than 1 hour) was primarily a motivational tool to stimulate involvement. Seventy-five percent of physicians and eighty percent of dentists in many COMMIT communities received no training beyond the basic session. It is likely that almost no changes in procedures followed these training events. (Analysis and reporting of the postintervention survey is under way.) However, it is possible that basic training raised awareness and motivation sufficiently that physicians and dentists started to pay more attention to what resources were available and began to mention smoking more frequently to their patients. It is also possible that after attending *basic* training, many physicians and dentists perceived no need to attend *comprehensive* training.

The quality of the comprehensive training, which included demonstration and practice opportunities, varied across the communities. Some health care providers trained to lead these sessions were highly committed and good educators. Others had strengths as community leaders but, in some cases, were not strong advocates of the COMMIT activities that they were representing. It was often difficult for dedicated leaders to remain enthusiastic and strong proponents of comprehensive training when they had such difficulty in attracting their colleagues to sessions.

Cessation counseling can be a frustrating process when a 15-percent quit rate is considered success in primary care settings. It may be unrealistic to expect health care provider leaders in the community to remain dedicated to this issue when there are many competing issues. Although it made sense from a cost perspective to train local health care providers to lead the educational activities, the presentations may have been more effective when a local leader was teamed with a cessation expert brought in for the training event. However, this strategy also met with mixed success. It is possible that by the time a community offered a session with an expert, those who had an interest in smoking cessation felt that they had already given this issue sufficient time.

COMMIT staff members across the study attempted many format variations in marketing, timing, speakers, location, and incentives to attract medical and dental care teams to training. There appears to be no ideal format. Because it is so difficult to attract health professionals to training session that is longer than 1 1/2 hours, it may be better to divide the program into bite-size pieces with realistic goals in each session for making changes in health care providers' interactions with smokers. However, it may be unrealistic to think that health care providers will attend more than one session. Another approach, when time is short, is to ensure that the audience is homogeneous in terms of its learning needs and then focus the approach on those needs. For example, if the participants are not convinced that they should bother with smoking cessation in their practices, presenters can provide a motivational approach that will move them closer to action. If audience members are ready to learn what to do, they should be told clearly and convincingly what they can do. This type of approach requires strong and versatile educational leaders. Therefore, ongoing training and support for these leaders are important.

The integrated approach to practitioners' offices taken by the COMMIT protocol appears to have been successful. COMMIT staff members reported good results when physician or dentist training was followed by a visit to offices to reinforce the training, train office staff, and introduce other COMMIT activities. This approach was labor intensive, and those who consider adopting it will need to consider its costs and benefits.

It is important to consider the large systemic forces that direct change in professional practices. For the medical profession, procedures that are perceived to be required for competency and demands from patients are two of these important forces (Fox, 1989). Changes at the level of policy within the professions were occurring before and continued throughout the COMMIT intervention period. In the medical profession, these changes were under way early in the study; however, change occurred at a much later stage in the dental care profession. The pacing of changes in professional standards of practice was beyond the control of this intervention. On the other hand, it was possible to promote patient demand. The attention given to Ask Your Doc campaigns and the availability of the nicotine patch increased this demand. The analysis of the final survey of smokers will demonstrate the effect of these approaches.

CONCLUSIONS   Support is growing within both the medical and dental professions to make smoking cessation a part of competent practice. This support from the professions is critical, and as more health care professionals perceive endorsement and support of this work as a standard of competent practice, there should be an increased openness to opportunities to learn more about smoking cessation interventions.

Dental and dental hygiene schools are adding tobacco issues to their undergraduate curricula and continuing education programs. Recently revised curriculum guidelines for all professional schools have incorporated tobacco topics. In 1993, the American Association of Dental Schools established a Tobacco-Free Initiatives Special Interest Group so that educators could share experiences and accelerate the process of developing student knowledge, skills, and interest in tobacco intervention services. In addition, the importance of the dental profession is recognized in fulfilling the national health objectives for the 1990's; tobacco objective 3.16 (U.S. Department of Health and Human Services, 1991) states: "Increase to at least 75 percent the proportion of primary care and oral health care providers who routinely advise cessation and provide assistance and follow-up for all of their tobacco-using patients."

The medical profession has established smoking cessation as an issue clearly within the jurisdiction of primary care providers as well as of many specialists. Indicative of this support is the recent dedication of a full issue of the *Journal of the American Medical Association* (1994) to the subject of smoking. Surveys indicated that physicians and dentists now clearly perceive smoking as a problem they should address. However, they are not yet applying state-of-the-art interventions in their practices. COMMIT offered training to medical and dental care teams who did not perceive the need to attend training on smoking cessation or who felt that the many demands on their continuing education time prevented making smoking a high priority. It is likely that there will be an increasing readiness to attend training as these professionals see this issue as a part of a competent practice and as their patients increasingly ask them for help.

Through COMMIT, many things have been learned about how to approach the medical and dental professions. It is time now to expand this learning through work with all health professionals in communities. An integrated approach to planning and implementing a communitywide approach to smoking cessation will create congruence and synergy among providers that should help more patients stop smoking.

REFERENCES

Anda, R.F., Remington, P.L., Sienko, D.G., Davis, R.M. Are physicians advising smokers to quit? The patient's perspective. *Journal of the American Medical Association* 257(14): 1916-1919, 1987.

Centers for Disease Control and Prevention. Physician and other health-care professional counseling of smokers to quit—United States, 1991. *MMWR. Morbidity and Mortality Weekly Report* 42(44): 854-857, 1993.

Cohen, S., Stookey, G., Katz, B., Drook, C., Smith, D. Encouraging primary care physicians to help smokers quit. *Annals of Internal Medicine* 110: 648-652, 1989a.

Cohen, S.J., Christen, A.G., Katz, B.P., Drook, C.A., Davis, B.J., Smith, D.M., Stookey, G.K. Counseling medical and dental patients about cigarette smoking: The impact of nicotine gum and chart reminders. *American Journal of Public Health* 77: 313-316, 1987.

Cohen, S.J., Stookey, G.K., Katz, B.P., Drook, C.A., Christen, A.G. Helping smokers quit: A randomized controlled trial with private dentists. *Journal of the American Dental Association* 49(3): 147-152, 1989b.

COMMIT Research Group. Community Intervention Trial for Smoking Cessation (COMMIT): Summary of design and intervention. *Journal of the National Cancer Institute* 83(22): 1620-1628, 1991.

Cummings, S., Coates, T., Richard, R. Training physicians in counseling about smoking cessation: A randomized trial of the "Quit for Life" program. *Annals of Internal Medicine* 110: 640-647, 1989.

Davis, D.A., Thomson, M.A., Oxman, A.D., Haynes, B. Evidence for the effectiveness of CME: A review of 50 randomized controlled trials. *Journal of the American Medical Association* 268(9): 1111-1117, 1992.

Fox, R.D. (Editor). *Change and Learning in the Lives of Physicians.* New York: Praeger, 1989.

Gerbert, B., Coates, T., Zahnd, E., Richard, R.J., Cummings, S.R. Dentists as smoking cessation counselors. *Journal of the American Dental Association* 118(1): 29-32, 1989.

Gilbert, J.R., Wilson, D.M., Singer, J.S., Lindsay, E.A., Taylor, D.W., Willms, D., Best, J.A. A family physician smoking cessation program: An evaluation of the role of follow-up visits. *American Journal of Preventive Medicine* 8(2): 91-95, 1992.

Hayward, R.A., Meetz, H.K., Shapiro, M.F., Freeman, H.E. Utilization of dental services: 1986 patterns and trends. *Journal of Public Health Dentistry* 49(3): 147-152, 1989.

Janz, N.K., Becker, M.H., Kirscht, J.P., Eraker, S.A., Billi, J.E., Woolliscroft, J.O. Evaluation of a minimal-contact smoking cessation intervention in an outpatient setting. *American Journal of Public Health* 77: 849-851, 1987.

Jones, R.B., Pomrehn, P.R., Mecklenburg, R.E., Lindsay, E.A., Manley, M., Ockene, J.K. The COMMIT dental model: Tobacco control practices and attitudes. *Journal of the American Dental Association* 124(9): 92-104, 1993.

Journal of the American Medical Association 271(8): 569-636, 1994.

Kottke, T.E., Brekke, M.L., Solberg, L.I., Hughes, J.R. A randomized trial to increase smoking intervention by physicians. *Journal of the American Medical Association* 261(14): 2101-2106, 1989.

Lichtenstein, E., Wallack, L., Pechacek, T.F. Introduction to the Community Intervention Trial for Smoking Cessation (COMMIT). *International Quarterly of Community Health Education* 11(3): 173-185, 1990-91.

Lindsay, E.A., Ockene, J.K., Hymowitz, N., Giffen, C., Berger, L., Pomrehn, P. Physicians and smoking cessation: A survey of office procedures and practices in the Community Intervention Trial for Smoking Cessation. *Archives of Family Medicine* 3(4): 341-348, 1994.

Lomas, J., Enkin, M., Anderson, G.M., Hannah, W.J., Vayda, E., Singer, J. Opinion leaders versus audit and feedback to implement practice guidelines. *Journal of the American Medical Association* 265: 2202-2207, 1991.

Manley, M., Epps, R.P., Husten, C., Glynn, T., Shopland, D. Clinical interventions in tobacco control: A National Cancer Institute training program for physicians. *Journal of the American Medical Association* 266(22): 3172-3173, 1991.

Mecklenburg, R.E., Christen, A.G., Gerbert, B., Gift, H.C., Glynn, T.J., Jones, R.B., Lindsay, E., Manley, M.W., Severson, H. *How To Help Your Patients Stop Using Tobacco: A National Cancer Institute Manual for the Oral Health Team.* NIH Publication No. 93-3191. Rockville, MD: U.S. Department of Health and Human Services, Public Health Service, National Institutes of Health, 1993.

Ockene, J., Lindsay, E.A., Manley, M. Tobacco control activities of primary care physicians in the Community Intervention Trial for Smoking Cessation, in preparation.

Ockene, J.K. Physician-delivered intervention for smoking cessation: Strategies for increasing effectiveness. *Preventive Medicine* 16: 723-737, 1987.

Ockene, J.K., Aney, J., Goldberg, R.J., Klar, J.M., Williams, J.W. A survey of Massachusetts physicians' smoking practices. *American Journal of Preventive Medicine* 4: 14-20, 1988.

Ockene, J.K., Kristeller, J., Goldberg, R., Amick, T.L., Penelope, P.S., Hosmer, D., Quirk, M., Kalan, K. Increasing the efficacy of physician-delivered smoking intervention: A randomized clinical trial. *Journal of General Internal Medicine* 6: 1-8, 1991.

Ockene, J.K., Lindsay, E., Berger, L., Hymowitz, N. Health care providers as key change agents in the Community Intervention Trial for Smoking Cessation (COMMIT). *International Quarterly of Community Health Education* 11(3): 223-237, 1990-91.

Orlandi, M.A. Promoting health and preventing disease in health care settings: An analysis of barriers. *Preventive Medicine* 16: 119-130, 1987.

Orleans, C.T., George, L.K., Houpt, J.L., Brodie, K.H. Health promotion in primary care: A survey of U.S. family practitioners. *Preventive Medicine* 14: 636-647, 1985.

Poland, B. "Concept and Practice in Community Mobilization for Health: A Qualitative Evaluation of the Brantford COMMIT Smoking Cessation Intervention Trial." Unpublished doctoral disseration, McMaster University, 1993. 402 pp.

Prochaska, J.O., DiClemente, C.C. Stages and processes of self-change of smoking: Toward an integrative model of change. *Journal of Consulting and Clinical Psychology* 51(3): 390-395, 1983.

Russell, M.A., Wilson, C., Taylor, C., Baker, C.D. The effect of general practitioners' advice against smoking. *British Medical Journal* 2: 231-235, 1979.

Secker-Walker, R.H., Solomon, L.J., Hill, H.C. A statewide survey of dentists' smoking cessation advice. *Journal of the American Dental Association* 118(1): 37-40, 1989.

U.S. Department of Health and Human Services. *Reducing the Health Consequences of Smoking: 25 Years of Progress. A Report of the Surgeon General, 1989.* DHHS Publication No. (CDC) 89-8411. Rockville, MD: U.S. Department of Health and Human Services, Public Health Service, Centers for Disease Control, Center for Chronic Disease Prevention and Health Promotion, Office on Smoking and Health, 1989.

U.S. Department of Health and Human Services. *Seventh Report to the President and Congress on the Status of Health Personnel in the United States.* DHHS Publication No. HRS-P-OD-90-1. Washington, DC: Supt. of Docs., U.S. Govt. Print. Off., 1990.

U.S. Department of Health and Human Services. *Healthy People 2000: National Health Promotion and Disease Prevention Objectives.* DHHS Publication No. (PHS) 91-50212. Washington, DC: Supt. of Docs., U.S. Govt. Print. Off., 1991, p. 153.

Wilson, D.M., Taylor, D.W., Gilbert, J.R., Best, J.A., Lindsay, E.A., Willms, D.G., Singer, J. A randomized trial of a family physician intervention for smoking cessation. *Journal of the American Medical Association* 260(11): 1570-1574, 1988.

AUTHORS

Elizabeth A. Lindsay, Ph.D.
Associate Professor
Community Health Research Unit
Department of Epidemiology and
    Community Medicine
University of Ottawa
Ottawa, Ontario K1H 8M5
CANADA

Norman Hymowitz, Ph.D.
Professor of Clinical Psychiatry
Department of Psychiatry and Mental
    Health Services
University of Medicine and Dentistry of
    New Jersey Medical School
Newark, NJ 07103

Robert E. Mecklenburg, D.D.S., M.P.H.
Oral Health Coordinator
R.O.W. Sciences, Inc.
Suite 400
1700 Research Boulevard
Rockville, MD 20850-3142

Linda C. Churchill, M.S.
Project Director
Department of Preventive and Behavioral
  Medicine
University of Massachusetts Medical School
Room S-7, 746
55 Lake Avenue North
Worcester, MA 01655

Blake Poland, Ph.D.
Scientist
Social Evaluation and Research Department
Addiction Research Foundation
33 Russell Street
Toronto, Ontario M5S 2S1
CANADA

Promoting Community Tobacco Control Through Worksites

Linda Nettekoven, Russell E. Glasgow, Robert H. Shipley, A.J. Roy Cameron, Lesa T. Dalton, Aleena Erickson, Sharon Ann Rankins-Burd, Sandy Tosti, Glorian Sorensen, and Kitty K. Corbett

INTRODUCTION   As the move toward health care reform focuses increasing attention on health promotion and disease prevention, the worksite becomes an increasingly attractive setting from which to influence health behaviors, such as tobacco use. Project designers identified worksites as one of four major "channels" for promoting smoking cessation within the Community Intervention Trial for Smoking Cessation (COMMIT). Because 70 percent of adults between ages 18 and 65 are employed (U.S. Bureau of the Census, 1986), worksites can provide access to many community residents who may not be reached through other means, including low-income and minority groups (Nathan, 1984; Shipley et al., 1988; Terborg and Glasgow, in press). Interest in worksite health promotion continues to increase; national surveys of a random sample of private sector worksites with 50 or more employees indicated that 65.5 percent of worksites surveyed offered at least one type of health promotion activity (Fielding and Piserchia, 1989), and by 1992 this figure had increased to 81 percent (U.S. Public Health Service, 1993).

Worksite health promotion often is viewed as a way to reduce company and employee health care expenditures through the provision of convenient, free or low-cost prevention and early detection interventions. Proponents also credit worksite health promotion efforts with improving labor-management relations, increasing employee productivity, decreasing absenteeism resulting from illness and injury, and reducing employee turnover and insurance costs (Glasgow et al., 1990; Sorensen et al., 1990).

Previous research suggests that worksites can offer special opportunities for the promotion and support of smoking cessation efforts, using both policies and programs. Multiple types of intervention can be offered repeatedly over time in worksites. By such continual contact, smokers at varying stages in the process of change, including those not yet contemplating change as well as those trying to quit, may be motivated to quit and to sustain cessation (Abrams et al., 1994; Rossi et al., 1988). This contact may include the promotion of communitywide cessation events or activities sponsored by other agencies.

Changes in worksite norms and in the social environment, such as those that may be fostered by no-smoking policies, can provide critical support for cessation and its maintenance (Sorensen et al., 1986). The percentage of companies with restrictive smoking policies has increased steadily in recent years. Whereas 27 percent of private worksites with

50 or more employees had policies that either banned or severely restricted smoking in 1985, 59 percent had such policies by 1992 (U.S. Public Health Service, 1993).

Those conducting reviews of the worksite health promotion literature (Fielding, 1984; Terborg and Glasgow, in press), including a meta-analysis of worksite smoking cessation studies, generally have concluded that worksite smoking cessation programs have been efficacious (Fisher et al., 1990) and cost-effective (Warner et al., 1988). However, a recent literature review concludes that positive effects are not always found in more highly controlled studies and that outcomes often vary across worksites (Jeffrey et al., 1993; Terborg and Glasgow, in press).

This chapter reviews the experiences of the 11 COMMIT intervention communities in implementing worksite-based activities and describes the following aspects of the workplace intervention effort: (1) goals for worksites and the assessment methods used to measure progress in this channel; (2) methods for planning worksite interventions; (3) intervention activities delivered to worksites throughout the trial, along with examples of the successes and challenges that accompanied the implementation process; (4) means used to deliver the intervention, including tailoring protocol activities to fit the cultures of the diverse localities and the role of staff, volunteers, and community structures; and (5) lessons learned from activities that seemed to work and those that did not, along with suggestions for approaches that might prove effective in other community settings. A more detailed description of the evaluation methods and results of the COMMIT worksite intervention can be found elsewhere (Sorensen et al., 1990-91; Glasgow et al., submitted for publication).

GOALS, ACTIVITIES, AND PROCESS OBJECTIVES

The COMMIT worksite intervention was designed to support smoking cessation by changing social norms both in individual worksites and in the overall business community. The emphasis was on reaching many community residents through repeated interventions that together would affect social norms as well as change individual behavior. Thus, the COMMIT worksite plan was guided by four intervention goals.

1. increase smoking cessation among workers who smoke;

2. produce changes in worksite norms to support no-smoking;

3. increase adoption and effective implementation of comprehensive worksite nonsmoking policies; and

4. enhance support for no-smoking in the business and labor sectors of the community.

The effectiveness of intervention efforts was measured by the extent to which specified impact objectives were achieved. The impact objectives related to the goals listed above for the worksite plan are presented in Table 1.

Achievement of these objectives was assessed through surveys of randomly selected community residents—the evaluation cohort (described

Table 1
Impact objectives, by 1993

1. Seventy percent of employed smokers will report that their worksites ban smoking completely or restrict smoking to designated areas.
2. Fifty percent of heavy smokers will report feeling pressure from coworkers to quit smoking.
3. Eight percent of heavy smokers will report having participated in stop-smoking programs or contests/lotteries to promote cessation at their workplace.
4. Seventy percent of targeted worksites will report offering, within the past 12 months, lectures, classes, materials, or other programs to help or encourage employees to quit smoking.

Source: Sorensen et al., 1990-91.

in Chapter 3)—and worksite respondents. In each community, measurement (intervention and comparison) at the worksite level was assessed with a survey of 30 worksites (or a census, whichever measurement number was smaller) in each of three size strata (50 to 99, 100 to 249, and 250 or more employees). Worksite respondents were asked about the level of company participation in several different types of smoking control activities as well as worksite characteristics potentially associated with different smoking control activities. These assessment procedures, described in more detail by Mattson and coworkers (1990-91) and Glasgow and colleagues (1992), are modeled after those used in previous national surveys of worksites (Fielding, 1991; U.S. Public Health Service, 1993).

To assist COMMIT project staff members and community volunteers in delivering a comparable intervention across all 11 communities, an intervention protocol was developed by the COMMIT Steering Committee. Additional information on the COMMIT protocol is contained in Chapter 4. For each of the nine mandatory worksite intervention activities listed in Table 2 and discussed later in this chapter, the protocol established standard process objectives and timelines to be met by all intervention communities when conducting that activity.

The process objectives established the minimum level of activities to be conducted annually in each intervention community. Compliance with these objectives was monitored by Program Records, a computerized database recordkeeping system (Corbett et al., 1990-91).

Table 2
Worksite activities and process objectives

Activities for Each Community	Cumulative Objectives (1988-1992)	Number Completed	Process Objectives Achieved (%)
Presentation to Business Groups	88 presentations	88 presentations	100
Annual Workshop for Worksites:	44 workshops	47 workshops	107
Large worksites	30%		133
Small worksites	20%		105
Compile Resource List for Smoke-Free Worksites	All communities	11 guides	92
Distribute Resource List to Worksites Annually	90%		92
Policy Consultations to:			
Large worksites	20%		145
Small worksites	165 sites	150 sites	91
Promotional Activities to:			
Large worksites	70%		140
Small worksites	50%		180
Distribute Incentive Guidebooks to:			
Large worksites	80%		118
Small worksites	50%		194
Three Between-Worksite Competitions	33 competitions	33 competitions	100
Distribute Self-Help Cessation Materials to:			
Large worksites	50%		180
Small worksites	20%		450
Promote Smokers' Network in:			
Large worksites	85%		113
Small worksites	20%		460

[a] *Average for combined communities.*

PLANNING WORKSITE INTERVENTIONS
To become familiar with the needs, resources, and organizational structures present in both the intervention and comparison communities, project staff members conducted an extensive community analysis in all COMMIT communities (see Chapter 5). Using nonreactive approaches, qualitative and quantitative sources, and discussion with key informants, staff members gathered information to help them begin to understand the two types of communities.

For the worksite channel, this community analysis served several functions. The analysis identified key community players and major employers, including business leaders, union representatives, and providers of smoking cessation programs (commercial as well as nonprofit). Many of these people were eventually invited to serve on the community Board or the Worksites and Organizations Task Force. To aid in program planning, information was compiled on community smoking policies and cessation resources available to worksites, and gaps in these services were identified. An attempt also was made to identify "early adopter" worksites that already had implemented exemplary policies or programs so that they could serve as role models for other workplaces.

The community analysis drew on a variety of archival information sources. These included lists of worksites and their characteristics (e.g., size, type of industry) from the chamber of commerce, State business census, or local business license records; newspapers and other public documents reviewing community and business concerns; and annual reports from local businesses and business organizations. Interviews with community representatives provided a more indepth picture, including information on the business and labor community's culture and history. For example, the following questions were asked.

- Do worksites have a history of promoting smoking cessation or other healthy behaviors?

- How extensively have the media covered worksite health concerns?

- Which health issues are of highest priority to the business and labor communities?

- What other community issues are of great concern to employers and workers?

- Are there regular meetings, networks, or other community structures that bring together representatives of various worksites?

In this way the community analysis identified potential barriers and opportunities, highlighted issues likely to compete with tobacco control as a priority for this sector of the community, and provided an assessment of the capability and readiness of local worksites to address the tobacco issue. The report also suggested ways to begin tailoring the intervention protocol to fit the unique configuration of needs and resources within each intervention community.

In Yonkers, NY, for example, the analysis report accurately anticipated that the many small worksites would require special strategies for implementing the large-scale protocol activities, such as the annual smoking policy workshops, between-worksite competitions, and recruitment for magnet events. However, several COMMIT sites reported that the community analysis was not totally reliable in identifying the business community's key players. In some communities the analysis overestimated the activity level of one or more of the voluntary health agencies; in Medford/Ashland, OR, the status (funding levels and staffing) of the voluntary agencies changed so rapidly that this portion of the report had to be updated before the Community Planning Group could begin its work. Some of these gaps and inconsistencies were immediately apparent to community volunteers who joined the project, and modifications were made; others emerged much later as activities were being planned and implemented.

INTERVENTION ACTIVITIES AND THEIR IMPLEMENTATION Worksites were viewed as a key natural channel for reaching less motivated or less educated smokers who might not volunteer for or be reached by other project activities. The worksite intervention offered a comprehensive, coordinated set of tobacco control activities designed to build on each other over time and to support the momentum being created in other sectors of the community. Worksite activities were based on a three-faceted approach: promotion of restrictive smoking policies, use of motivational and incentive techniques to encourage participation and cessation, and provision and promotion of smoking cessation and maintenance resources. A description of the activities and examples that illustrate the experiences of communities in implementing each activity are given below.

Decisions about which worksites to target in a communitywide initiative like COMMIT are often influenced by two considerations: (1) how to achieve the maximum intervention effect (in this case, impact on tobacco use) and (2) how to make the best use of the limited staff time and other project resources that are available for this purpose. After weighing these concerns, project designers came to view larger worksites as a more efficient setting for the delivery of worksite intervention activities. Worksites were categorized according to size, and the protocol defined which worksites would be targeted in each community. Large targeted worksites were defined as those employing 100 or more persons, and initially, small targeted worksites included only those that employed 50 to 99 persons. These categories included all worksites in which at least 30 percent of the work force lived within the boundaries of the intervention community. In some communities this meant that additional worksites located in proximity to, but outside of, intervention community boundaries were also targeted for intervention. However, this emphasis changed somewhat during the second half of the intervention.

The initial COMMIT evaluation cohort survey indicated that 60 percent of smokers were employed in workplaces with fewer than 100 employees; 37.6 percent of smokers in the intervention communities worked in settings with fewer than 25 employees, and another 22.4 percent were employed in companies with between 25 and 99 workers (Glasgow et al., 1992). After the first 2 years of the intervention, the protocol was modified, and COMMIT sites were encouraged to expand their efforts to include smaller worksites (those employing 25 to 49 people) in some workplace intervention activities.

Promotion of Worksite Smoking Policies Adopting policies to restrict or ban smoking was the type of smoking control activity undertaken at worksites according to recent national studies (Fielding and Piserchia, 1989; U.S. Public Health Service, 1993). In addition, some workplaces removed cigarette vending machines from their premises.

Smoking control policies are important for several reasons. First, their primary purpose is to protect employees from exposure to environmental tobacco smoke (ETS). Second, they serve an educational function, sending messages to smokers about the seriousness of the health risks involved in smoking and the impact their smoking may have on others. Third, restrictive policies create a no-smoking environment that may stimulate quit attempts and increase opportunities for long-term cessation by reducing exposure to smoking situations.

Some recent studies have reported an increase in smoking cessation following a worksite's adoption of a restrictive smoking policy (Emont and Cummings, 1990; Millar, 1988; Sorensen et al., 1989; Stave and Jackson, 1991), although others have found no effect on cessation but have reported a decrease in the number of cigarettes smoked at work (Biener et al., 1989; Borland et al., 1990; Petersen et al., 1988; Rosenstock et al., 1986). Adopting a restrictive smoking policy also may stimulate interest in smoking cessation classes (Martin, 1988; Sorensen et al., 1989; U.S. Department of Health and Human Services, 1986) and may support norms that promote cessation and the maintenance of a smoke-free lifestyle (Sorensen and Pechacek, 1989).

Within the COMMIT worksite effort, four intervention activities promoted the adoption of restrictive smoking policies: (1) smoking policy presentations; (2) annual smoking policy workshops; (3) onsite smoking policy consultations; and (4) development of a Worksite Smoking Policy Network Guide. When writing their final reports, all intervention communities pointed to an increase in the number of worksites and restaurants with restrictive smoking policies as one of their major successes. However, many intervention sites also reported some difficulty in achieving one or more of the following smoking policy objectives.

Smoking Policy Presentations

To begin to raise awareness of smoking policy issues within the business community, staff members and volunteers made presentations on health of at least 15 minutes to worksite groups, such as chambers of commerce or other business groups, during their regular meetings. Presentations focused on effects of ETS, health and legal issues pertaining to smoking policies, national and local trends, and policy and program options. During the first intervention year, a minimum of one presentation was given in each COMMIT community; in subsequent years, at least two presentations were made annually.

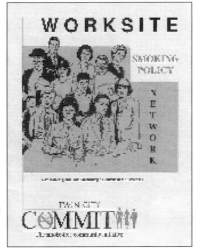

The underlying strategy was for COMMIT to join with the groups that the project hoped to reach and to become part of the agenda in their usual settings before attempting to involve them in COMMIT activities. The interest of local business groups in tobacco control information varied over time across COMMIT sites. Nearly two-thirds of COMMIT intervention communities (64 percent) met the process objective for this activity, but some reported difficulty in involving business groups in worksite efforts. Many local COMMIT organizations became card-carrying members of one or more of these business groups during the course of the project. Some communities, Paterson, NJ, for example, enjoyed a highly supportive relationship with the local chamber of commerce. At least one of Paterson's annual awards dinners to honor COMMIT project volunteers was held in conjunction with a chamber meeting.

Finding an active member who was also concerned about the tobacco issue seemed central to success in this area. Despite resistance from a key chamber officer, Fitchburg/Leominster was able to develop strong ties with its chamber group by building a strong relationship with an active member who had recently lost a relative to lung cancer and became a COMMIT volunteer. On the other hand, without a key contact, Medford/Ashland struggled for 4 years to arrange for space on a chamber meeting agenda, despite being a chamber member in good standing from the beginning of the project. Because staff members could not arrange to give a presentation to the full chamber membership until near the end of the intervention, they chose an alternative strategy of becoming active in the early morning "Chamber Greeters' Group," which allowed them to informally publicize project activities to those members who attended these drop-in, get-acquainted sessions.

Annual Smoking   Annual smoking policy workshops were conducted in each
Policy Workshops   intervention community. Workshop agendas included information on smoking as a public health issue, ETS, laws and regulations, and policy options and recommended procedures for implementing new policies. Smoking policy workshop guides, one each for large and small worksites, were developed for COMMIT to assist project staff members and community representatives in planning workshops (Institute for the Study of Smoking Behavior and Policy, 1989a and 1989b). These guides and COMMIT promotional efforts emphasized the advantages of smoke-free facilities over segregated smoking arrangements that do not completely eliminate exposure to ETS.

COMMIT communities adopted different strategies in presenting the annual workshop, which was to run 2 to 3 hours. For example, some communities elected to offer a workshop in conjunction with another worksite issue, such as alcohol and drug education. Others targeted one of their annual workshops toward unions or small businesses. In many COMMIT sites, the workshops were cosponsored by local chapters of the American Lung Association, American Cancer Society, or local chamber of commerce. Brantford, Ontario, Canada, capitalized on the business community's interest in "sick building syndrome" by sponsoring a workshop on that topic. It became evident to participants that the major source of pollution in buildings where smoking occurred was ETS. This served to educate those attending about the health risks of ETS and the need for restrictive smoking policies.

There was general agreement among staff members that the workshops were well designed and beneficial for those attending. Although most communities were successful in reaching the required number of targeted worksites, worksite smoking policy workshops received mixed reviews from staff and volunteers: Some found them to be well attended and well received; others described them as costly in terms of staff effort and project dollars, with a low response rate from the community. The investment of significant project resources to bring in outside experts did not necessarily lead to increased attendance. During the early phases of the intervention, only a few COMMIT sites exceeded their participation target levels. However, a few sites canceled workshops because of low registration despite extensive publicity and preparation.

Smoking policy workshop attendance appeared to be linked to three factors: (1) environmental or external support for policy change, (2) number of larger worksites in the community available to attend such presentations,

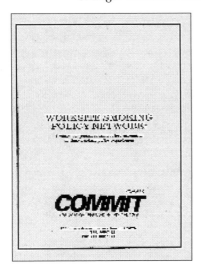

and (3) promotional strategies used. Foremost was the influence of external events within the larger environment, such as the passage or consideration of clean indoor air legislation at the State or local level. The enactment of the New York State Clean Indoor Air Act in January 1990 provides an example of the impact of external events. After workplace smoking policies were mandated by law, Utica and Yonkers, NY, found their worksites to be much more interested in assistance in formulating policy and more receptive to cessation resource materials from COMMIT and voluntary health agencies. Yonkers reported that its policy workshops "created additional visibility, allowed COMMIT to attract media attention, receive free publicity, and reach large numbers of worksites (53 percent during the 4 years of the trial) all at the same time." Utica had similar success, reaching 44 percent of large and 17 percent of small worksites.

One external event on which COMMIT sites had planned to capitalize from the outset of the project was the release of the Environmental Protection Agency's (EPA) report labeling ETS as a Class A carcinogen.[1] After repeated delays, the report was finally released in January 1993 (U.S. Environmental Protection Agency, 1992), 1 month after the COMMIT

---

[1] A Class A carcinogen designation is used "when there is sufficient evidence from epidemiologic studies to support a causal association between exposure to the agents and cancer" (U.S. Environmental Protection Agency, 1986).

intervention ended. One COMMIT site managed to exploit the situation despite the delays. By highlighting the controversy surrounding the draft report's key findings, staff members and volunteers from Cedar Rapids/ Marion, IA, were able to generate additional interest in worksite policies during the final year of the project.

A second factor was the size of the COMMIT community and the number of worksites potentially available to attend policy workshops. For example, Cedar Rapids/Marion, one of the largest intervention communities and one with a large number of worksites, attracted 45 participants to its first smoking policy workshop. Three television stations, four radio stations, and a newspaper provided coverage of the event. Some of the smaller COMMIT communities (with few worksites of more than 100 employees) reported difficulty generating sufficient interest in policy workshops, especially on an annual basis. As the project continued, more worksites already had policies in place, had attended an earlier workshop, or were not willing to devote a half day of company time to a workshop devoted exclusively to smoking policy.

A third factor, the type of promotional strategies used, proved critical to workshop success, regardless of community size and number of large employers present. With workshops required on an annual basis, program planners worked hard to avoid offering what might appear to be repetitious events. They attempted to capitalize on new or timely angles for their policy workshops and varied their promotion strategies to attract new attendees as well as repeat participants. For example, in Raleigh, NC, workshops in 1989 and 1990 focused on health and safety (e.g., "Avenues to a Safe and Healthy Workplace: Exploring Worksite Policy Options"). Later workshops emphasized the costs to business owners of workplace smoking (e.g., "Is Smoking Affecting Your Bottom Line?") and included information on fine-tuning existing policies.

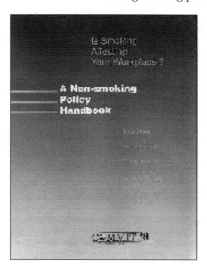

Even those communities experiencing lower than anticipated turnouts reported participant satisfaction with the content and format of their workshops. Medford/Ashland, one of the smaller communities, used a format that included presentations from multiple speakers followed by a panel discussion involving representatives from local worksites that had implemented policies. Panel members then joined participants for lunch, which provided further opportunities to interact informally and share information. In Raleigh, the largest site, COMMIT staff members developed a similar format based on feedback from workshop participants.

Many project personnel recognized the importance of reaching out to smaller worksites, and COMMIT developed a policy workbook geared to their concerns (Institute for the Study of Smoking Behavior and Policy, 1989b). However, several COMMIT sites noted additional needs in such settings in terms of both policy and cessation activities. Many smaller worksites felt they could not afford the time away from work necessary to send employees to attend a worksite policy workshop or felt such policies were not relevant to their settings. Consultations, written materials, or small-group sessions may be more effective ways to reach some small worksites.

Onsite Smoking Policy Consultations COMMIT staff members and volunteers in each intervention community also provided worksites with onsite smoking policy consultations in which information and materials were provided to assist worksites in adopting and implementing smoking policies. Building on external events was seen as critical to ensuring the success of these free policy consultations. In addition to the demand for consultations generated by new State legislation mandating policies (e.g., New York State), COMMIT staff members also found that companies tended to be more receptive to consultations when they were opening a new facility, remodeling, overhauling general company policies, or adjusting health benefits or when the media focused substantial attention on rising health care costs.

Worksite smoking control policies, long seen as a potential source of conflict between management and labor, sometimes improved relations between the two sectors when consultations were handled sensitively and were tailored to the needs of the specific setting. One consultation at a local grocery store was so successful in this respect that a group of employees who smoked sent flowers to Cedar Rapids/Marion's worksite specialist to acknowledge her care in representing their concerns while negotiating their new smoking policy. Another success involved a unionized company in Bellingham, WA; however, in other instances, the stance of union officials hindered efforts to develop a smoking policy. Even the expectation of union resistance was enough to cause some worksites to defer action.

In some cases, the needed policy information was provided in a single meeting, whereas for other worksites, multiple meetings were necessary. For small targeted worksites, small-group consultations with representatives from two or three worksites were sometimes conducted. Some communities relied on project staff members to conduct consultations; others subcontracted this activity to a local agency with expertise in this area. Some also provided special training for community representatives in the hope that they might be encouraged to continue consultations after the project ended.

The experience of the Vallejo, CA, site with worksite consultations is especially interesting because the project used two subcontractors, and each used a different approach in delivering onsite consultations (California COMMIT staff, 1992). Both approaches were effective in meeting the process objectives for this activity. The first subcontractor viewed a policy consultation as an opportunity to accomplish multiple project objectives during a single visit by offering an array of tobacco control information and resources to the "client." During a 1-hour visit, the consultant attempted to accomplish several of the following process objectives: (1) present information and advice about how to design and implement a no-smoking policy, (2) discuss how to set up onsite cessation classes and describe other community cessation resources, (3) distribute tobacco cessation self-help materials and cessation resource guides, (4) explain the Smokers' Network and deliver registration materials, (5) outline the value and strategies for utilizing incentives for employees trying to quit, (6) generate interest in participating in a stop-smoking competition with another worksite, and (7) deliver promotional materials for any communitywide cessation events that may be planned for the near future.

The second subcontractor's approach was to make "cold calls" by knocking on doors of businesses all day if necessary. For this subcontractor, the focus of the visit was to convince the client of the need for a restrictive smoking policy using whatever motivational strategies might be appropriate in that workplace. The multipurpose mindset used by the first subcontractor was assumed not to be optimal for the customer. Business representatives might be overwhelmed with too much information on cessation and be unable to concentrate on policy. Using this strategy, a 1-hour block of time for a policy consultation (as required by the protocol) was often too long; many employers were not willing to allocate that much time for an initial visit. A series of 15- to 20-minute visits discussing overall policy issues and strategies with a busy worksite contact, while using followup telephone calls to deal with specifics, also proved to be an effective way to advance worksite smoking policy efforts.

Regardless of which approach a consultant used initially, the process of developing and implementing a worksite smoking policy often required ongoing support from COMMIT personnel. For example, in Bellingham, staff members worked with a hospital for 2 years, carefully prompting without pushing, amid personnel turnovers and competing issues until the institution finally became smoke-free.

Development of Worksite Smoking Policy Network Guide   Each intervention community developed a Worksite Smoking Policy Network Guide, which was updated annually, and attempted to promote the use of existing smoking policy resources within the community. The guide identified local worksites with different types of smoking control policies and a contact person who was willing to serve as a "peer counselor" and confer with people from other companies about the worksite's experiences in developing and implementing its policy. The network was designed to facilitate the diffusion of smoking control innovations by identifying early adopters—individuals and companies that had been successful in implementing a smoking ban or restrictions. A few communities were able to identify a wide cross-section of businesses; others either had trouble identifying places with strong policies or, as in the case of

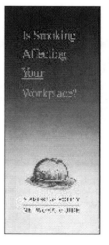

Raleigh, located in the heart of tobacco country, encountered some reluctance among worksites about receiving such publicity because of concern for repercussions from the tobacco industry. The number of companies on the first Worksite Smoking Policy Network Guide lists ranged from 6 (Yonkers and Vallejo) to approximately 30 (Bellingham). By the end of the intervention these numbers had increased greatly across all communities. For example, Brantford, which began with 23 businesses (24 percent of targeted worksites), reported that 97 (98 percent) targeted worksites were part of the network at the end of the project.

Although the basic list of worksites with policies was similar, the amount and format of additional information (rationale for policies, implementation guidelines, sample policies, cessation resources, case studies) contained in the network guide varied. Early versions of the guide often involved multiple pages of information contained in a folder or small notebook. By the end of the project, some sites sensed that the network guides were not being widely used and resorted to a trifold pamphlet format, which was less cumbersome and seemed more readable. Staff members and subcontractors frequently used the guide when doing consultations as a way to point to local policy exemplars. In addition, a list of local worksites with policies already in place seemed to encourage other worksites to take action. However, several COMMIT community final reports indicated the guides had failed to generate the projected level of independent networking among businesses, and the process of updating the guides on an annual basis involved a significant amount of time for an already busy staff.

Motivational and Incentive Activities To Encourage Smoking Cessation This category includes three major types of activities: (1) promotional activities, (2) incentive programs, and (3) between-worksite competitions. These activities were designed to encourage employees to initiate smoking cessation attempts, maintain recent changes in smoking behavior, and provide increased support to coworkers for cessation attempts. Promotional activities served to increase participation in worksite-based or communitywide cessation events. Incentive programs required little professional time to administer, could be used to encourage participation in educational or skills-training activities, and may address issues of long-term behavior change and maintenance (Sorensen et al., 1990). Incentives also can encourage those not yet ready to quit smoking to consider doing so (Winett et al., 1989) and may help those who have already quit not to start again (Mattson et al., 1993). Use of various types of incentives have been reported, including the use of guaranteed incentives to reinforce workers' attempts to quit for a specified period (Jeffrey et al., 1988; Shepard and Pearlman, 1985), contests or lottery drawings within a given worksite (Emont and Cummings, 1990), and competitions between organizations (Brownell and Felix, 1987; Klesges et al., 1986). Three worksite intervention activities involved the use of motivational and incentive activities: (1) promotion activities in the worksite accompanying magnet events; (2) promotional of worksite stop-smoking incentives; and (3) between-worksite challenges and competitions.

Promotional Activities in the Worksite Accompanying Magnet Events

Promotional activities were conducted in targeted worksites to foster participation in communitywide magnet events, such as "Quit and Win" contests, the GASO, Non-Dependence Day, and other events designed to encourage cessation attempts and attract attention to the smoking issue. COMMIT sites reported success in promoting these events in worksites through display of materials, registration at the worksite, or other activities, such as expired carbon monoxide testing. Worksite promotions were designed to enhance the impact of community-wide events by integrating activities across channels and by increasing the likelihood of multiple exposures to a given event. Process objectives defined a cumulative increase over time in the number of worksites to be personally contacted about these events. Several sites relied on worksite task force members and other volunteers to assist with the delivery of promotional materials to identified worksite contacts. For example, Medford/Ashland's task force members agreed to "adopt" specific worksites; each member took responsibility for developing contacts and delivering materials to a given number of community workplaces.

Promotion of Worksite Stop-Smoking Incentives

Because the use of stop-smoking incentives was expected to be a new strategy for many worksites, the COMMIT project developed a workbook to explain this approach. The COMMIT Incentives Programs Workbook (Glasgow and McRae, 1989) was distributed in person to worksites to provide information about how to use incentives in the workplace to encourage smoking cessation and maintenance activities. It included guidelines on selecting awards, setting contest rules, and promoting and evaluating an incentive program and contained an overall timeline and several activity planning worksheets to facilitate implementation. Consultation on implementing the plans was provided on request. Many communities reported that employers viewed support for cessation as an extracurricular activity, not as a priority item. These attitudes made it difficult, especially during the hard economic times many communities were experiencing, to persuade employers to devote resources, or even experiment with incentives, to encourage cessation among their employees. The workbook also provided information on between-worksite challenges and competitions, which intervention sites were expected to conduct each year.

Between-Worksite Competitions

Between-worksite competitions proved more challenging to implement than expected in many COMMIT communities, despite plentiful resource materials. Such contests often generated excellent media coverage for worksite tobacco issues as well as the COMMIT project. Competitions were easiest to arrange and implement when staff members were able to identify a committed "champion" within each company. Such a person was able to generate real enthusiasm from within that helped foster participation and support from others in the worksite. For example, the COMMIT project in Brantford enlisted senior executives from the two local hospitals, who were already friends, to arrange a highly successful between-worksites competition. In Bellingham the co-owner of an auto parts business arranged a competition among the divisions of her company and offered to cook a gourmet dinner in her home for the winners and their spouses.

The amount of staff member and volunteer effort devoted to the competition did not seem to correlate directly with the level of smoker participation, as examples from Vallejo and Medford/Ashland illustrate. In Vallejo volunteers and staff members carried out a successful worksite challenge among five local auto dealerships (involving 40 participating smokers) in June 1990. A young project subcontractor working closely with COMMIT staff and task force volunteers arranged for auto mechanics and salespersons to launch a successful competition. Careful communication with all constituencies involved was critical to the success of the event and helped sensitize the subcontractor to the barriers and limitations facing dealerships and their employees. Face-to-face meetings with dealership owners or managers provided information about what motivated them to support and encourage participation by their employees. Meetings with employees who smoked helped determine what incentives would motivate them to quit. During the competition, labor-intensive, one-to-one check-ins with competing participants helped to sustain motivation. Participants later reported that the support provided by these personal contacts "made the difference in their ability to remain smoke-free." Sharing the results of the competition with the rest of the community had a positive, ripple effect. The media coverage was a "win-win" situation: Auto dealerships received positive publicity (a key incentive for their participation) and successful participants received public recognition. People who had never heard of COMMIT heard about the worksite challenge, which enabled COMMIT staff members and volunteers to take further pride in their projects and increased local awareness of the tobacco issue.

Medford/Ashland also carried out a competition involving auto dealerships. The effort here also generated extensive publicity and was well executed and labor intensive. However, weeks of work resulted in only a few participants; only 13 smokers entered from across the 6 participating dealerships. Seven of the eight people successful in quitting for the 1-month contest also completed a special Freedom From Smoking clinic, a program of the American Lung Association, held in conjunction with the competition.

Fitchburg/Leominster used a competition among fire stations to enhance participation in a Quit and Win contest. Project staff members made regular visits, sometimes at rather strange hours, to recruit and later provide support and encouragement to participating firefighters. Besides increasing participation in the Quit and Win contest, the event helped encourage firefighters to begin talking more constructively about smoking restrictions in the fire stations where they lived and worked.

However, despite these successes, most COMMIT final reports indicate that staff members viewed these competitions as among the most difficult to accomplish and least efficacious worksite activities. The large amount of staff and volunteer effort involved often did not seem justified by the few smokers who participated. For example, a report from Yonkers summarizes the frustrations common to many COMMIT communities:

Each year our task force brainstormed new ways to recruit worksites to engage in competitions. Many companies were approached through key contacts within each workplace, but most declined for a variety of reasons such as time restrictions, poor economic climate, or not enough smokers in the company. One worksite actually worked with COMMIT for several months to plan a competition, met extensively with project staff and the task force chair, set up a planning committee, and asked COMMIT to purchase pro-health buttons with the company's name on them. At the last minute the company canceled the competition citing economic constraints.

Promotion of Self-Help Materials and Cessation Services

Activities and materials teaching the skills needed to quit smoking were generally available in most communities prior to COMMIT's arrival on the scene. Therefore, the project sought to enhance the reach and effectiveness of these existing community resources through two activities designed to bring them into the workplace: (1) distribution of self-help materials and (2) promotion of a Smokers' Network.

Distribution of Self-Help Materials

Tobacco cessation self-help materials available through voluntary or governmental health agencies were personally distributed to targeted worksites. Staff members or volunteers from local voluntary agencies, representatives of the Smoking Cessation Resources Task Force or Worksites and Organizations Task Force, or COMMIT project staff delivered materials to a worksite representative willing to take responsibility for the dissemination of the information within that worksite. To generate additional interest in these self-help resources, some intervention sites used special promotional materials, such as buttons, posters, mugs, and desk accessories, to gain access to companies either for initial visits or followup activities.

Promotion of a Smokers' Network

The Smoking Cessation Resources Task Force also established a Smokers' Network, a voluntary list or registry of smokers in each community who received mailings and materials several times a year to encourage cessation and its maintenance (see Chapter 8). This network was promoted in worksites through posters, flyers, and other informational materials distributed in conjunction with the promotion of communitywide and worksite events. Many of these materials contained stamped, self-addressed network registration cards that allowed a smoker to join the network simply by completing the card and returning it to the local COMMIT office. Smokers could also request Spanish-language materials as part of the network registration process.

Project staff members stressed the need to stagger visits to worksites and to coordinate efforts with other organizations doing worksite health promotion to ensure continued business community cooperation. The need to coordinate visits sometimes created new opportunities for collaboration with the voluntary health organizations. For example, in one COMMIT site the worksite specialist helped to orient an American Heart Association volunteer interested in the Heart at Work project so that they could share the work of delivering health materials to worksites.

The worksite activities described above were designed to be incorporated into the communitywide intervention implemented by the COMMIT project. By building ongoing relationships with local worksites and voluntary health organizations, COMMIT was able to provide multiple and sustained interventions rather than single programs. Prior research suggests that no one treatment strategy can guarantee success; the more successful programs use multifaceted, multicomponent interventions. Such programs tend to be highly flexible and are designed to reach employees at various points on the "stages of change continuum" (Abrams et al., 1994; DiClemente et al., 1991; Prochaska and DiClemente, 1983).

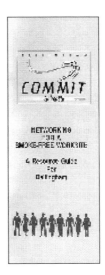

DELIVERING THE INTERVENTION TO THE COMMUNITY   Effective delivery of intervention activities to worksites was contingent on each COMMIT site's ability to convince workplace personnel of the relevance and importance of community tobacco control efforts. The COMMIT project relied on a community Board and task forces to assist field staff in reaching out to the many businesses and labor organizations in each community.

Participation of Board and Task Force Members   The design of the COMMIT project called for a community Board accountable for the overall goals—how to increase quit rates in the community at large—and task forces responsible for the planning and implementation of activities specific to a given channel—in this case, the worksite channel. The Worksites and Organizations Task Force was charged with overseeing activities involving civic and religious organizations as well as worksites. Each community was responsible for reaching many diverse organizations, and most COMMIT sites experienced significant difficulties in achieving the objectives established for these groups. Efforts directed toward other organizations are described in Chapter 11. The impact of this dual focus on task force functioning is discussed in more detail in the "Lessons Learned" section below. In brief, given that there were more objectives under "Other Organizations" than under "Worksites" and that the organizational objectives proved difficult to achieve, considerable task force effort was devoted to organizations other than worksites.

The roles played by the community Boards and task forces in the worksite channel included the following (Kizer, 1987; Sorensen et al., 1990):

- *catalyst* for the support and involvement of community leaders;

- *key informant* on ways to tailor the intervention to community needs and available resources;

- *liaison* with community service providers and service vendors;

- *information clearinghouse* on health information, community resources, and effective implementation models of health promotion;

- *coordinator* in sponsoring communitywide health promotion activities; and

- *supporter* of ongoing program implementation.

Some worksite task forces experienced significant turnover in membership and found the mobilization of community leaders for worksite endeavors to be an ongoing effort. In several COMMIT sites, the task force had to be rebuilt, sometimes more than once, after resignations of key members and significant member attrition. Turnover occurred for many reasons: For instance, in the Brantford and Raleigh sites, several Board and task force members resigned because of expected pressure from the local tobacco industry. Other communities had difficulty filling the position of task force chair; therefore, the task force lacked the leadership it needed to move ahead.

Brantford's experience highlights the importance of recruiting effective leadership for worksite efforts. For the first 2 years the project was unable to develop a viable worksite task force. The initial worksite chair, a local union leader, was highly regarded in the community. However, his time was limited, his employer discouraged him from attending meetings during working hours, and smoking was not high on his list of priorities. A second chair, also highly regarded in the community, had a leadership style that others perceived as autocratic and not good for the project.

The turning point came when management personnel from two local hospitals (the chief executive officer from one and the director of education from the other) agreed to serve as cochairs of the task force. Each had good leadership and organizational skills and a commitment to smoking control that included a personal as well as professional dimension. Both were well connected to the business community and used their contacts to assemble an effective team. The task force cochairs, both senior executives, also used their worksites as models. For instance, they quickly organized a Quit and Win competition between the two hospitals in town, a successful, high-profile event that encouraged staff and provided a model for other worksites.

Another cornerstone of effective leadership, according to several COMMIT communities, was the ability of task force chairs to involve task force members in activity planning. Meetings devoted to recitation of activity reports with little opportunity for volunteers to engage in creative thinking were less likely to maintain member interest and produce results. When volunteers could see that their ideas and opinions were a vital part of the intervention process, their creativity and productivity increased.

During the second half of the project, Brantford elicited so many good ideas from its task force that not all of them could be implemented. To keep track of these ideas for future consideration, the essence of the idea was captured in a few words and posted on the wall of the meeting room where the Board and task forces met. The "idea bank" was embraced, and ideas from many sources were accepted and saved for possible later implementation. Individuals who contributed these ideas felt they were recognized, the visible idea bank helped establish a "culture of creativity," and new brainstorms occurred as ideas posted on the walls stimulated further thinking by participants.

Gaining Access to Worksites   COMMIT staff members and volunteers were expected to work first with high-profile and early adopter worksites to build community awareness and confidence in program efforts, thereby laying the groundwork for efforts with worksites less ready for change (Abrams et al., 1994). Although the community analysis identified business and labor leaders targeted for membership on the community Board and its various task forces, recruitment of these individuals often proved more difficult than anticipated. In many cases the early adopter worksites did not have high profiles in the community. Often, business and labor leaders with the most extensive histories of community volunteer work did not view smoking control as a high priority. In many communities potential task force members had to be convinced first of the extent of the tobacco problem and then of the merits of the COMMIT project. Initially, the worksites most often represented on the task force were those already providing health promotion programs or otherwise supportive of smoking control efforts. These worksites sometimes served as role models for other businesses, enhancing the attractiveness of participating in the effort (Orlandi, 1986; Rogers, 1983), but this did not occur as readily as expected.

COMMIT personnel used a variety of approaches for engaging worksites in COMMIT efforts. All agreed that having a "well-connected" employee or employees committed to tobacco control inside a workplace who could serve as a program or issue champion was critical for effective implementation. However, the definition of a well-connected employee varied across intervention communities.

Some COMMIT sites felt that the project's original emphasis on recruiting chief executive officers and top-level management was misplaced. These sites saw occupational health nurses, human resource managers, or worksite health and safety committees as key to obtaining worksite involvement. For example, Brantford informants reported notable success with some of these groups. They obtained their best results by working with human relations officials. Canadian health and safety officers also expressed interest in the smoking issue and invited COMMIT representatives to speak to large audiences at their regional events, but those officers were less well positioned to provide entree into individual worksites. Other sites reported frustrations in working with these midlevel contacts because although they were often knowledgeable and highly motivated, the contacts were less successful in getting worksite decisionmakers to implement activities. Most intervention sites agreed that efforts to work through unions were unsuccessful or slow to provide results.

After reaching out to human relations officers, health and safety representatives, and union officials, Brantford reported that the best results were obtained by working with human relations officials. Although health and safety officers were interested in smoking and invited COMMIT to speak to large audiences at regional events, they were less well positioned to provide access to individual worksites. However, others felt they were unable to obtain access through such contacts because they could not capture the attention of worksite decisionmakers when it was time to implement activities.

Tailoring Project Activities
The community Board and the Worksites and Organizations Task Force, working with project staff, were responsible for tailoring the intervention activities to fit the community, which happened in several ways. In most communities, the COMMIT Board reviewed the priorities set by individual task forces through the development of annual action plans. These plans described how the intervention activities would be implemented during the coming year, outlined the tasks necessary to implement each intervention activity, identified who would carry out each task, established a timeline for task completion, and specified the money and other resources required. The development of the annual action plans helped to encourage community partnership in implementing the mandated protocol activities. The amount of resources allocated and the number of community members involved in implementing a given activity depended primarily on local staffing patterns as well as the makeup of the community, especially the configuration of worksites and cessation services.

In addition to the activities mandated by the protocol, some COMMIT sites conducted optional activities that were designed to take advantage of special opportunities present at a given time in the community. For example, in Santa Fe, NM, community analysis showed that the business sector had an unusual configuration, dominated by State government offices and a large tourist industry. Therefore, the task force assembled a booklet called "Santa Fe's Guide to Dining and Lodging," which included information on the smoking policies of restaurants and hotels. This was the only restaurant guide available in Santa Fe and was in great demand. Paterson, one of the most racially and ethnically diverse of the COMMIT communities, was especially concerned about reaching blue-collar workers. A useful strategy involved teaming COMMIT with other health promotion efforts in the community. For example, expired carbon monoxide testing and feedback to smokers and ex-smokers were offered regularly in conjunction with blood pressure screenings provided at worksites by a local hospital. One of the challenges facing Fitchburg/Leominster was lack of participation from labor groups. COMMIT staff members met with representatives of several unions during a regular union meeting to make a brief presentation and to conduct a focus group discussion. The focus group allowed them to begin to identify labor's concerns about tobacco control and to devise strategies to encourage union involvement.

Worksite Implementation Structures
COMMIT Boards and task forces tended to use two types of staffing arrangements to deliver worksite activities. In eight COMMIT sites, a decision was made to hire and use a half-time or full-time COMMIT staff member (e.g., an "intervention specialist," "task force

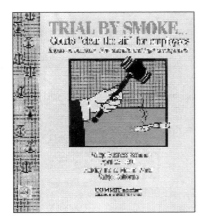

coordinator," or "worksite specialist") who devoted from 20 to 40 hours per week to worksite activities. Such staff members were often responsible for publicizing worksite events; arranging for dissemination of cessation information and promotional materials; planning worksite smoking policy workshops, sometimes in collaboration with one or more of the local voluntary organizations; and providing worksite policy consultations. Another site also used a paid staff member for worksite activities, but this person provided support to several of the task forces.

In the two remaining sites, Utica and Vallejo, the COMMIT leadership opted to subcontract many or all the worksite activities to a local agency. In both instances staff members learned from experience how to work effectively with subcontractors and found that subcontracting, although a well-intentioned strategy and an excellent use of community resources, brought its own set of challenges. There was general agreement that substantial supervision was required, especially during the first year of a contract, if activities were to be implemented effectively by subcontractors who often had a lesser commitment to the tobacco issue than did COMMIT staff and volunteers. Initially, Utica set up two subcontracts with community agencies, one for a "worksite policy consultant" and one for a "worksite liaison," to carry out most of the task force's directives. A year's experience taught that overlaps between the subcontracts resulted in duplicate contacts to worksites. This, along with subcontractor reporting problems, led the Board to combine all worksite activities the next year and rebid the subcontract to a single agency.

After subcontracting some worksite activities, Vallejo found that project staff members and worksite task force members were becoming insulated from contact with the employers and employees who were targeted for participation in worksite activities. They found themselves forced to depend on the subcontractor for a picture of the business climate and the concerns and needs of employers. When the accuracy of this picture was called into question, the task force responded by developing more measurable outcomes, clarifying lines of accountability, and extending the timeline for activities. These actions increased opportunities for collaborative planning between the subcontractor and COMMIT staff and volunteers, allowed for more timely feedback, and left time for fine-tuning the plans prior to implementation. Both Utica and Vallejo reported difficulty in maintaining task force interest when meeting agendas focused on reports from subcontractors with no opportunity for creative planning by members. Whether worksite activities were implemented by subcontractors or project staff, COMMIT participants stressed the importance of bringing in these individuals early in the project. Most intervention sites did not hire staff members or subcontractors to handle worksite activities until well into the second year of the intervention, which delayed progress in the worksite channel.

LESSONS
LEARNED
Workplaces can be ideal for reaching smokers, and initial COMMIT survey findings indicated there was substantial opportunity for intervention in all three of the following targeted areas—smoking policies, incentive and motivational programs, and the provision of cessation resources to employees—especially in smaller worksites (Sorensen et al., 1989).

To optimize these opportunities for intervention, COMMIT personnel stressed the need to take advantage of external changes and link tobacco control activities to larger events such as clean indoor air laws or the release of information at the national level (such as the EPA report on ETS [U.S. Environmental Protection Agency, 1992]). A well-publicized smoking policy change by a major employer also could be used to generate interest among other worksites. For example, Paterson reported that policy changes by school districts, changes in standards by hospital accreditation agencies, and passage of more stringent youth access laws all generated further interest in worksite smoking policy consultations.

The value of time was one of the lessons from Vallejo. COMMIT staff members reported that long seminars, offsite trainings that took people away from their work, usually did not draw as high attendance as brief trainings or lunch-time gatherings. Brief materials were more likely to be read by busy employers than large, elaborate packets of information.

COMMIT interventionists quickly learned or remembered the old adage, "if they won't come to you, then go to them," and attempted to incorporate their programs, materials, and information within settings where targeted individuals and worksite representatives gathered for other purposes. For example, in Medford/Ashland where it proved difficult to attract significant numbers of worksite representatives to annual worksite smoking policy workshops, staff members began to incorporate their smoking policy information within the agenda of the community's "drug-free workplace" workshops. These workshops were held several times a year and drew many worksite representatives. The substance abuse awareness group in turn began to incorporate tobacco use into its ongoing agenda. Staff members from Cedar Rapids/Marion indicated they might have been even more effective in reaching worksites had they begun to work with substance abuse prevention groups earlier in the process.

Most communities reported that the expected synergistic effect among intervention channels did bolster worksite efforts. Cedar Rapids/Marion found that Quit and Win contests, radio advertisements, billboards, and media spots publicizing other COMMIT activities all generated name familiarity for the project and made it easier for the worksite specialist to get management's attention about the tobacco issue. The project in turn used worksite successes to generate additional media coverage by creating a public education campaign based on testimonials from a wide variety of workplaces.

Using worksites as a setting to recruit for community events and distribute cessation materials was recognized by all COMMIT sites as a highly successful approach. Magnet events such as Quit and Win contests and the GASO or National Non-Smoking Week (Canada) reached many smokers across communities, and worksites often played an integral part in these efforts. Publicly recognizing worksites that went smoke-free via newspaper advertisements, plaques, or decals often encouraged others to emulate their decisions and created a sense of growing momentum in the community. Building on this awareness, staff members and volunteers were better able to use a peer approach to sell no-smoking policies in their worksite consultations.

Although smoking policy interventions were recognized as a key strategy, they did not receive as much consistent emphasis across the trial as planned because of difficulties encountered in generating interest from worksites in some communities. This apparent lack of interest in policies at the worksite level prompted some communities to suggest that efforts be devoted to passing municipal, county, or State clean indoor air ordinances before trying to convince worksites to establish or strengthen their policies. Such actions created opportunities in States where such regulations were passed.

Despite the recognized importance of worksite smoking policy interventions in shaping community smoking norms, staff members from one site questioned whether:

> from a quitting smoker's point of view, the workplace is the most opportune place to receive cessation services. Onsite cessation classes were often not well attended, and "public" team events, like cessation competitions, were problematic, i.e., didn't appeal to the numbers anticipated by project designers—many of those smokers who remain do not seem interested in quitting in groups or do not necessarily want to quit at the same time.

In their final reports, most COMMIT communities pointed to the implementation of no-smoking policies by worksites and restaurants as one of their most significant accomplishments. One community asserted that the institutionalization of smoking control through worksite policies was the most effective way to bring about lasting change in the smoking behavior of the community.

Although smoking control efforts through workplaces seem to hold great promise for reducing the burden of smoking in communities, achieving process objectives in this arena required exceptional effort from several COMMIT communities. The process objective data indicate that the majority of objectives were achieved (see Table 2). However, most COMMIT sites found that successfully involving smokers was not simply a function of the level of effort invested. There were several reasons for this.

First, businesses were selected and contacted according to the protocol for targeting worksites, but they often had to be convinced to endorse and carry out smoking control activities. Resistance may have stemmed from the ideas or smoking habits of powerful individuals in a worksite, organizational culture, perceptions by company leadership of the larger community culture as unsympathetic to smoking control activities, potential for aggravating relations between labor and management, threat or actuality of economic downturn, or existence of competing priorities. Few worksites in any community were recruited easily, and even when management cooperated fully, workers, especially heavy smokers, often did not come forth in large numbers to participate in programs.

Unlike most prior research involving worksites, the COMMIT project ultimately involved *all* those worksites in the community that satisfied project basic inclusion criteria, rather than concentrating on a relatively few motivated worksites selected and "cultivated" by the researchers. Most worksite research has taken place in major metropolitan areas with activities designed for large worksites (often more than 500 employees) with considerable resources. The scope of the COMMIT effort and the inclusiveness of its sample of large worksites presented special challenges, especially for some of the smaller size intervention communities.

The many small worksites in most COMMIT communities also required special efforts. Collectively, these worksites may employ more people than large workplaces, but staff resources limited the amount of outreach that could be done. Small businesses often felt they could not afford to send someone to a half-day policy workshop. Yet, they often benefited from extra attention in the form of special materials, incentives, and encouragement. To meet these needs, communities worked through chambers of commerce, small business associations, educational institutions serving small business, and other settings where small businesses sought information and support. The structure and financing of health care reform may help to shape future efforts to reach small businesses.

COMMIT's focus on a single health risk factor—in this case, tobacco use—may have been an impediment to forming ongoing relationships with worksites. In Brantford one cochair of the worksite task force went on to become a volunteer with the Heart and Stroke Foundation and, in this capacity, became involved in its worksite programs. He found worksites much more receptive to him when he was tied to an organization that was interested not only in smoking but also in broader lifestyle issues, which meant he was able to generate interest among a higher proportion of worksites. It also meant that it was easier for him to establish ongoing relationships and repeat business.

Some COMMIT researchers stress the efficacy of approaches used in other worksite interventions. For example, using a health risk appraisal as a tool for gaining entree to worksites might have allowed project staff members and volunteers to generate more involvement in activities. The health risk appraisal could have provided special feedback to smokers and shown the unique role of smoking as a risk factor for heart disease and cancer, while generating more widespread interest in the project among nonsmoking employees. Giving something to managers for their employees at the onset might have generated a greater willingness to participate in other project activities. The demands of the protocol limited the ability of staff members to join with worksites to carry out other health promotion goals, but establishing workplace steering committees in some worksites to tailor activities and provide options might create a greater sense of ownership as well as opportunity for more frequent contacts with the worksites (Sorensen et al., 1992).

Finally, the decision to combine worksite activities with efforts directed toward other community organizations within the same task force resulted in an awkward, sometimes totally unworkable, structure. In some intervention sites the structure diverted scarce volunteer energy from the business community away from worksite activities or away from the project altogether. In other cases community organizations were neglected in favor of worksites where chances of success seemed greater. The two types of settings are different; the sheer numbers of worksites and organizations to be reached were overwhelming for staff and volunteers, especially when combined. Task force members became frustrated and were often uninterested in one or the other half of this two-part task force agenda. By the end of the intervention, several COMMIT sites had established separate task forces for involving organizations or had reached agreements with existing community structures to take on some of the activities targeting other organizations.

A participant from Brantford summed up his site's struggles to balance the demands of science with the demands of the community by speaking of the "opportunity costs" associated with implementing the worksite intervention. All the worksite activities were effective in reaching some smokers or policymakers in some communities at some times. However, with limited resources, staff members and volunteers sometimes were frustrated at having to carry out protocol activities that they suspected (based on recent experience) were likely to have limited impact in their community. The task force found itself struggling to avoid tying up too many of its resources in required "good" activities when those resources might be invested in a few "better or best" activities, all of which were part of the COMMIT protocol.

REFERENCES

Abrams, D.B., Emmons, K.M., Linnan, L., Biener, L. Smoking cessation at the workplace: Conceptual and practical considerations. In: *Interventions for Smokers: An International Perspective*, R. Richmond (Editor). Baltimore: Williams & Wilkins, 1994, pp. 137-169.

Biener, L., Abrams, D.B., Follick, M.J., Dean, L. A comparative evaluation of restrictive smoking policy in a general hospital. *American Journal of Public Health* 79: 192-195, 1989.

Borland, R., Chapman, S., Owen, N., Hill, D. Effects of workplace smoking bans on cigarette consumption. *American Journal of Public Health* 80(20): 172-180, 1990.

Brownell, K.D., Felix, M.R. Competitions to facilitate health promotion: Review and conceptual analysis. *American Journal of Health Promotion* 77: 28-36, 1987.

California COMMIT staff. "Conducting a Successful Worksite Consultation: Lessons Learned." Case study CAL-SP92. COMMIT Project Archives and Quarterly Reports, Oakland, CA, 1992. pp. 18-20.

Corbett, K., Thompson, B., White, N., Taylor, M. (for the COMMIT Research Group). Process evaluation in the Community Intervention Trial for Smoking Cessation (COMMIT). *International Quarterly of Community Health Education* 11(3): 291-309, 1990-91.

DiClemente, C.C., Prochaska, J.O., Fairhurst, S.K., Velicer, W.F., Velasquez, M.M., Rossi, J.S. The processes of smoking cessation: An analysis of precontemplation, contemplation, and preparation stages of change. *Journal of Consulting and Clinical Psychology* 59: 295-304, 1991.

Emont, S.L., Cummings, K.M. Organizational factors affecting participation in a smoking cessation program and abstinence among 68 auto dealerships. *American Journal of Health Promotion* 5: 107-114, 1990.

Fielding, J.E. Health promotion and disease prevention at the worksite. *Annual Review of Public Health* 5: 237-265, 1984.

Fielding, J.E. Health promotion at the worksite. In: *Work, Health and Productivity*, G.M. Green and F. Baker (Editors). New York: Oxford University Press, 1991, pp. 256-276.

Fielding, J.E., Piserchia, P.V. Frequency of worksite health promotion activities. *American Journal of Public Health* 79(1): 16-20, 1989.

Fisher, K.J., Glasgow, R.E., Terborg, J.R. Work site smoking cessation: A meta-analysis of long-term quit rates from controlled studies. *Journal of Occupational Medicine* 32(5): 429-439, 1990.

Glasgow, R.E., Hollis, J.F., Ary, D.V., Lando, H.A. Employee and organizational factors associated with participation in a worksite incentive program for smoking cessation. *Journal of Behavioral Medicine* 13: 403-418, 1990.

Glasgow, R.E., McRae, S. *Incentives Programs Workbook*. Community Intervention Trial for Smoking Cessation. Bethesda, MD: National Cancer Institute, 1989.

Glasgow, R.E., Sorensen, G., Corbett, K. (for the COMMIT Research Group). Worksite smoking control activities: Prevalence and related worksite characteristics from the COMMIT study, 1990. *Preventive Medicine* 21(6): 688-700, 1992.

Glasgow, R.E., Sorenson, G.G., Giffin, C., Shipley, R., Corbett, K., Lynn, W. (for the COMMIT Research Group). Promoting worksite smoking control policies. The COMMIT experience. *Preventive Medicine*, submitted for publication.

Institute for the Study of Smoking Behavior and Policy. *COMMIT Guide to Running a Worksite Smoking Policy Workshop*. Community Intervention Trial for Smoking Cessation. Bethesda, MD: National Cancer Institute, 1989a.

Institute for the Study of Smoking Behavior and Policy. *COMMIT Guide to Nonsmoking Policies for Small Businesses*. Community Intervention Trial for Smoking Cessation. Bethesda, MD: National Cancer Institute, 1989b.

Jeffrey, R.W., Forster, J.L., French, S.A., Kelder, S.H., Lando, H.A., McGovern, P.R., Jacobs, P.R., Baxter, J.E. The healthy worker project: A worksite intervention for weight control and smoking cessation. *American Journal of Public Health* 83: 395-401, 1993.

Jeffrey, R.W., Pheley, A.M., Forster, J.L., Kramer, M., Snell, M.K. Payroll contracting for smoking cessation: A worksite pilot study. *American Journal of Preventive Medicine* 4: 83-86, 1988.

Kizer, W.M. *The Healthy Workplace: A Blueprint for Corporate Action*. New York: Wiley, 1987.

Klesges, R.C., Vasey, M.W., Glasgow, R.E. A worksite smoking modification competition: Potential for public health impact. *American Journal of Public Health* 76: 198-200, 1986.

Martin, M.J. Smoking control—policy and legal methods. (Letter.) *Western Journal of Medicine* 148(2): 199, 1988.

Mattson, D.M., Lee, J.W., Hepp, J.W. The impact of incentives and competitions on participation and quit rates in worksite smoking cessation programs. *American Journal of Health Promotion* 7(4): 270-280, 295, 1993.

Mattson, M.E., Cummings, K.M., Lynn, W.R., Giffen, C., Corle, D., Pechacek, T. Evaluation plan for the Community Intervention Trial for Smoking Cessation (COMMIT). *International Quarterly of Community Health Education* 11(3): 271-290, 1990-91.

Millar, W.J. *Smoke in the Workplace: An Evaluation of Smoking Restrictions*. Health and Welfare Canada. Ottawa, Ontario: Minister of Supply and Services Canada, 1988.

Nathan, P.E. Johnson & Johnson's Live For Life: A comprehensive positive lifestyle change. In: *Behavioral Health: A Handbook of Health Enhancement and Disease Prevention*, J.D. Matarazzo, S.M. Weiss, J.A. Herd, N.E. Miller, and S.M. Weiss (Editors). New York: John Wiley and Sons, 1984, pp. 1064-1070.

Orlandi, M.A. The diffusion and adoption of worksite health promotion innovations: An analysis of barriers. *Preventive Medicine* 15: 522-536, 1986.

Petersen, L.R., Helgerson, S.D., Gibbons, C.M., Calhoun, C.R., Ciacco, K.H., Pitchford, K.C. Employee smoking behavior changes and attitudes following a restrictive policy on worksite smoking in a large company. *Public Health Reports* 103: 115-120, 1988.

Prochaska, J.O., DiClemente, C.C. Stages and processes of self-change of smoking: Toward an integrative and model of change. *Journal of Consulting and Clinical Psychology* 51: 390-395, 1983.

Rogers, E.M. *Diffusion of Innovations*. (3rd edition.) New York: The Free Press, 1983.

Rosenstock, I.M., Stergachis, A., Heaney, C. Evaluation of smoking prohibition policy in a health maintenance organization. *American Journal of Public Health* 76: 1014-1015, 1986.

Rossi, J.S., Prochaska, J.D., DiClemente, C.C. Processes of change in heavy and light smokers. *Journal of Substance Abuse* 1: 1-9, 1988.

Shepard, D.S., Pearlman, L.A. Health habits that pay off. *Business Health* 2: 37-41, 1985.

Shipley, R.H., Orleans, C.T., Wilbur, C.S., Piserchia, P.V., McFadden, D.W. Effect of the Johnson & Johnson Live For Life Program on employee smoking. *Preventive Medicine* 17: 25-34, 1988.

Sorensen, G., Glasgow, R., Corbett, K. Involving worksite and other organizations in health promotion. In: *Organizing for Community Health Promotion: A Guide*, N. Bracht (Editor). Newbury Park, CA: Sage, 1990, pp. 158-184.

Sorensen, G., Glasgow, R.E., Corbett, K. Promoting smoking control through worksites in the Community Intervention Trial for Smoking Cessation (COMMIT). *International Quarterly of Community Health Education* 11(3): 239-257, 1990-91.

Sorensen, G., Hsieh, J., Hunt, M.K., Morris, D.H., Harris, D.R., Fitzgerald, G. Employee advisory boards as a vehicle for organizing worksite health promotion programs. *American Journal of Health Promotion* 6: 443-450, 1992.

Sorensen, G., Pechacek, T., Pallonen, U. Occupational and worksite norms and attitudes about smoking cessation. *American Journal of Public Health* 76: 544-549, 1986.

Sorensen, G., Pechacek, T.F. Implementing nonsmoking policies in the private sector and assessing their effects. *New York State Journal of Medicine* 89(1): 11-15, 1989.

Sorensen, G., Rigotti, N., Rosen, A., Pinney, J. "The Effects of a Worksite Nonsmoking Policy: Evidence for Increased Cessation." (Abstract.) Paper presented at the annual meeting of the American Public Health Association, Chicago, IL, October 1989.

Stave, G.M., Jackson, G.W. Effect of a total worksite smoking ban on employee smoking and attitudes. *Journal of Occupational Medicine* 33(8): 884-890, 1991.

Terborg, J.R., Glasgow, R.E. Worksite interventions: A brief review of health promotion programs at work. In: *Cambridge Handbook of Psychology, Health and Medicine*, A. Baum, C. McManus, S. Newman, J. Weinman, and R. West (Editors). London: Cambridge University Press, in press.

U.S. Bureau of the Census. *Statistical Abstract of the United States, 1986*. Washington, DC: Supt. of Docs., U.S. Govt. Print. Off., 1986.

U.S. Department of Health and Human Services. *The Health Consequences of Using Smokeless Tobacco. A Report of the Advisory Committee to the Surgeon General*. NIH Publication No. 86-2874. Bethesda, MD: U.S. Department of Health and Human Services, Public Health Service, 1986.

U.S. Environmental Protection Agency. Guidelines for carcinogen risk assessment. *Federal Register* 51: 33992-34003, 1986.

U.S. Environmental Protection Agency. *Respiratory Health Effects of Passive Smoking: Lung Cancer and Other Disorders*. EPA 600/6-90/006F. Washington, DC: Office of Research and Development, Office of Health and Environmental Assessment, 1992.

U.S. Public Health Service. 1992 National Survey of Worksite Health Promotion Activities: Summary. *American Journal of Health Promotion* 7(6): 452-464, 1993.

Warner, K.E., Wickizer, T.M., Wolfe, R.A., Schildroth, J.E., Samuelson, M.H. Economic implications of workplace health promotion programs: Review of the literature. *Journal of Occupational Medicine* 30: 106-112, 1988.

Winett, R.A., King, A.C., Altman, P.G. *Health Psychology and Public Health: An Integrative Approach*. New York: Pergamon, 1989.

ACKNOWLEDGMENT   The authors wish to acknowledge Tom Weldon, Community Board Chair and Chair of the Worksites and Organizations Task Force, Medford/Ashland, OR, for his helpful comments.

AUTHORS

Linda Nettekoven, M.A.
Project Coordinator
Oregon Research Institute
1715 Franklin Boulevard
Eugene, OR 97403

Russell E. Glasgow, Ph.D.
Research Scientist
Oregon Research Institute
1715 Franklin Boulevard
Eugene, OR 97403

Robert H. Shipley, Ph.D.
Department of Psychiatry
Duke University Medical Center
Box 3964
Durham, NC 27710

A.J. Roy Cameron, Ph.D.
Professor
Department of Health Studies and
  Gerontology
University of Waterloo
BMH, Room 2311
Waterloo, Ontario N2L 3G1
CANADA

Lesa T. Dalton
Project Director
Division of Health Promotion Research
American Health Foundation
Fifth Floor
800 Second Avenue
New York, NY 10017

Aleena Erickson
2117 Washington Avenue, S.E.
Cedar Rapids, IA 52403

Sharon Ann Rankins-Burd
Box 99
North Winfield Road
West Winfield, NY 13491

Sandy Tosti, M.A.
7335 Franco Lane
Vacaville, CA 95688

Glorian Sorensen, Ph.D., M.P.H.
Associate Professor
Department of Epidemiology and Cancer
  Control
Dana Farber Cancer Institute
Harvard School of Public Health
44 Biney Street
Boston, MA 02115

Kitty K. Corbett, Ph.D., M.P.H.
Adjunct Investigator
Division of Research
Kaiser Permanente Medical Care Program
3505 Broadway
Oakland, CA 94611
and
Assistant Professor
Health and Behavioral Sciences, CB-103
Department of Anthropology
University of Colorado at Denver
P.O. Box 173364
Denver, CO 80217

Involving Diverse Community Organizations in Tobacco Control Activities

Kitty K. Corbett, Linda Nettekoven, Linda C. Churchill, Lesa T. Dalton, Carolyn L. Johnson, Lysha Dickinson, Glorian Sorensen, and Beti Thompson

THE RATIONALE FOR INVOLVING COMMUNITY ORGANIZATIONS In the Community Intervention Trial for Smoking Cessation (COMMIT), the active participation of multiple sectors of the community was a fundamental vehicle for comprehensive changes in the "tobacco control environment" in communities. In addition to focusing on the workplaces, clinical settings, and school-based organizations so necessary to health promotion, the COMMIT project from the outset recognized that community and civic organizations were important targets of and channels for pursuit of health promotion objectives (Sorensen et al., 1990; Lasater et al., 1986). Some organizations representing employees and employers, medical care practitioners and clinical settings, and schools were considered so necessary to COMMIT's goals that from the outset they warranted separate, dedicated channels (and are discussed in separate chapters in this monograph). Miscellaneous remaining community organizations were handled within the separate and more amorphous channel of "other organizations." This chapter summarizes the experiences of the 11 COMMIT intervention communities in working with diverse civic and community organizations to accomplish tobacco control objectives. The rationale for such involvement is compelling. However, the process of engaging such organizations in tobacco control was highly challenging for participants.

All community-based health promotion efforts use community organizations in many ways (Cuoto, 1990; Hatch et al., 1993; Nickens, 1990; Shea, 1992). Organizations are points of access to targeted individuals for planned interventions. Many organizations are involved in publicity, magnet events, assistance with logistics for activities, and provision of expertise for health promotion efforts. When hospitals, other clinical settings, educational institutions, and worksites are enlisted in multifaceted community projects, staff members are recruited from organizations with a health promotion or social service focus. Representatives of organizations that have implemented smoking bans have been involved in conferences and other educational forums throughout the country. Voluntary agencies (e.g., American Lung Association [ALA], Canadian Cancer Society [CCS]) and health departments have sponsored many health promotion activities. Community organizations also have been useful in efforts to secure funding of health promotion efforts, for example, through written endorsements of and involvement in specific projects.

Community organizations offer opportunities for identifying smokers and others at risk from tobacco, and they also are sources of persons and resources for fostering change and its maintenance (Roncarati et al., 1989; DePue et al., 1987; Eng et al., 1985; Carlaw et al., 1984). Community organizations are important local institutions through which to implement policy changes, publicize project activities, offer programs, provide education, and otherwise create an environment supportive of health. Organizational policies and opinions of leaders may have considerable influence on members' attitudes and behaviors. Networks of organizations in the form of coalitions may wield considerable influence in a community, and their activities and policies are often well covered by local media. Some types of community organizations have a long history of community service, outreach, and participation in

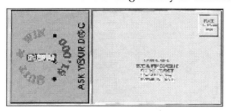

health promotion and education. Many such groups already regard health-related social service as part of their mission. Organizational facilities, many of which are in neighborhoods, are centers for their members and often for other people and functions. They allow dissemination of information to people outside usual health promotion settings (i.e., educational and medical care settings). Some community organizations (e.g., church groups, community centers) also deal with families, which is another important sector infrequently addressed as a unit elsewhere and which may not be readily reached via other channels. Programs such as a Salvation Army mission, those dealing with employment and training, and the Women, Infant, and Children's program (WIC) also can be seen as organizations providing important access to diverse special populations.

Religious organizations appear to have enormous potential as a channel for smoking control messages and activities. They are central social and cultural institutions in American and Canadian communities. Membership in a religious organization in 1990 was reported by 69 percent of American adults in a Gallup Poll, and 40 percent said they had attended a church or synagogue in the past 7 days (Princeton Religious Research Center, 1993). Many religious organizations already take part in health-related activities, such as education, treatment, and screening programs dealing with subjects such as diet and nutrition, fitness, alcohol and substance abuse, mental health, stress management, AIDS (acquired immunodeficiency syndrome), heart disease prevention, and CPR (cardiopulmonary resuscitation), to name a few (Corbett et al., 1991; Elder et al., 1989). Many religious organizations also are interested in prevention programs, have restrictive smoking policies, and have become involved in a variety of programs for their members (Emory University, Carter Center and Park Ridge Center, 1990; Foege, 1990; Hatch and Lovelace, 1980; Hatch and Johnson, 1981; Lasater et al., 1986; Levin, 1984; Saunders and Knog, 1983; Smith, 1983; Wiist and Flack, 1990; Stillman et al., 1993). It is reasonable to assume that clerics, who have seen members die of smoking-related diseases and counseled them and their grieving families, would be receptive to tobacco control. In addition, many members of religious organizations may live with a smoker, have a child who smokes, work with smokers, or have friends who smoke; nonsmokers who become informed and involved through a religious (or other) organization may be useful channels of tobacco control messages and information to smokers they encounter in their daily lives. Even in those religious organizations with few members who are smokers, nonsmokers could endorse community-wide nonsmoking norms and communicate information about tobacco control and cessation resources to their family members, friends, associates, and acquaintances who are smokers.

The developers of the COMMIT protocol recognized that success required having enduring, influential community organizations endorse the project's goals, steer interventions over the period of Federal funding, enhance their own smoking control policies, participate in tobacco control activities, and provide access to targeted smokers (Lichtenstein et al., 1990-91; Thompson et al., 1990-91). Community organizations beyond health care, worksite, and educational institutions needed to be incorporated into COMMIT's plan, but which ones, and how?

OTHER ORGANIZATIONS IN COMMIT
In COMMIT's protocol, organizational entities dealing with health care, public education, and cessation resources were targeted through channels handled separately from other organizations. Worksites were structurally linked with other organizations into a single channel but also were dealt with separately in the delineation of activities and process objectives. Other organizations, by virtue of the nebulous character of the channel as well as their diversity, became in effect the stepchild of the worksites and organizations channel.

Community organizations are diverse and complex, with no standard configuration across communities. They vary in type, mission, values, structure, leadership, demographic representation, sheer numbers, charter, rules, and relationships with members. A nonexhaustive list of types of community organizations would include religious organizations, service and fraternal organizations, coalitions (e.g., for health promotion, drug use prevention, community beautification), ethnic organizations, voluntary agencies, business

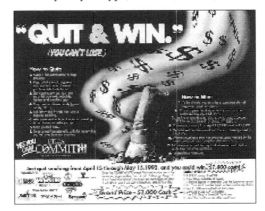

groups, unions, veterans' organizations, social service locales (e.g., WIC program offices, employment development offices), self-help and support groups, and other local groups such as recreational, neighborhood, and social clubs. Membership or affiliation in community organizations is voluntary, and in many, leadership is short term or rotating. Organizational rules often are derived from tradition and consensus and are adhered to or enforced internally and informally, without support from formal legal sanctions. In most organizations, participation is occasional, optional, or sporadic. The manner of implementation of activities must be responsive to the special and diverse characteristics of organizations. In addition, specific organizations vary in their potential for assisting with the achievement of COMMIT's objectives. Some organizations were clearly less appropriate for COMMIT activities than others.

The 11 COMMIT intervention communities had diverse constellations of organizations that appeared appropriate for tobacco control activities. The visibility, influence, and penetration of specific organizations were different in various sites. Organizations varied greatly in size in a community. An initial tally of other organizations in the 11 sites (from a review of telephone book classified listings [e.g., "Yellow Pages"] and chamber of commerce lists and modified by other sources, including staff members' knowledge of the community) was more than 1,500 groups, of which about 56 percent were religious organizations and 24 percent were civic and fraternal organizations (Table 1). The number of religious organizations serving the communities totaled more than 800.

All communities contained a wide range of organizations, such as those listed above. In addition, various communities mobilized less traditional organizations such as Drug Abuse Resistance Education (DARE), WIC agency offices, the Puerto Rican Day Committee, and summer youth programs to implement successful intervention activities. In one site, Medford/Ashland, OR, there was no local health voluntary association presence at all, whereas in another, there was a small operation dedicated to preserving its existing mandate and tasks rather than expanding its role. In the Vallejo, CA, and Raleigh, NC, sites, health voluntary associations were the most powerful,

Table 1

Initial tally[a] of other organizations in the COMMIT intervention sites, by type of organization

Type	Number	Percent
Religious Organizations	843	55.7
Business/Professional Groups	101	6.7
Fraternal/Sorority Groups	80	5.3
Civic Groups	281	18.6
Trade/Labor/Union Groups	105	6.9
Groups With Health Mandate[b]	80	5.3
Miscellaneous Groups	23	1.5
Total	1,513	100.0

[a] These numbers reflect the specific organizations generated by staff in each site in the preliminary community analysis from review of telephone book classified listings, chamber of commerce lists, and other local sources prior to final trialwide adjustment of operational criteria for interventional and promotional organizations.

[b] This category includes organizations beyond those that would be targeted through the health care providers or worksites channels.

best funded, and most visionary tobacco control advocates. Both well-known, longstanding groups (e.g., health voluntaries, the Rotary Club) and local, shorter term, grassroots coalitions (e.g., Minority Coalition for Cancer Prevention, Coalition for Health and Responsible Public Policy, Healthy Mothers/Healthy Babies, Community Partnership for Substance Abuse, neighborhood coalitions) played central roles in COMMIT's attempts to meet its objectives.

A typology of community organizations was developed in response to cross-community diversity and COMMIT's varied needs. The activities mandated by the COMMIT protocol for organizations were designed on the premise that community organizations tend to play one or both of two basic roles in tobacco control efforts: (1) acting as institutions through which smokers can be contacted directly or (2) serving as a source of volunteers and other resources that can be engaged in tobacco control efforts directed broadly at the community. In the first case, the organizations were expected to provide a locale where smokers periodically gathered or through which smokers might be reached with mailings, organizational policies, activities, special events, and cessation programs. Organizations so identified were designated as "interventional" organizations. Particular organizations such as large churches and business-related groups such as chambers of commerce, unions, and service organizations were designated interventional organizations when they met the following criteria:

- Active membership of at least 50 adults as evidenced by:

  — size of attendance at meetings;

  — size of attendance at organization-sponsored events; and

  — number of dues-paying members (persons committed enough to send in dues are likely to be accessible through an organization's mailouts).

- Meet at least six times a year.

- Have a regular meeting place.

- Have a number of members who smoke, as determined by available information (e.g., key informant, informal conversations with one or more members).

- At least 30 percent of membership are estimated to be community residents.

In addition to those criteria, limits were placed on the size of religious organizations targeted for intervention activities. Given the many religious organizations in some COMMIT sites, limited resources did not permit that interventions be directed at all of them. Reasoning that religious organizations with 250 or more members would be likely to reach more smokers than those with fewer than 250 members, the size of the religious organization became an additional eligibility criterion.

Other targeted organizations were designated as "promotional" organizations, although some fit in both promotional and interventional categories. Promotional activities were those that were held to contribute to community smoking control efforts in one or more of the following ways:

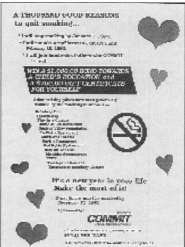

- generating community recognition of, interest in, and sanction for the COMMIT project;

- providing greater access to the socioeconomically disadvantaged and other nonmainstream groups likely to include heavy smokers;

- increasing the amount of information available in the community regarding smoking cessation/control efforts and resources;

- generating volunteer support for COMMIT activities;

- providing material resources (e.g., money, supplies, equipment, meeting space);

- enhancing media coverage, publicity, and other public relations activities related to smoking control;

- contributing to community mobilization for smoking control through the creation or enhancement of local networks; and

- helping to increase the number of quit attempts made by community residents.

This approach was designed for organizations that did not necessarily include a substantial number of smokers within their membership yet might be willing because of their mission or role in the community to involve volunteers or other resources to the tobacco control cause.

Once revised operational criteria were employed, the number of organizations designated for assessment of progress toward process objectives totaled 726 interventional and 702 promotional organizations across the 11 sites (Table 2). Beyond the challenge posed by the sheer numbers involved, the numbers by community illustrate the diversity existing among the sites: The number of interventional organizations ranged from a low of 46 to a high of 138, and promotional organizations ranged from a low of 21 to a high of 256. Site ratios of the number of organizations targeted for intervention activities to the total population ranged approximately from .0005 to .001, with only slight agreement between size of community and number of organizations identified for intervention.

Table 2

Numbers of interventional and promotional organizations for assessing annual achievement of process objectives, by site, for the initial 3 years of intervention[a]

Sites	Interventional	Promotional	Both
Site A	50	77	127
Site B	57	78	135
Site C	47	27	74
Site D	103	53	156
Site E	138	256	394
Site F	54	69	123
Site G	46	21	67
Site H	67	105	172
Site I	86	34	120
Site J	85	24	109
Site K	50	36	86
Total	726	702	1,428

[a] Adjusted totals for the final intervention year summed only a few more: 727 and 713 for interventional and promotional organizations, respectively. Sites are listed in random order.

The emphasis in the channel of other organizations shifted early in the COMMIT project. In the planning phase, a wide variety of organizations were featured as potentially equivalent, with the relative importance of their diverse types to be determined locally. However, as the evaluation requirements of the overall project were articulated into mandated activities and concrete process objectives, religious organizations emerged as the sole type of organization in the channel that could be formally evaluated in standardized fashion (Mattson et al., 1990-91; Corbett et al., 1990-91). In light of the considerable diversity of organizations in communities and the difficulty of generating comparable sampling frames of organizations across communities, a decision was made to use a survey of religious organizations as a kind of proxy for assessing the penetration and

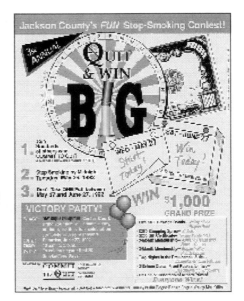

efficacy of COMMIT activities in diverse organizations. The articulation of this in the mandates expressed in the COMMIT protocol (i.e., required activities and process objectives) and the recognition of the survey of religious organizations as a critical evaluation tool resulted in a shift in local understandings of priorities in the channel. In most sites there was also a corresponding shift in activities implemented in the channel. Religious organizations came to preeminence in this channel at a trialwide level and in most communities. Requirements for evaluation data drove the intervention to a degree unforeseen by COMMIT's designers.

The mandated activities of this channel are given in Table 3 and reflect the difference between interventional and promotional organizations.

Presentations on Smoking Issues   To increase awareness of the tobacco problem, COMMIT staff members and volunteers made short presentations of at least 15 minutes to organizations targeted for intervention during the groups' regular meetings. Presentations included information on smoking cessation, the health implications of tobacco use and secondhand smoke, policy and program resources, and national as well as local trends in tobacco control. If appropriate, COMMIT speakers also provided information on legal issues and publicized upcoming smoking policy and cessation seminars and workshops. Organizations likely to include a high proportion of smokers on their membership rolls, such as labor unions or veterans' groups, were emphasized. Promotional organizations also were contacted in an effort to strengthen local tobacco control networks.

Table 3
Activities and process objectives for organizations

Activities for Each Community	Cumulative Objectives (1988-1992)	Number Completed	Process Objectives Achieved[a] (%)
Short Presentations to Organizations Targeted for Intervention	30%		83
Comprehensive Seminars to Organizations Targeted for Intervention	44 seminars 30%	40 seminars	91 77
Promotional Activities in Organizations Targeted for Intervention	50%		152
Distribution of Self-Help Materials in Organizations Targeted for Intervention	50%		160
Distribution of Promotional Materials to Organizations Targeted for Intervention	50%		172
Annually Involve Organizations Targeted for Promotion in Magnet Events	440 organizations	497 organizations	113

[a] *Average for combined communities.*

**Seminars
on Smoking
Issues**
Seminars or policy presentations of at least 1 hour in length were offered to representatives of organizations targeted for intervention. The longer format allowed presenters to cover tobacco control topics in more detail. Workshop content included the health implications of tobacco and secondhand smoke, cessation resources and strategies, national and local trends, legal issues, and policy and program options. Examples of nonsmoking policies and cessation efforts from local organizations were highlighted. In some communities separate seminars were held, for example, for religious groups or labor organizations. In other cases, tobacco control issues were covered as part of a larger workshop agenda on a related topic, such as substance abuse, that was designed to reach larger numbers of participants.

**Activities
Promoting
Magnet Events**
To foster member participation in communitywide cessation events, COMMIT staff members and volunteers conducted promotional activities in organizations targeted for interventional and promotional activities. In conjunction with "magnet events" such as "Quit and Win" contests, The Great American Smokeout (GASO), and Non-Dependence Day, COMMIT staff members distributed event materials, solicited signups, displayed information, and conducted other activities such as carbon monoxide testing.

**Promotion
of Self-Help
Materials
and Cessation
Services**
Although activities and materials teaching the skills needed to quit smoking were already available in most communities, the COMMIT project sought to enhance the effectiveness and penetration of these cessation resources by directly targeting interventional organizations. Posters, flyers, brochures, pamphlets, and other information were delivered directly to organizations for distribution to their members who smoke. In addition, materials encouraged smokers to join the Smokers' Network. The network, created by COMMIT, was a voluntary list of smokers in each community who were interested in receiving mailings designed to provide information on how to quit smoking and remain smoke-free (see Chapter 8 [Lichtenstein and colleagues]).

**SUCCESSFUL EFFORTS
WITH COMMUNITY
ORGANIZATIONS**
Community groups already existed in most sectors of the community and, consequently, provided useful structures for enlisting smokers on the network, reaching diverse populations, and bringing about restrictive tobacco control policies and bans. To recruit smokers to COMMIT's Smokers' Network, communities enlisted the support of groups as diverse as the Girl Scouts of U.S.A., WIC providers, ethnic organizations, sports groups, and the American Red Cross. Activities ranged from health fairs, materials dissemination, and a "Butt-out Party," including a display of the domino effect of 720 cigarette packages. Diverse populations were reached through DARE in Bellingham, WA, the Puerto Rican Day Parade in Paterson, NJ, and food distribution at neighborhood health centers. Community grants also were given to various organizations to reach diverse populations in creative ways, thereby promoting cessation and maintenance. The Vallejo site provided a positive, high-energy experience in tobacco prevention and cessation through its

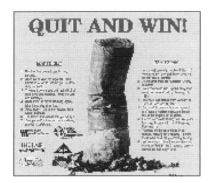

"African-Americans Celebrate Life" event. In sites that achieved restrictive tobacco control policies and bans (e.g., local ordinances banning vending machines), success resulted from the collaboration of tobacco control advocates with other coalitions, such as substance abuse prevention groups, community organizations such as the Boy Scouts of America, and police and health departments. Communities used sports and recreational events; for example, Utica, NY, disseminated a tobacco-free message to 1,500 fans of the Champion Boomerang Team in a "Throw Tobacco Out of Sports Campaign." Medford/Ashland and Bellingham each held a "Smoke-Free Night" with local baseball teams, and Yonkers, NY, promoted a "Nix to Nicotine" basketball game. Paterson held a rally against cigarette billboards in collaboration with the National Coalition of Negro Women.

Organizations involved in promotional activities included groups with a health orientation (e.g., American Red Cross, American Dietetic Association, American Chiropractic Society, community hospital auxiliaries), service and civic organizations (Big Brothers/Big Sisters, Hispanic Community Progress Foundation, Rotary Club, Soroptimists), and business and professional organizations (e.g., chambers of commerce, downtown merchants' associations, personnel directors' associations). Examples of their "promotional" involvements with COMMIT included assisting with the development of local tobacco control events; staffing the GASO and Tobacco Free Young America activities; generating publicity for smoking control efforts and specific events through meeting announcements, networking, newsletters, and bulletin boards; providing volunteers, local staff, and Board members for smoking control efforts; and providing other resources, advice, and expertise for the implementation staff.

In all sites, representatives of community organizations were integrally involved in local COMMIT planning, program design, and decisionmaking. Health-related organizations such as local health departments and health voluntary agencies, such as the American Cancer Society (ACS), ALA, and American Heart Association (AHA), played key roles in many communities. Members of civic and service clubs were mobilized to assume promotional roles as the project's leaders sought broader participation and outreach by citizens. From the outset COMMIT sought existing coalitions for health promotion or substance abuse prevention and joined with them or encouraged them to participate in COMMIT's efforts. In many communities, civic task forces and community coalitions that addressed drug-related issues were encouraged to add smoking control and educational efforts. In Brantford, Ontario, Canada, town forums were called to foster grassroots ideas and involvement in the initial stage of the project; these events also generated some volunteers for the project. In a few communities, COMMIT formally subcontracted with local organizations to carry out mandated activities, thereby capitalizing on a local agency's experience and creativity with, for instance, smoking cessation resources or media advocacy. In Utica, the Summer Youth Employment Program trained and employed young people from low-income families to counsel smokers to quit while those smokers were attending community centers (e.g., health clinics or WIC clinics) or community sponsored programs (e.g., blood pressure screening programs).

Cooperating with existing groups in public events was a creative way to foster partnership with the community as well as gain publicity. A youth theater group in Vallejo, eager for an opportunity to be involved, produced skits that humorously illustrated the fact that smoking is not at all glamorous or sophisticated. In Bellingham, COMMIT participants paraded publicly in

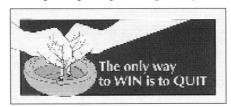

a turkey costume, to promote "quitting cold turkey," and in cigarette costumes in an annual parade. Vallejo and Medford/ Ashland used a Statue of Liberty and "Statue of Liberation from Tobacco" theme, one site for Halloween and the other for a Fourth of July parade. In Cedar Rapids/Marion, IA, Girl Scouts marched in a parade along with a COMMIT float, and the entry won second prize. Publicity through such activities may well have assisted in establishing the legitimacy of COMMIT efforts in the community as well as furthering smoking control goals.

COMMIT communities' successes included an "Adopt-A-Tavern" campaign, as in Bellingham and Fitchburg/Leominster, MA, in which volunteers became responsible for keeping taverns, bars, bowling alleys,

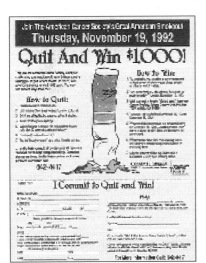

and other facilities where smoking is prevalent supplied with materials about tobacco control and cessation. Paterson found it beneficial to work through youth groups in religious organizations to get information about tobacco control to the entire membership.

The primary emphasis in COMMIT's other organizations arena was on large religious organizations. Although this was found by all communities to be a difficult channel, several experienced successes using a variety of innovative approaches. In Cedar Rapids/Marion, a coalition of representatives from the U.S. Attorney's Office, Substance Abuse Free Environment (SAFE) coalition, Iowa Substance Abuse Information Center, and COMMIT Cedar Rapids sponsored "Congregations for a Substance-Free Environment: A Conference for Clergy and Lay Leaders." The conference was attended by 150 people representing a broad spectrum of religious and ethnic groups. As one of the financial sponsors for this conference, COMMIT was able to contact difficult-to-reach organizations and encourage religious organizations and social service organizations to think of tobacco use as an addiction. Specifically, the conference asked attendees to consider the following issues: (1) tobacco as a drug along with alcohol and drugs, (2) the dangers of passive smoking, (3) the need for education and cessation interventions, (4) the establishment of smoke-free policies at places of worship as well as worksites, and (5) the continuing efforts of tobacco companies to thwart these efforts through extensive advertising. This event led to a half-day strategic planning conference to discuss possible interventions and a workshop to train ministers and lay leaders in intervention skills.

To involve churches in more than just the provision of self-help materials and information about local cessation resources, Paterson implemented a proactive "adopt-a-smoker" campaign aimed at nonsmoking church members who were asked to do the "morally right thing," that is, help someone in need: a smoker. Working through the Paterson Pastor's Workshop, an organization composed of about 32 area ministers, a "Smokeless Sabbath" program was initiated. It was a day of religious observance that would be declared by the congregation as a day during which smoking issues would be the focus of the sermon, educational materials would be disseminated, and available community resources would be identified.

COMMIT in Vallejo reported some success in this channel. An ecumenical focus group of local ministers was convened to develop strategies for effectively involving religious organizations in tobacco control. The focus group generated one consensus issue that they believed would be of universal concern to religious organizations: They did not want young people to start smoking. Based on shared information from recent research about tobacco use and youth, the clergy members recommended moving away from the "tired and worn" health education approach to tobacco prevention and suggested highlighting instead the youth-oriented marketing efforts of the tobacco industry (Fischer et al., 1991; DiFranza et al., 1991; Pierce et al., 1991). COMMIT staff members reported that once they understood churches' perceived role in promoting ethical standards among their congregations (and especially with youth), staff members were able to engage them in advocating against the tobacco industry marketing strategies. Staff members designed a biblically based curriculum using discussion and visual aids to encourage youth to discuss how to assess claims to truth made in tobacco advertising, how such marketing affects youth, the health effects of smoking, and potential advocacy opportunities to combat the efforts of the tobacco industry. The foundation for the 1-hour curriculum was the story of King Solomon's gift of wisdom that enabled him to discern right from wrong. The "Mission Possible: Target YOUth" curriculum was reviewed and approved by a panel of teachers, ministers, and health educators and is still being used in some Sunday school programs.

CHALLENGES ENCOUNTERED WITH COMMUNITY ORGANIZATIONS

The key process objective for this channel, making presentations to at least 30 percent of organizations targeted for intervention activities, was not achieved on a trialwide basis. The average across sites was 25 percent, and only four sites met the goal of 30 percent. Although one community succeeded in in reaching 52 percent of rostered organizations, two sites reached only 10 percent of the organizations. Problems were experienced by all the communities in using other organizations.

A few problems were linked to the protocol's definitions and specifications. For the initial 2 years of COMMIT's intervention phase, staff members across the 11 sites struggled with the protocol's nebulous distinction between interventional and promotional organizations. Definitional ambiguities across the trial were not resolved until late 1990. Gathering the necessary information for categorizing specific religious organizations was a burdensome task. Once designated as promotional, an organization may not have been targeted for attention until late in the intervention. Although it may have been logical to present an informational talk to a promotional organization before requesting cooperation or resources, staff members reported that such a step was often neglected because, by the protocol's mandates, only presentations to interventional organizations "counted" toward process objectives (see Table 3). Many communities expressed greater success, or greater optimism, only in the final year or two of the intervention period.

COMMIT's designers underestimated the difficulty COMMIT staff members and volunteers would experience in establishing contact with and gaining access to interventional organizations that were assumed to have smoking members. Although some activities were as simple as the delivery of cessation information and materials, many fraternal, service, and labor-related organizations such as the Elks, Lions, Masons, Veterans of Foreign Wars groups, and unions had no one onsite during business hours. In many organizations, access to meetings was restricted to members only. Often, it was only after repeated return visits that contact was established with a member or staff person. In at least one site, gatekeepers were then found to be protective of members who smoked and resistant to smoke-free policies or dissemination of cessation information. Many groups met only for social gatherings and business meetings and had no forum for outside speakers to present programs.

There were also multiple challenges in dealing with promotional organizations such as parent-teacher associations (PTAs), substance abuse prevention programs, and service clubs (e.g., Rotary, Lions, Soroptimists). These organizations were diverse, each with its own established mission and full agenda. Many did not perceive community tobacco control activities as a priority. Staff members typically found that getting to know organizations well was labor intensive, and they questioned the efficacy of the time spent making these contacts. Likewise, in many communities the ideas of reciprocity, linking with organizations' existing agendas, or expanding beyond a single-issue approach were not developed until late in the project. Finding a "hook" with which to involve organizations with COMMIT required knowledge of their missions and structures. One potential hook was to highlight concerns about youth (everyone wanted to help young people), but with COMMIT's focus on adult smokers, staff members and volunteers were reluctant to use children's issues as "bait."

COMMIT's most logical ally among community organizations was thought to be the health voluntaries (ACS, CCS, AHA, ALA), but experiences with them varied across sites. In six sites (Bellingham, Medford/Ashland, Fitchburg/Leominster, Santa Fe, NM, Paterson, and Yonkers), the local voluntaries were found to be struggling for volunteers and funds. In these sites COMMIT became responsible for the smoking problem and the local health voluntaries focused their resources on programs targeting other risk factors or diseases, such as breast cancer, high cholesterol, asthma, and tuberculosis. In a few communities where the voluntaries were strong, COMMIT Boards and staff members had to deal with competition, conflict-of-interest, and turf issues. Recruitment of volunteers for COMMIT through other organizations was sometimes viewed as competition in a shrinking community pool of potential volunteers. Four communities (Utica, Vallejo, Cedar Rapids/Marion, and Raleigh) contracted with or gave grants to the voluntaries to carry out some required activities. Developing requests for proposals and reviewing them, plus monitoring progress toward achieving process objectives, took a great deal of COMMIT staff time.

As the intervention progressed, several sites added community organizers to the staff to concentrate their efforts to achieve process objectives. Sites began to recognize that combining worksites and organizations under one task force was not effective because outreach to organizations tended to become a low priority on an already crowded task force agenda. The sheer numbers of organizations in some communities was daunting (see Table 2); for many staff members and volunteers, there seemed to be barely enough time to say hello as flyers and informational materials were delivered to organizations. Paterson set up a separate community task force to target this channel.

In the last 2 years of intervention, most COMMIT sites designed new strategies to reach heavy smokers. Although the protocol did not specifically target low-income, minority, or high-risk populations, there was a growing awareness of their importance as targets and messengers for tobacco control. Staff members and volunteers focused on agency settings such as employment offices, job training programs, WIC food voucher distribution clinics, American Red Cross blood drives, gospel mission shelters, and community centers serving minority populations. Special events were targeted at places smokers frequent, including outdoor sports stadiums, bowling alleys, bingo halls, and bars/taverns. At the same time communities used umbrella organizations such as human services coalitions, minority coalitions, and community action agencies to promote intervention activities.

Although some COMMIT communities experienced successes in working with their community's religious organizations, many reported facing a multitude of problems in forming partnerships with this sector. Pursuing clerics as intermediaries in smoking control seemed to be a natural course because bonds often are formed between congregations and clerics who are, in general, respected members of the community. However, many clergy were not receptive to COMMIT's attempts. For some, resistance was passive; clergy did not respond to verbal or written attempts to enlist their support. Others explained that tobacco control was not a priority issue. The Brantford site had an involved and helpful minister on the community Board, but as its final report stated, "even with his help" they were unable to "crack" religious organizations. Smoking was not common among parishioners, and it was not a priority issue.

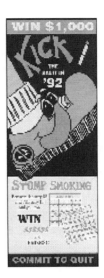

The failure of some clerics to view smoking as an important issue had several explanations. In some sites clerics immersed in the issue of substance abuse and other social problems did not acknowledge the connection between smoking and other drug use. Others felt that churchgoers were not involved in drug use. Often, staff members heard that smoking is not an issue because "no one smokes in church." Some who did acknowledge the problem of smoking and nicotine addiction resisted outside intervention efforts, relying on the religious organization to provide answers. Some clerics, especially smokers, expressed skepticism as to their ability to help people quit. Other reasons for resistance included the clergy's already taxing workload and an unwillingness to take on another burden or join one more community organization. Some congregations were concerned that implementing smoking policies would conflict with income-producing church functions such as wedding receptions and bingo games. One church was reluctant to implement a smoking policy for fear of alienating a church board member who smoked.

Resistance also was fostered by the diversity of religious denominations. In some communities religious organizations or clergy were responsive to umbrella organizations that often had different agendas. For example, in Yonkers, two of the four umbrella groups were involved in the city's struggle to introduce desegregated housing. In Cedar Rapids/Marion, plans for a clergy conference were complicated by competing events, including the actions of an ecumenical clergy group (spanning Christian denominations) that sought to exclude non-Christian faiths from participating in the planning committee and refused to change its name to an interfaith council.

Work with religious organizations relative to other efforts within COMMIT was often so labor intensive that staff members wondered whether results were worth the level of effort and resources invested. Because most

churches had few or no paid staff members, many attempts were made
to reach the cleric before receiving a response. In Medford/Ashland, staff
members reported that it took an average of six attempts before contact was
made. Staff members became frustrated with unreturned telephone calls
and having to leave messages on machines. When a staff person was reached,
he or she was frequently unwilling to act as a representative for the church.
At least two communities reported that some church staff members refused
to accept materials while the pastor was out.

Despite difficulties, communities continued to develop strategies to
include religious organizations in smoking control activities. In some
cases, task forces developed activities specifically to elicit clergy support
and address their issues. Based on feedback from a presentation to the clergy,
Yonkers COMMIT developed a seminar on addiction to educate clergy on

the problems of nicotine and other drug
addiction and to give them specific tools
for identifying and addressing this
problem. A planning committee
was established, and outreach efforts
were extensive; however, only two
clerics participated in planning the
event. The clergy's lack of response
prompted the committee to broaden
the seminar's focus to include other
community intermediaries as well as
the general public. In Raleigh, a
seminar incorporating nicotine with
substance abuse was designed for clergy.
Staff members felt challenged to keep
peace within planning meetings and
were disappointed by the limited clergy
turnout. Other issues arose regarding
the view by some major religious
denominations that alcohol and drug

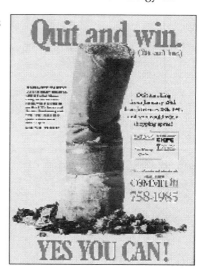

use is a sin; thus, an individual smoker's need for the church's help would be
viewed as an admission of sinning. Although a similar conference in Cedar
Rapids was mostly successful, staff members faced challenges in maintaining
the issue of tobacco use on the program because the conference planners and
audience had more interest in alcohol and drugs. Staff members had to
repeatedly remind the planning committee to include tobacco in each
part of the event.

Making presentations to church groups also proved to be challenging.
In Fitchburg/Leominster, three staff members repeatedly contacted religious
organizations to schedule presentations, with little response. In Medford/
Ashland, the community involvement coordinator focused much of her
energy on reaching clergy through presentations but had little return on
her time and effort. Similarly, in Yonkers, staff members devoted many
hours to reaching targeted churches but made minimal progress. Although

presentations were made at two meetings of the community's largest umbrella group, attendance was poor, and staff members felt that participants were merely being polite. At the second meeting, clergy admitted that smoking was not a priority issue; housing, desegregation, and substance abuse were their primary concerns. When offered suggestions for prohealth activities that would involve the congregation, attendees stated that they could only post informational and cessation materials. However, when following up on the attendees' willingness to display cessation information, staff members found that, in reality, few were willing to help.

Overall, COMMIT communities had to overcome many obstacles to accomplish objectives with religious organizations. Staff members and task forces often redefined objectives to make progress in enlisting support and involvement. Eventually, communities were gratified by even minimal successes, and project reports packaged these achievements in a positive light, perhaps to help maintain morale. Regardless of the individual experiences, staff members learned a valuable lesson in attempting to work with religious organizations on the issue of smoking control: Be prepared for a challenge.

EXPERIENCES WITH OTHER ORGANIZATIONS ACROSS THE COMMUNITIES

Overall, the community organizations channel was reported to be the most problematic, difficult, and frustrating of the intervention channels. In most instances even high levels of staff and volunteer effort did not produce much return on their investment. Communities were concerned that they did less well than they would have liked in reaching blue-collar workers, ethnic minority groups, and low-income smokers.

The development of relationships with existing organizations was a critical task at each site. Involving existing community organizations in the local definition, refinements, and governance of the project was a basic strategy for community mobilization in COMMIT, and community groups were a prime source of grassroots support, volunteers, and staff. Community groups provided an extensive network of local

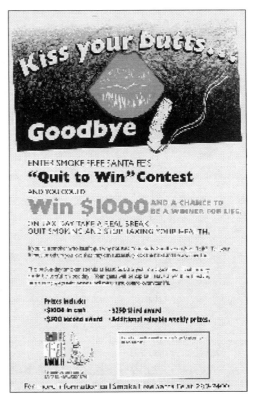

persons from multiple backgrounds and with a great variety of affiliations. Working with or joining existing organizations and coalitions was valued over creating new, competitive, or exclusive structures or replacing activities that were within another group's domain. However, gaining entree into much of the other organizations channel was inordinately time consuming for representatives of all the COMMIT communities. As several sites' final reports explicitly stated, community organizations may have been a more useful target for the dissemination of information than for direct involvement in activities. "The payoff isn't worth it," said Raleigh's report, "unless it's already part of their agenda. Otherwise the most impact you get is to become 'speaker of the week'" (Community Intervention Trial for Smoking Cessation, 1993a, p. 8). Medford/Ashland staff members summarized their experiences, "No real successes here" (Community Intervention Trial for Smoking Cessation, 1993b, p. 10), and Bellingham COMMIT said it was "never able to convince organizations to be concerned about this issue" (Community Intervention Trial for Smoking Cessation, 1993c, p. 2).

Why were so many organizations, across all the communities, difficult to penetrate? Some staff members speculate that they may have been besieged already with requests from nonprofit organizations and community causes. Organizational "gatekeepers" may have been protecting the organization from outsiders' requests. Some organizations were inaccessible by telephone or in person; presumably, some were without a paid staff, street address, regular office location, or telephone-answering machine. The meetings of some organizations included no forum open to outside speakers or issues. Most key organizations already had full agendas, and tobacco may not have been a logical add-on. COMMIT recognized also that smoking and health issues were often seen as unrelated to the group's purpose. The charter of organizations with regard to such issues varied widely, and whereas one group (e.g., the high school PTA) might have been eager to emphasize smoking control and prevention, another seemed to regard it as counterproductive interference with their principal objectives. Yet another organization might have seen smoking as irrelevant to their activities. Finally, and importantly, COMMIT brought a single-issue, time-limited mission into intervention communities that had many existing, longstanding organizations, and COMMIT was a new, "outsider" organization with no local history, name recognition, or promise of longevity.

Productive relationships required knowledge of organizations individually as well as existing coalitions, networks, and other umbrella organizations. To be successful, COMMIT intervention activities had to be congruent with the contexts and cultures of each community (Bracht and Gleason, 1990). Community analyses developed in the first months of the project (see Chapter 5 [Thompson and colleagues]) were essential sources of information for later programs (Bracht, 1988). They were based on review of media, secondary sources, and interviews with informants from the communities and described community organizations, leaders, and historical considerations that acted as potential facilitators of or barriers to COMMIT efforts. The trial also required that a local Community Planning Group be formed to nominate and recruit

COMMIT Board members. The planning group was to recruit members who were representative of the various key local organizations as well as to modify the community analysis so that good decisions about involving various groups could be made. However, the planning did not predict the amount of time and ongoing interpersonal interaction with organizations that most sites believed would have been essential to success in this channel.

The COMMIT protocol called for a Worksites and Organizations Task Force. The task force was a means of involving organizations in tailoring and implementing the specifics of intervention activities in the communities. The task force, under the direction and guidance of the COMMIT Board, prepared an annual action plan to specify how activities would be implemented in its community. In some communities, other groups were used or formed to target organizations more effectively. For instance, Vallejo drew on the community's minority coalition, and Paterson established a separate community task force.

Activities mandated by health promotion projects needed to be flexible, creative, and sensitive enough to reflect varied needs of diverse situations. Significant time and resources were needed to identify sites, develop creative ideas, and maintain individuals' involvement throughout the project with an issue whose relative priority was low to begin with or was threatened by other issues. Communities noted that being put on organizations' agendas was often difficult and labor intensive and staying on the agendas and producing results required ongoing "nurturing." Many organizations had no forum available for presentations on tobacco issues. Decisions had to be made about the level of participation to be solicited from different groups, taking into account the level of effort necessary for recruitment, training, and coordinating activities. In some situations, despite COMMIT staff members' allegiance to principles of cooperation and the enhancement of local resources, COMMIT was perceived by persons in other organizations as a competitor for local resources, such as volunteers or funding.

All communities found it useful to localize and tailor their approaches with community organizations based on the staff members' and task forces' knowledge of the group's goals, needs, structure, and general mode of operation. The level of participation solicited varied along a continuum of involvement from little to extensive and intensive. Between those poles were activities such as one-time involvement on a specific activity (e.g., posting flyers about the GASO on a bulletin board, speaking out at a city council meeting), to regular

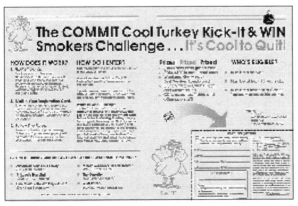

information dissemination (e.g., publishing notices each month about smoking cessation classes in the organization's bulletin), to central involvement in an event (e.g., designing and riding on a theme float in a parade), to an ongoing role on a task force.

Many organizations had little interest in participating in assessing needs, designing elements of the project, setting smoking control agendas, or otherwise taking on leadership roles. Their representatives may have had little experience with, understanding of, or interest in several optional activities around tobacco control or were not interested in adding another item to an already full agenda. However, many appeared to be comfortable with small roles in specific activities. A typical mode for addressing social issues that fell outside the organization was to respond to specific requests from other groups or people for concrete, time-limited help. Consequently, it was a sound, appropriate strategy for COMMIT task force members and their staffs to decide how they could best use the services of selected organizations and to make specific, direct requests of them.

Given the different nature, size, and history of communities and their associations, a major focus on a particular type of organization (e.g., religious organization) was deemed wise in some communities but not in others. For instance, in the COMMIT sites situated in metropolitan areas, the membership of some organizations contained many nonresidents, so targeting them for interventions was not thought to be as useful as emphasizing other organizations or even other intervention channels. For example, a community where a ministerial association already included innovators in church-based health promotion warranted a different approach and expectations than a community where major religious institutions were only marginally involved in communitywide social concerns or where competing agendas overwhelmed the attention of the leaders.

With only a few exceptions, the COMMIT communities questioned whether pursuing religious organizations as a means to reach smokers was a productive use of staff time and resources. A Cedar Rapids/Marion informant described churches as "the most difficult of the difficult" groups to reach, and a staff member from Raleigh said, "Forget them; they might not have been worth the effort." Field staff members in Brantford rated their religious organizations' involvement and use of resources as low and the difficulty of working with them as high. Although in these sites the field staffs attempted to maintain a minimum level of contact with these target groups, they often redirected energies to other channels where the anticipated effect was greater. For those communities able to overcome some obstacles, progress was made through hours of staff time and one-on-one contacts. The key to Vallejo's moderate success was reported to have been a staff person's being a practicing Christian. As that site reported, "Once religious organization leaders learned this, doors started to open." But just as having the right person among the staff members or volunteers was critical, so was finding the right counterpart in the religious organization.

Overall, few religious organizations were perceived by staff members to have participated in COMMIT's motivational, educational, or cessation activities. Attendance by representatives of religious organizations at workshops or seminars on smoking issues was reported to be low. A few religious organizations already prohibited smoking by members (e.g., Seventh-Day Adventists, Mormons), and some seemed to regard a smoking control focus as unnecessary, unless like some Seventh-Day Adventist congregations they regard tobacco control and education as part of their mission.

Special skills were needed by the COMMIT staff members charged with conducting mandated activities in the diverse organizations found in the sites. Knowledge was needed of current and past activities of local organizations in health and smoking issues and of organizations' histories of working with other groups. Staff members needed special skills for encounters and meetings with people of different education, class, and ethnic backgrounds, including chief executive officers, union representatives, blue-collar workers, grassroots activists, and representatives of ethnic groups. They needed to understand the benefits and problems of working with volunteers and to be able to work effectively with them. Staff members also needed to recognize that some citizens and organizations (e.g., unions, blue-collar smokers) objected to smoking control activities and had to be prepared to address these objections with clarity and sensitivity. They needed to attend to media coverage as well as promotional activities of local organizations. Staff members' efforts required creativity in tailoring or designing activities for local organizations and in enlisting support for promotional activities. They also needed to be committed to recruiting diverse persons and organizations, especially underserved groups and those with a high prevalence of heavy smokers.

RETHINKING HOW TO WORK WITH COMMUNITY ORGANIZATIONS
With the benefit of hindsight, what should or could have been done differently with community organizations? To meet its objectives, COMMIT needed to generate community recognition of, interest in, sanction for, and practical support of the project and its goals among all sectors. COMMIT required more time to nurture relationships with organizations, to address smoking appropriately within local and parent organizations, and to tailor activities to them. Community groups and organizations presented unique opportunities and stages for information dissemination and enhancement of project visibility in the community. Nevertheless, the consensus was that this was a time-consuming and often thankless channel where few "victories" occurred.

If the protocol were rewritten with the benefit of hindsight, the mandates for handling other organizations would need to define better which constellation of organizations and which specific organizations in the communities should have highest priority. Perhaps an innovative way to map and visualize community organizations and the sectors they serve could be developed, and the Program Records onsite data management system could be expanded to allow for better cross-referencing and tracking of organizations. That other organizations were linked with worksites in the Worksites and Organizations Task Force probably contributed to most communities' lesser emphasis on organizations through much of the trial. It may have been productive to tie organizations more explicitly to the Cessation Resources Task Force, or a task force dedicated only to organizations might be considered. Finally, the protocol's nature may have inhibited pursuit of some needed but neglected onsite activities. Concrete numbers specified in process objectives became targets, and the concern for evaluation data outcomes may have unwittingly driven decisions in the field. Although communities were encouraged to tailor the protocol to the local context, as one staff member said, "Instead, we let it creep in and color our thinking about the smoking problem. The protocol encouraged us to think like managers (civil servants) counting off numbers of organizations contacted instead of thinking like entrepreneurs, being creative about how to work effectively with those that might be most important to our success."

Experiences affirmed the need for fitting COMMIT's agenda and plans into those of targeted community organizations. To implement activities for COMMIT's other organizations channel, special skills, information, creativity, and access to expertise were needed. This included information about the structure, goals, formal and informal modes of operation, means of economic support, management practices, governing bodies, and decisionmaking mechanisms of diverse individual organizations. Activities may be more effectively and efficiently implemented when there is a period of ongoing involvement during which trust can be built, when there is regular attendance at community events, and when collaboration among participants and of agendas occurs between organizations.

COMMIT staff members and volunteers found that having a person supportive of COMMIT's goals working inside a community organization was useful. The personal ties of task force, Board, and staff members with leaders in other organizations opened many doors. Where these bonds did not already exist, entrée often required a high personal investment of time and energy, commodities that were sometimes in short supply.

In working with religious organizations, communities usually proceeded from the assumption that the largest, most prominent religious organizations in communities should be the primary targets for COMMIT because they had the greatest potential for affecting the most people. In hindsight, a better strategy would have been to initially target the religious organization with which a staff or task force member had a personal affiliation or which had a clergy member known in the community for social activism involvement in health promotion. Where it is determined that religious organizations should be brought into smoking cessation and control activities, emphasis should be placed on strategies for reaching and engaging them.

Discussions late in the project with Christian clerics in COMMIT-related focus groups generated suggestions for approaching religious organizations with tobacco control messages. Two key variables emerged: (1) moral codes regarding smoking and (2) the size of the organization. First, churches with strong moral codes (i.e., smoking regarded as a "sin" and unlikely to be discussed openly by smokers) should be approached with an outreach ministerial program to offer to other family members, friends, or coworkers. The basic assumption is that although the church members may not smoke, they may live next to, work with, or know people who do. The program can focus on how individuals can help others quit smoking. In churches without clear moral codes around smoking and where smoking is often allowed during social gatherings, the approach of having a smoke-free activity and offering an educational program around passive or secondhand smoke can be used. In such a setting it would then be possible to offer self-help materials and possibly a smoking cessation class. Given that a program taking place in a religious organization already has a certain moral tone, care should be taken to ensure that any smoke-free message be as positive and nonblaming as possible. In developing a program for any size church (moral code or not), a packaged approach would be best. If the message is directed toward youth, prevention education programs can be offered to both types of churches during Sunday School or youth education classes.

Second, church size and type should inform program implementation. For the purposes of developing intervention strategies, knowledge of the relationship between the size and characteristics of religious organizations would be useful. Local church leaders readily supply ideas of categories and critical features of different organizations, as in Vallejo where a focus group generated a set of types, including family churches, pastoral churches, program churches, and corporate churches. A shortage of research in this area precludes firm recommendations, but it is important that approaches to churches be carefully tailored to general and local considerations.

Seminars and workshops designed to attract representatives of diverse organizations should address topics relevant to them, based on careful needs assessment and groundwork. If tobacco is not immediately recognized as an important issue, it may be more productive to add it to whatever agenda is already a central theme in the organization, whether family life, substance abuse, or social outreach.

Was specifically targeting community and civic organizations, clubs, churches, and other local associations for interventional activities worth the substantial effort involved? Significant problems were reported in every community. Given the limited resources and the competing priorities of other trial activities, it remains unclear whether the energy needed to mobilize these diverse groups was well spent.

In sum, the other community organizations channel was more nebulous and equivocal in COMMIT than the more conventional channels relating to health care, worksites, cessation resources, and the media. It may have considerable potential for targeting smokers, reinforcing smoking control messages and policies in the wider community, and disseminating smoking cessation information, but strategies for efficient and effective cooperation still need work.

REFERENCES

Bracht, N. Community analysis precedes community organization for cardiovascular disease prevention. *Scandinavian Journal of Primary Health Care* August (Suppl 1): 23-30, 1988.

Bracht, N., Gleason, J. Strategies and structures for citizen partnership. In: *Health Promotion at the Community Level*, N. Bracht (Editor). Newbury Park, CA: Sage, 1990, pp. 109-124.

Carlaw, R.W., Mittlemark, M.B., Bracht, N., Luepker, R. Organization for a community cardiovascular health program: Experiences from The Minnesota Heart Health Program. *Health Education Quarterly* 11: 243-252, 1984.

Community Intervention Trial for Smoking Cessation. "COMMIT Intervention Final Report." Raleigh, NC, site, 1993a.

Community Intervention Trial for Smoking Cessation. "Final Report for Project Archives and Quarterly Report (PAQR)." Medford/Ashland, OR, site, 1993b.

Community Intervention Trial for Smoking Cessation. "COMMIT Final Report." Bellingham, WA, site, 1993c.

Corbett, K., McGranaghan, R., Sorensen, G., Glasgow, R. "The Secular, the Sacred, and Smoking Control: Reflections on COMMIT's Findings on Churches." Paper presented at the annual meeting of the American Public Health Association, Atlanta, GA, November 1991.

Corbett, K., Thompson, B., White, N., Taylor, M. Process evaluation in the Community Intervention Trial for Smoking Cessation (COMMIT). *International Quarterly of Community Health Education* 11(3): 291-309, 1990-91.

Cuoto, R.A. Promoting health at the grass roots. *Health Affairs* 9(2): 144-151, 1990.

DePue, J.D., Wells, B.L., Lasater, T.M., Carleton, R.A. Training volunteers to conduct heart health programs in churches. *American Journal of Preventive Medicine* 3(10): 51-57, 1987.

DiFranza, J.R., Richards, J.W., Paulman, P.M., Wolf-Gillespie, N., Fletcher, C., Jaffe, R.D., Murray, D. RJR Nabisco's cartoon camel promotes Camel cigarettes to children. *Journal of the American Medical Association* 266(22): 3149-3153, 1991.

Elder, J.P., Sallis, J.F., Jr., Mayer, J.A., Hammond, N., Pelinski, S. Community-based health promotion: A survey of churches, labor unions, supermarkets, and restaurants. *Journal of Community Health* 14(3): 159-168, 1989.

Emory University, Carter Center and Park Ridge Center. *Healthy People 2000: A Role for America's Religious Communities. A Joint Publication of the Carter Center of Emory University and the Park Ridge Center for the Study of Health, Faith, and Ethics.* Chicago: Park Ridge Center, 1990.

Eng, E., Hatch, J., Callan, A. Institutionalizing social support through the church and into the community. *Health Education Quarterly* 12(1): 81-92, 1985.

Fischer, P.M., Schwartz, M.P., Richards, J.W., Jr., Goldstein, A.O., Rojas, T.H. Brand logo recognition by children aged 3 to 6 years. *Journal of the American Medical Association* 266(22): 3145-3148, 1991.

Foege, W. The vision of the possible: What churches can do. *Second Opinion: Health, Faith, and Ethics* 13: 36-42, 1990.

Hatch, J., Moss, N., Saran, A., Presley-Cantrell, L., Mallory, C. Community research: Partnership in black communities. *American Journal of Preventive Medicine* 9(6)[Suppl]: 27-31, 1993.

Hatch, J.W., Johnson, C.N. Carolina Baptist Church program. *Urban Health* 10: 70-71, 1981.

Hatch, J.W., Lovelace, K.A. Involving the southern rural church and students of the health professions in health education. *Public Health Reports* 95: 23-25, 1980.

Lasater, T.M., Wells, B.L., Carleton, R.A., Elder, J.P. The role of churches in disease prevention research studies. *Public Health Reports* 101(2): 125-131, 1986.

Levin, J.S. The role of the black church in community medicine. *Journal of the National Medical Association* 26: 477-483, 1984.

Lichtenstein, E., Wallack, L., Pechacek, T. Introduction to the Community Intervention Trial for Smoking Cessation. *International Quarterly of Community Health Education* 11(3): 173-185, 1990-91.

Mattson, M.E., Cummings, K.M., Lynn, W.R., Giffen, C., Corle, D., Pechacek, T. Evaluation plan for the Community Intervention Trial for Smoking Cessation. *International Quarterly of Community Health Education* 11(3): 271-290, 1990-91.

Nickens, H.W. Health promotion and disease prevention among minorities. *Health Affairs* 9(2): 133-143, 1990.

Pierce, J.P., Gilpin, E., Burns, D.M., Whalen, E., Rosbrook, B., Shopland, D., Johnson, M. Does tobacco advertising target young people to start smoking? *Journal of the American Medical Association* 266(22): 3154-3158, 1991.

Princeton Religious Research Center. *Religion in America, 1992/1993 Report*. Princeton, NJ: Princeton Religious Research Center, 1993.

Roncarati, D.D., Lefebvre, R.C., Carleton, R.A. Voluntary involvement in community health promotion: The Pawtucket Heart Health Program. *Health Promotion* 4(1): 11-18, 1989.

Saunders, E., Knog, B.W. A role of churches in hypertension management. *Urban Health* 12: 49-55, 1983.

Shea, S. Community health, community risks, community action. *American Journal of Public Health* 82(6): 785-787, 1992.

Smith, D.H. Churches are generally ignored in contemporary voluntary action research: Causes and consequences. *Review of Religious Research* 24: 295-303, 1983.

Sorensen, G., Glasgow, R., Corbett, K. Involving worksites and other organizations. In: *Health Promotion at the Community Level*, N. Bracht (Editor). Newbury Park, CA: Sage, 1990, pp. 158-184.

Stillman, F.A., Bone, L.R., Rand, C., Levine, D.M., Becker, D. Heart, body, and soul: A church-based smoking cessation program for urban African-Americans. *Preventive Medicine* 22: 335-349, 1993.

Thompson, B., Wallack, L., Lichtenstein, E., Pechacek, T. Principles of community organization and partnership for smoking cessation in the Community Intervention Trial for Smoking Cessation. *International Quarterly of Community Health Education* 11(3): 187-203, 1990-91.

Wiist, W.H., Flack, J.M. A church-based cholesterol education program. *Public Health Reports* 105(4): 381-388, 1990.

AUTHORS

Kitty K. Corbett, Ph.D., M.P.H.
Adjunct Investigator
Division of Research
Kaiser Permanente Medical Care Program
3505 Broadway
Oakland, CA 94611
and
Assistant Professor
Health and Behavioral Sciences, CB-103
Department of Anthropology
University of Colorado at Denver
P.O. Box 173364
Denver, CO 80217

Linda Nettekoven, M.A.
Project Coordinator
Oregon Research Institute
1715 Franklin Boulevard
Eugene, OR 97403

Linda C. Churchill, M.S.
Project Director
Department of Preventive and Behavioral
    Medicine
University of Massachusetts Medical
    School
Room S-7, 746
55 Lake Avenue North
Worcester, MA 01655

Lesa T. Dalton
Project Director
Division of Health Promotion Research
American Health Foundation
Fifth Floor
800 Second Avenue
New York, NY 10017

Carolyn L. Johnson, R.N.
Program Manager
Healthy Start Program
Jackson County Department of Health and
    Human Services
Building A
1005 East Main Street
Medford, OR 97504

Lysha Dickinson
Research Associate/Project Coordinator
Division of Research
Kaiser Permanente Medical Care Program
3505 Broadway
Oakland, CA 94611

Glorian Sorensen, Ph.D., M.P.H.
Associate Professor
Department of Epidemiology and Cancer
    Control
Dana Farber Cancer Institute
Harvard School of Public Health
44 Biney Street
Boston, MA 02115

Beti Thompson, Ph.D.
Associate Professor
University of Washington School of Public
    Health and Community Medicine
Associate Member
Fred Hutchinson Cancer Research Center,
    MP-702
1124 Columbia Street
Seattle, WA 98104

Promoting Communitywide Tobacco Control Activities by Involving Schools

Deborah Bowen, Lesa T. Dalton, Rosemary Walker, Susan Crystal, and Mario A. Orlandi

INTRODUCTION   Tobacco use among youth is a critical public health problem. National surveys from high school classes from 1975 to 1990 indicate that smoking rates among adolescents had not declined in comparison with adult smoking rates (Johnston et al., 1991). Recently, rates of lifetime use, use in the past 30 days, and half-pack daily use have not declined from 1991 and 1992 to 1993 among 8th, 10th, and 12th graders (National Institute on Drug Abuse, 1994). Trends in smoking prevalence among high school seniors of both sexes are presented in Figure 1. These data indicate clearly that cigarette use rates among adolescents have changed little over the past decade and also suggest that smoking could be on the increase among those in this age group. Similar findings have been reported by others, including reports in a series of nationally representative estimates of smoking among U.S. youth ages 12 to 18 conducted by the U.S. Public Health Service since 1968 (U.S. Department of Health and Human Services, 1994). The trend for teens is directly opposite that for adults, whose smoking rates have declined steadily among both men and women since the mid-1970's (Shopland, 1995).

The data presented in Figure 1 represent an older, in-school population and do not include those youth who dropped out of school before their senior high school year and who have higher smoking rates than those who stay in school. Thus, the magnitude of the youth smoking problem is likely to be higher than the figures for high school students suggest. The lack of progress in reducing youth tobacco use on a national level has led researchers and community health experts to search for opportunities to influence youth smoking behavior. The Community Intervention Trial for Smoking Cessation (COMMIT) has provided several of these opportunities. This chapter describes COMMIT intervention activities to reduce youth tobacco use that were connected with schools. It describes the rationale for including youth and schools in COMMIT and the intervention and evaluation strategies related to schools. It also includes the field experiences in implementing the school-based youth tobacco use interventions and discusses some of the lessons learned about working with schools in the hope that the knowledge of those experiences might help others working with school-based public health tobacco programs.

Rationale for Including Youth in COMMIT   As discussed in Chapter 2, the main goal of COMMIT is cessation among adults who are heavy smokers, with the primary intervention targets being adult smokers who smoke more than 25 cigarettes per day. The initial reaction of investigators to including youth as a focus within COMMIT was that it was inappropriate. Youth are not

Figure 1

**Prevalence of daily smoking among high school seniors, by gender, 1976-93—
percentage smoking one or more cigarettes per day during previous 30 days**

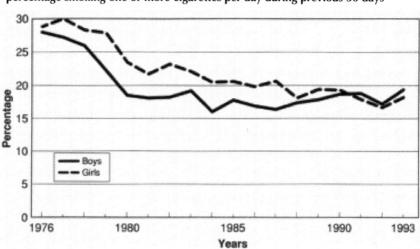

Source: Lynch and Bonnie, 1994.

likely to be found in the target group (i.e., heavy smokers) of COMMIT.
Many members of the steering committee thought that including a focus on
youth would detract from the focus on adults and on heavy smokers. Some
further thought that all available resources should be spent on heavy smokers
and that there were not enough funds for targeting youth. Over time, the
scientific groups realized that COMMIT would enhanced the likelihood of
change in the communities by including youth, so a youth intervention
and evaluation component was added.

The decision to broaden the intervention and evaluation targets to
include youth was based on several arguments. First, it was hoped that
youth could serve as a conduit to reach heavy smokers. Anecdotal evidence
from school-based smoking prevention programs indicates that many
parents are pressured to quit by their children. There is a consistently
positive relationship between parent and youth smoking, indicating that
influencing youth smokers may help reach adult smokers. It was hoped
that targeting youth would prove an additional source of both pressure
on and encouragement for heavy smokers to quit. Second, and equally
important, it was hoped that communitywide intervention targeting adults,
especially heavy smokers, would increase awareness of smoking as a public
health problem among young people and those who deal with them in their
daily activities. Such awareness could reduce youth smoking as well. If adults
are actively involved in trying to quit smoking, they might present smoking
in a negative light to their children and other youth. This could result in

fewer adolescents starting to smoke. In a larger perspective, youth as well as adults should be aware of several components of the COMMIT intervention, including communitywide media intervention, advertising bans, and interventions in public places. These communitywide interventions theoretically should change community norms about smoking and make it more difficult for youth to begin using tobacco.

Rationale for Recommending School-Based Interventions in COMMIT Schools are an excellent channel for reaching youth and have received much research attention. There is an extensive body of knowledge about the most efficacious school-based smoking prevention curriculum to implement at the junior high school level (Flay et al., 1983). School-based curriculum programs have been evaluated in previous vigorous research programs and are widely available. There is evidence that these programs have consistent short-term effects (Best et al., 1988) and therefore should form part of a comprehensive communitywide effort to reduce smoking. Many schools across the country have mandates to include or mention smoking as part of general health education or drug abuse prevention, although this varies by region and locale. However, few schools provide focused attention and curriculum time to tobacco control without guidance and support from experts, and it is in this expert role that COMMIT staff members could collaborate with schools to implement appropriate curricula.

School policy regarding tobacco, and subsequent policy enforcement, is another area of school-based intervention, with support for efficacy in preventing onset. Policy alters health behavior when the policy is clearly and simply stated, when it is fairly and consistently enforced, and when the means for following it are available to all whom it affects (Sabatier and Mazmanian, 1979). Most COMMIT schools had a policy limiting smoking in some fashion (Bowen et al., in press). Many schools had a smoking area or allowed smoking outside the school building. However, few schools disseminated the policy clearly, enforced it consistently, or provided full resources for students to follow it. The limited data on the effects of policy on smoking rates indicate that school policy, when clearly stated and enforced in a positive manner rather than a punitive one, is related to lower levels of youth smoking (Penz et al., 1989).

Youth are essentially a captive audience at school for several hours per day. To affect youth smoking it is essential that the school be used as a channel for providing clear, strong messages against smoking and other tobacco use. Policies involving no smoking on school grounds or at school events could be one strong message, provided it is enforced and supported. Other ways to provide messages at school include the policies that govern teachers' smoking behavior. Community activities that involve youth in the planning or the activities are appropriate for increasing the visibility of smoking as a social problem. COMMIT interventions attempted to include all these strategies in their arsenal.

INTERVENTION ACTIVITIES AND PROCESS OBJECTIVES FOR SCHOOLS   The goals for this channel were to (1) increase the percentage of public schools that are tobacco-free, (2) increase the percentage of heavy smokers in the community who perceive social pressure from their children to quit smoking, and (3) decrease the prevalence of smoking among youth. To achieve those objectives, several mandated activities (see Table 1) were developed. The interventions were based on the previously cited literature on school-based intervention where available (e.g., Glynn, 1989 [see below]). Where other information was not available, interventions were based on examples of tobacco-related youth activities that, in the experience of the intervention teams, had been successful in involving youth. The major strategies are described below.

Curriculum Initiatives   Each site was given several resources to encourage schools to initiate tobacco use prevention curricula in schools or to improve on existing efforts. These included an article by Thomas Glynn, then program director for smoking research at the National Cancer Institute, called "Essential Elements of School-Based Smoking Prevention Programs" (Glynn, 1989), which discussed strategies within existing programs that seem most critical for successful smoking prevention packages, including prices, descriptions, and ordering information. The field staff members at each site were encouraged to use these and other available materials.

School Policy   Policy changes of all types were a major focus of COMMIT, in keeping with the community and public health nature of the intervention focus. Influencing school policies on smoking was thought to be different from influencing State or community law about smoking because of the process by which organizations such as schools make decisions about their internal rules and functioning. However, some COMMIT communities sought to make changes in school policy at the State level (e.g., Oregon). Although knowing that clear, enforced school smoking policies could prevent tobacco use, COMMIT staff members used care in coming from outside the school system to alter policy. To promote policies, many communities used a manual created by the National School Board Association on creating

Table 1
Activities and process objectives for schools

Activities for Each Community	Cumulative Objectives (1988-1992) (%)	Process Objectives Achieved[a] (%)
Distribute Smoking Policy Materials to School Boards	100	94
Annually Contact Schools Not Smoke-Free	100	96
Provide Tobacco Curriculum Information to Educators	85	104

[a] *Average for combined communities.*

212

and implementing school policies. This well-written manual includes a description of types of nonsmoking policies, methods of deciding on and implementing the policies, examples of policies that have been implemented and all the supporting legal and other documents used in the implementation process, and a list of school districts nationally that were willing to provide technical assistance. Again, COMMIT field staff members were encouraged to use these documents to assist schools in forming strong, restrictive tobacco use policies.

School-Based Activities That Target Youth   Other activities involving schools were not clearly defined in a protocol and were left up to the field staff and schools to negotiate. These included using schools to publicize community events involving youth and recruiting youth from schools to help with covert tobacco-buying adventures (see Chapter 13). The accessibility of youth through schools enabled many community-based activities to involve youth more fully.

School Activities That Target Adults   Youth were used as a conduit to reach the adults in their lives, both passively and actively. The school student is a conduit for information to smokers or potential smokers at home. Young people can be organized into groups to seek out and recruit adults into antismoking activities. These adults can be relatives, other community members, or even members of the press, who can send a powerful message about smoking's harm. COMMIT interventionists were encouraged to consider using youth to "hook" adults whenever they could.

IMPLEMENTING SCHOOL-BASED INTERVENTIONS

Community Board Membership   In many of the 11 COMMIT intervention sites, community Boards included representation from the education sector, such as district personnel (e.g., superintendents, assistant superintendents), health educators specializing in drug abuse prevention, teachers, and parent-teacher association (PTA) members. Although sites with school gatekeepers (i.e., those who could "open doors" to individuals) on their Boards expected to have fairly easy access to the school system, that was not necessarily the case. Some sites were hampered by uncooperative key contacts whose individual personalities or smoking status created difficulties in working with the schools. At sites with school decisionmakers in a COMMIT leadership role, there was occasional conflict between the task force and the Board over youth or school activities, thus reducing some of the task force's autonomy. In one site this occurred so frequently that the uncooperative COMMIT member was bypassed whenever possible by directly approaching the targeted schools or teachers to plan activities.

Boards were generally enthusiastic about youth activities and, in particular, activities with an educational focus. However, there was criticism from Boards about the protocol's minimal focus on youth tobacco use prevention education. Project staff members often struggled to explain the reasoning behind the protocol's relatively minimal focus on youth activities and to involve schools in cessation activities. Activities like the American Heart Association's (AHA) Save a Sweet Heart (SASH) campaign were embellished to increase their educational focus; for example, in some sites teachers were given educational materials for classroom use.

Task Force   Youth and school activities fell under the jurisdiction of the public education task force; however, a few sites divided the public education task force into a media task force and a youth task force, thereby creating five task forces to carry out COMMIT activities in those communitites. Many communities formed formal subcommittees within the public education task force to carry out youth- or school-based activities and planned activities under their general task force agendas; other sites established ad hoc subcommittees. Many sites had some school personnel representation on task forces or subcommittees, although these individuals were not necessarily decisionmakers. Even individuals holding high-level positions within the school system often acted more as liaisons to COMMIT than as representatives of the schools. In sites where there was no school representation on the task force, planning for activities that were either promoted or conducted through the schools was complicated; task forces had to negotiate several tiers of decisionmakers to obtain approval for implementation. Some sites established separate task forces comprising youth. These task forces then took on the responsibility of ensuring that mandated and other activities within schools were implemented.

Volunteers   Teachers, guidance and peer assistance counselors, school nurses, PTA members, students, and others played key roles in implementing school-based youth activities. Volunteerism was essential for implementing policy initiatives, "magnet events," and promotional activities within the schools. Without the dedication and enthusiasm of these volunteers, task forces would have had little support for implementing or promoting activities for youth within the complex structure of most sites' school systems. Volunteers from the schools were also essential when youth attempted to recruit adults into programs, as was done in New York in Yonkers' second "Quit and Win" contest and other campaigns.

In addition, volunteers played a key role in promoting school-based youth activities. For instance, in Brantford, Ontario, Canada, teachers were supportive of a poster campaign based on the themes "How to get your friends to quit smoking." They incorporated the campaign into a classroom activity and made nominations for a poster contest. Many students in grades 1 through 8 entered the contest, and the 18 winners of free tickets to the Toronto Blue Jays baseball game on "World No Tobacco Day" arrived in chauffeured limousines. In Yonkers, teachers were instrumental in the implementation of two annual "No Proof, No Puffs" campaigns within the schools. These campaigns focused on activities to encourage stores to ask for age identification before selling tobacco products to adolescents. Teachers who are also COMMIT volunteers worked with staff and students to incorporate smoking prevention and cessation education into classroom activities. The first year, after writing to local area merchants, students went with their teachers from store to store to deliver their letters and other information regarding legislation on youth access to tobacco. The second year, teachers helped students write letters to merchants about youth access and to magazine publishers asking them to stop accepting tobacco advertisements. There were other classroom activities on the issues of smoking, and teachers developed a "Smoke-Free for a Week Partnership" campaign in which students encouraged the adults of their choice to quit smoking for a week. In all these examples, volunteer support provided the mechanism for educating youth and helped to foster good will for tobacco control efforts throughout the community because of the publicity these activities received.

Other types of volunteer support included stuffing envelopes, staffing booths, distributing survival kits, disseminating materials, and promoting activities. Sometimes gatekeepers provided access for volunteer support by appointing staff members within the schools to assist with a given activity or by identifying personnel interested in smoking control activities. Gatekeepers also helped COMMIT by directing staff

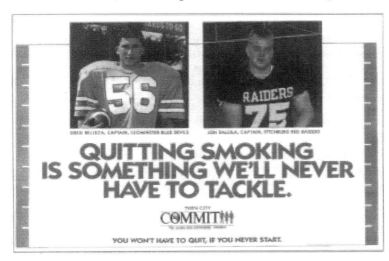

or task forces through appropriate channels for implementing smoking control activities within the schools. At other times, staff members and task forces enlisted volunteers through personal and professional contacts.

PATTERNS OF SCHOOL-BASED INTERVENTIONS

The types of activities implemented by COMMIT interventionists that focus on schools are summarized in Table 2. This list of activities was obtained from quarterly reports submitted by each study center (Corbett et al., 1990-91). This table does not represent all activities for each community but only the most salient for the data collection staff. The four categories (activities For Youth, To Influence Youth, Involving Youth, and Through Youth) represent the four common methods of targeting youth, each with different purposes, potential efficacy, and commitment of staff and other resources.

Intervention Activities

The first category of activities, For Youth, included those types of activities that were relatively easy to do and included information provided to students in the context of an existing meeting, class, or structure. Many schools produced displays about smoking and quitting. Curricula were

Table 2
Types of youth-related activities in COMMIT

For Youth	To Influence Youth	Involving Youth	Through Youth
School displays	School policies	Art, theater	Outreach to other youth
Classes/curricula	Teacher exposure	Special events	Outreach to adults
Substance abuse focus	School staff exposure	Advertising	
Events during school	Public statements	Contests	
Events after school	Resources		
Social events	Projects		

offered as part of health or physical education classes. Although COMMIT sites were mandated to provide state-of-the-art educational materials to schools, there was little opportunity for task forces and staff members to work one on one with educators to expand this activity beyond the mandated material dissemination process. Most sites were able merely to supply their school district with curriculum materials. However, some States like Iowa and Massachusetts held teacher training workshops, or as in Brantford, staff members were given the opportunity to schedule a workshop. Many times these curricula were integrated with a drug abuse prevention program, such as Drug Awareness Resistance Education (DARE) or SASH. For example, in Yonkers field staff members worked with the AHA and the Yonkers Pulse Healthy Heart Project to disseminate educational packets promoting SASH to more than 12,000 students' homes. The packets contained interactive materials for parents to use in talking about smoking with their children, AHA SASH pledge cards to quit smoking for a specified time, activity sheets, and COMMIT smoker registration cards in English or Spanish. Students were asked to encourage their smoking parents to return the registration cards by mail. In addition, part of the intervention was to have parents and students work on the activities together at home, and students were expected to bring completed sheets back to school for class discussion. Unfortunately, few smoker registration cards were returned through the mail, and few activity sheets were returned through the schools.

However, COMMIT staff members were able to work onsite with SASH youth volunteers and student assistance counselors at information booths in the schools on SASH days. Staff members performed expired carbon monoxide testing on adult smokers; distributed self-help brochures, cessation guides, and survival kits; and registered some faculty and school personnel in the Smokers' Network.

As a result of these efforts, the issue of smoking is permanently integrated into a community organization in the form of sessions, movies, and ongoing discussions. Events that occurred during or after school hours, such as assemblies and club meetings, were used as vehicles for getting word about smoking to youth. Speakers at classes and gatherings were included to emphasize a motivating aspect of quitting smoking. Social activities, such as adopt-a-younger-student days and career days, were used to include an antismoking message. Special antismoking activities, such as puppet shows, rallies, and theater presentations, were used to increase awareness about smoking in an enjoyable and entertaining manner.

The second category of activities, To Influence Youth, was conducted on the social and environmental structures that can promote or reduce smoking in the youth environment. Contact with teachers was used as a consistent way to indirectly influence youth. Teachers attended special COMMIT-led training sessions as an in-service requirement and received advice from COMMIT staff on the choice of curricula and other teaching devices. Other school personnel and youth-oriented staff members were exposed to COMMIT messages via staff discussion, training, and encouragement. Counselors at schools received special training in helping students quit smoking. PTAs and school boards received presentations and encouragement from COMMIT staff. Officials from schools were encouraged to take a public stand on the problem of tobacco use. Coaches at schools and in the community were urged to treat tobacco use as a health problem. Several local restrictions on access, including 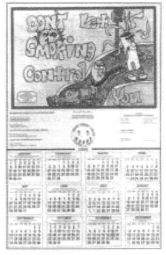 sales to minors, were organized first through schools and school personnel. Enforcement of existing school policies with positive supportive approaches and penalties was encouraged. These broadbrush intervention strategies probably helped to reach students who would not have been reached by the more traditional curriculum-based interventions.

The third category of activities, Involving Youth, involved youth as players in the planning or execution of the activity. Several different types of art projects and drama projects were developed, written, staged, or played by youth as part of class or school projects. Contests were held to get the messages of COMMIT out to youth, including contests in art, kite making, floats, athletics, essays, rap music, and photographs. In addition, youth in several communities attempted to counter the tobacco companies by creating counteradvertising. These activities often were sponsored by COMMIT staff, but young people were asked to plan and create the activities and often became involved in the final products.

Finally, for the fourth category of activities, Through Youth, young people served as a conduit to other youth groups and to adult heavy smokers. Individual COMMIT sites used this option in different ways. For example, some sites distributed cessation flyers and materials for youth to take home to give to family and community members. Some sites organized youth to speak to other young people, often to groups of younger or disadvantaged youth. Some sites had youth recruit and enroll adult smokers in the COMMIT Smokers' Network. Students wrote to local officials, tobacco companies, and their school personnel. Most sites found youth willing to participate actively in helping others to stop smoking.

Successes and Failures Across Communities   In general, communities wanted to do more in prevention than the protocol provided for; in fact, in many communities task force members were more interested in prevention than cessation and had difficulty understanding why the project did not have a stronger prevention focus. Communities thought that youth are important as a channel to reach adult smokers. Youth also provided a channel to the media when they were involved in newsworthy activities.

Most sites found schools to be fairly difficult to work with compared with other groups in the community. Field directors believed that a comprehensive approach was needed to involve schools, which COMMIT did not have a clear mission to provide. The amount of effort for COMMIT staff members to get schools involved varied from site to site, ranging from one site reporting that it took little effort to three sites reporting that it took a great deal of effort. The tendency of schools to leave tasks to the COMMIT staff was not as great as that of some other groups, but this also varied greatly from site to site. The extent to which schools used COMMIT information was high, with nearly half the sites reporting they used it a lot.

Schools collaborated willingly with COMMIT at most sites. Often, they showed some ownership of COMMIT activities or the project as a whole. Several sites found that schools showed innovation in implementing or institutionalizing COMMIT activities. There was considerable variation in the extent to which schools showed leadership or creativity in designing activities. There was also considerable variation in the provision of resources; several sites reported that schools provided many resources and in-kind donations, especially for poster contests and flyers, whereas other sites reported that few resources were provided.

Two communities had smokers on the school board who opposed smoke-free school policies. In one community, this barrier was not overcome. In the other, a COMMIT letter to the editor in a local newspaper initiated a public dialog that resulted in the policy's being implemented successfully. When no-smoking policies were implemented, schools in some communities became more amenable to COMMIT activities. For instance, in Brantford the school board enlisted COMMIT's assistance in handling the logistics of implementing its new smoke-free buildings policy. Oregon held a successful school and law enforcement summit following the passage of an antismoking ordinance.

Some communities felt constrained in their approach to schools, either because there were limited entry points to schools—they required a formal approach through appropriate administrative channels—or because other groups already were involved in selecting and providing school smoking curricula.

An Example of a Successful Youth Activity Brantford held a poster contest with the theme "How to get your friends to quit smoking" in early 1991. There were 18 prizes—tickets to a Toronto Blue Jays baseball game on World No Tobacco Day—with the winners to be driven to the game by limousine. Two prizes were allocated for each grade (1 through 8), and two prizes were to be allocated by a random draw from early entrants. On the advice of a task force member, prizes were awarded randomly as opposed to through a judging process. Task force members obtained the necessary school board approval, with the assistance of two COMMIT Board members (an elementary school principal and a superintendent) who were familiar with the system. A letter was sent to each school principal, and if the principal agreed to participate, classroom packages were sent to each teacher in the school through the board's mail system. Each child was given a flyer and an entry form to take home, both describing the contest and containing educational information on smoking. A parent's signature was required to allow the poster to be displayed publicly and to indicate that the child was permitted to accept the prize if he or she won. Several classroom teachers supported the contest enthusiastically, and there were several instances where a whole class submitted an entry as well as the anticipated individual entries. In addition to creating a focus on smoking cessation in the schools, the contest also provided some publicity opportunities. There was press coverage of the winners heading to the baseball game, and a selection of the posters was subsequently displayed in the community at the public library and at a health fair mall display.

Youth Activities With Some School Involvement (and Mixed Success) in Brantford, Ontario, Canada Across Ontario in winter 1992, a petition for a smoke-free planet was circulating and collecting names, with the objective of being able to measure the length of the petition in miles. The activity was sponsored by the Council for a Tobacco-Free Ontario (CTFO), which at that time functioned primarily as a coalition of the various agencies involved in smoking reduction and focused on events for National Non-Smoking Week and, to a lesser extent, World No Tobacco Day. COMMIT was one of the partner organizations in the CTFO. The petition was launched during National Non-Smoking Week and was to be presented to a government official in a ceremony to take place in Brantford on World No Tobacco Day. In almost all involved communities, the petition was circulated through the schools. Brantford public health nurses, who had contact with the schools, led the effort. However, a resident from the nearby tobacco-growing area objected to the antitobacco information that accompanied the petition, and as a result, the Brant County Board of Education recommended that each principal decide whether to allow the petition to circulate in his or her school. Some allowed it, and some did not. The final petition was two and a half times as long the Canadian National tower (the world's tallest freestanding building) in Toronto.

In another example, the worksite task force held a video contest. The theme was smoking cessation, and one objective was to obtain some short videos that could be used in conjunction with presentations. One place targeted for contest entries was the schools. Getting appropriate administrative approvals proceeded smoothly, but because of either an administrative problem or lack of interest, the contest registration and information materials did not get distributed in the schools for several weeks. When COMMIT staff members noticed this, they succeeded in arranging distribution, and there were several excellent entries from students. Audiovisual staff and teachers at the schools were supportive of the students who prepared entries.

Examples of Successful School Policy Initiatives   Some COMMIT sites achieved success in promoting changes in school smoking policies. For instance, in Cedar Rapids/Marion, IA, the public education task force formed a smoke-free schools subcommittee in September 1989 to change the school district's smoking policy. Although the standing policy prohibited youth from smoking on school grounds, it allowed teachers and employees to smoke in designated areas. The proposed change was complete ban in all district buildings and vehicles, but no restriction on smoking outside the buildings.

The smoke-free schools subcommittee wrote letters and disseminated policy information to the PTA presidents and school board members. They also obtained 300 signatures from individuals supporting smoke-free schools and presented their proposal to the school board. In response to the proposal, the school board scheduled two public hearings. At the first hearing, which was not well attended, there was no opposition to the proposal. The only two people to address the school board were members of the subcommittee. The second hearing received greater publicity and attracted more than 20 individuals. Opposition to the proposed policy changes was evident from the statements of several teachers and other school employees. A counterpetition with 281 signatures opposing the change was submitted to the school board. Despite opposition, almost 6 months after the initial presentation to the school board, the smoke-free schools proposal was approved on a 4-to-2 vote. The new policy was instituted at the beginning of the next calendar year, and cessation classes were offered to help smokers quit.

Another successful school policy initiative occurred in Yonkers. In response to the New York State Clean Indoor Air Act, the Yonkers school district decided to institute a restrictive smoking policy. After the school board approved the policy, administrators worked with legal counsel to develop a written policy and distributed a lay version to all employees. Friendly reminders were disseminated to all district personnel over the 3-month planning phase informing them of the number of days until the implementation of the new policy. Concern over employee welfare prompted the formation of a wellness committee that COMMIT joined. Although the district wanted to set an example for students and the community, it also hoped to minimize tensions among school district employees.

COMMIT worked with district personnel and the Yonkers Pulse Healthy Heart Program to provide materials for the district's approximately 950 smokers at the initiation of the new policy. Heart-healthy snacks, bottled water, and cessation referral information as well as self-help materials were given to each of the 37 schools to help support smokers during the first week of the policy's implementation. Volunteers were recruited to prepare materials, and school nurses assisted by staffing tables and counseling smokers. These supportive efforts helped to minimize employee hostility over the new policy and maintained a feeling of good will between the district and its employees. It also helped to promote smoking as a public health issue and educated nonsmokers about the difficulties smokers face in quitting.

Using Youth and Schools as a Channel   Although some youth channel activities were conducted within school systems, others were only promoted there. The Yonkers second annual quit-smoking campaign, called "A Thousand Good Reasons," used youth as a draw or hook to motivate adults to quit. The event matched an adult smoker with "an adopted child" in a 6-week campaign resulting in a grand prize of a $1,000 savings bond for the youth's education and a $250 supermarket gift certificate for the adult smoker. This effort sought to entice community participation by children, ages 5 to 18, encouraging adult smokers to quit. Promotion of this event occurred throughout the community in a variety of sectors, including the public schools. COMMIT was able to enlist the support of the school district through the district's public relations director, principals, and teachers. The public relations director contacted all elementary school principals, requesting their support in the dissemination of information promoting the contest. Through the schools, COMMIT was able to reach the parents of 12,000 students by having the students distribute flyers. In addition, through the district's central office, registration forms were sent to 1,360 teachers, administrators, and maintenance personnel. Posters were hung in each school, and the assistant superintendent was interviewed on the local cable television station to promote the campaign. One teacher who registered allowed her quitting progress to be followed throughout the 6-week period by the community's major daily newspaper and the cable station.

Yonkers' COMMIT field staff members also helped to organize two annual "No Proof, No Puffs" campaigns. The first-year elementary students went to local merchants to distribute information regarding the New York State law prohibiting the sale of tobacco products to minors, statistics on youth smoking, and display signs promoting the law. COMMIT staff members arranged for publicity, helped prepare materials, and provided a luncheon for students and teachers. Teachers enhanced this activity by planning a week's worth of lessons on smoking issues and helped students develop a song about preventing youth smoking that was performed for the entire school. Likewise, field interventionists played a significant part in the implementation of the second annual No Proof, No Puffs campaign. Field staff members worked with teachers to develop and plan activities as well as to coordinate the intervention. Staff members provided resource materials, collated "survival kits" for the Smoke-Free Partnership participants, gave T-shirts to student participants, arranged publicity, and even served pizza to students, teachers, and parents at the culminating celebration.

In the above examples, the schools were an effective vehicle for promoting smoking control activities. However, there were other instances throughout the trial where local districts hampered COMMIT's efforts to promote change, ignoring the fact that adults are critical role models for children. For example, in Vallejo, CA, the local school board sought to obtain a $700,000 grant for the school district from RJR Nabisco Foundation. A vocal group of COMMIT volunteers organized to block the school board's efforts to obtain the grant because of the "tainted" funding source. The COMMIT volunteers chose to frame the issue as a problem of insufficient school funding and an increase in the tobacco companies' handouts for youth projects, rather than reflect negatively on the school board's actions. The volunteers met, formulated plans, and presented resolutions to the school board and other community groups. Fortunately, the school district was not awarded the grant, although its attempts forced COMMIT volunteers into action to enlighten the school board about the hypocrisy of accepting money from the tobacco industry. Another example of a school district hampering COMMIT efforts occured in Brantford, as discussed above. The Council for a Tobacco-Free Ontario sponsored a petition for a smoke-free planet to coincide with World No Tobacco Day and National Non-Smoking Week; its goal was to measure petition length in miles. Almost all Ontario communities circulated the petition through the schools, but the Brantford school district would not permit the petition to be circulated even though the community was one of COMMIT's intervention sites.

In other cases, individuals presented barriers to change. For example, although administrators in Utica, NY, were supportive of implementing a smoke-free school district, they were not ready to fight the school board and local unions, which had smoking members. This resistance became even more frustrating to COMMIT when another school district outside the intervention community asked for help in initiating a smoke-free policy.

LESSONS LEARNED FROM COMMIT SCHOOL-BASED ACTIVITIES

Several lessons were learned from implementing COMMIT school-related activities, although these lessons were not completely understood until the end of the intervention project. For example, distributing materials to schools is relatively easy, but getting schools to use the materials and institute projects is more difficult. Often, materials would sit forgotten on a shelf until a COMMIT volunteer found them and reminded someone to use them. School personnel have many issues and activities to deal with, and a smoking prevention curriculum was sometimes not high enough on the list of priorities to move forward. Most COMMIT sites would have liked more direct input into planning school-based intervention activities, but the role of COMMIT field staff members was often restricted by the school administration. Field staff members found the dissemination process for curriculum and school policy information frustrating because they were allowed only minimal contact with individual school decisionmakers and had little information about how (if at all) COMMIT materials were used in most cases.

Another difficulty was a difference in the definition of the role of the school in children's lives. Some school administrators and teachers (and parents) saw themselves as the purveyors of knowledge and not as the conveyance for the solutions to social problems. Smoking, by COMMIT's definition a social problem, sometimes did not fit under what was perceived as the school's mandate. The COMMIT interventionists thought that they needed more time to work with school personnel to help them see themselves as health promotion agents and as well as educators. This translated into a need for more followup on delivery of curriculum and policy recommendations regarding smoking.

Some COMMIT interventionists found that encouraging the enforcement and implementation of school policy is more difficult than setting policy. Enforcement of policy often requires resources and constant monitoring, sometimes beyond the strained limits of schools today. At times the enforcement of policies limiting smoking in schools put teachers and staff in awkward positions (i.e., the role of the cop or "bad guy" rather than the students' friend). The issue of enforcing smoking or tobacco policy when other seemingly more important policies go unenforced is a difficult choice for officials who are overworked and whose schools are understaffed. The COMMIT teams believed that there was much more to be done to enforce current policies in schools.

Most COMMIT field staff members found that youth could function well within the structure of COMMIT. The caution for the field staff was not to underestimate the effectiveness of teenagers, because they can be incredibly competent. In many sites, youth identified activities, planned the strategies, and participated fully in community organizing. Youth need "hands-on" projects with lots of activities for them to do. Youth of all ages participated in COMMIT, from elementary school children to college artists who designed some of the projects, logos, and other materials. Involving youth in as many activities as possible was encouraged and can be increased in an intervention like COMMIT.

Youth smoking is a highly visible issue in a community and draws attention from many groups and constituencies. Prevention is a high-profile media issue. Print and broadcast media writers and photographers will use information from youth in addition to expert or community testimony. Schools can help community organizers by providing good access to media for students. Youth can be coached to respond well to the limelight and can testify before local and State governing bodies with effectiveness.

Young antismoking advocates can be effective for prevention *and* cessation. Adults can be pressured by their children or by any children to quit smoking, and older children can influence younger children not to start smoking. In addition, prevention is a more compelling concept for volunteers than cessation. Many people want to help keep children from smoking, whereas some feel uncomfortable pushing adults to quit. Community Boards felt that organizing a community for prevention could help to encourage adults to quit as a side benefit. In some cases, community interest in youth antismoking efforts threatened to overshadow adult cessation activities. It took a great deal of planning and encouragement for interventionists to redirect the focus and energy on youth smoking to a broader one of tobacco control in the community.

REFERENCES

Best, J.A., Thompson, S.J., Santi, S.M., Smith, E.A., Brown, K.S. Preventing cigarette smoking among school children. *Annual Review of Public Health* 9: 161-201, 1988.

Bowen, D.J., Kinne, S., Orlandi, M. School policy in COMMIT: A promising strategy to reduce smoking in youth. *Journal of School Health*, in press.

Corbett, K., Thompson, B., White, N., Taylor, M. Process evaluation in the Community Intervention Trial for Smoking Cessation (COMMIT). *International Quarterly of Community Health Education* 11(3): 291-309, 1990-91.

Flay, B.R., D'Avernas, J.R., Best, J.A., Kersell, M.W., Ryan, K.B. Cigarette smoking: Why young people do it and ways of preventing it. In: *Pediatric and Adolescent Behavioral Medicine*, P. McGrath, and P. Finestone (Editors). New York: Springer-Verlag, 1983, pp. 132-183.

Glynn, T.J. Essential elements of school-based smoking prevention programs. *Journal of School Health* 59: 181-186, 1989.

Johnston, L., O'Malley, P.M., Bachman, J.G. *Drug Use Among American High School Seniors, College Students, and Young Adults, 1975-1990. Volume 1. High School Seniors.* DHHS Publication No. (ADM) 91-1813. Rockville, MD: U.S. Department of Health and Human Services, Public Health Service, Alcohol, Drug Abuse, and Mental Health Administration, National Institute on Drug Abuse, 1991.

Lynch, B.S., Bonnie, R.J. (Editors). *Growing Up Tobacco Free: Preventing Nicotine Addiction in Children and Youths.* Committee on Preventing Nicotine Addiction in Children and Youths. Washington, DC: Institute of Medicine, National Academy of Sciences, 1994, p. 10.

National Institute on Drug Abuse. *NIDA Notes.* Vol. 9, no 1. NIH Publication No. 94-3478. Rockville, MD: U.S. Department of Health and Human Services, Public Health Service, National Institutes of Health, National Institute on Drug Abuse, 1994, p. 19.

Penz, M.A., Brannon, B.R., Charlin, V.L., Barrett, E.J., MacKinnon, D.P., Flay, B.R. The power of policy: The relationship of smoking policy to adolescent smoking. *American Journal of Public Health* 79(7): 857-862, 1989.

Sabatier, P.A., Mazmanian, D.A. The conditions of effective implementation: A guide to establishing policy objectives. *Public Policy Journal* 5: 481-504, 1979.

Shopland, D.R. Effect of smoking on the incidence and mortality of lung cancer. In: *Lung Cancer*, B.E. Johnson and D.H. Johnson (Editors). New York: Wiley, 1995, pp. 1-14.

U.S. Department of Health and Human Services. *Preventing Tobacco Use Among Young People: A Report of the Surgeon General.* Atlanta, GA: U.S. Department of Health and Human Services, Public Health Service, Centers for Disease Control and Prevention, National Center for Chronic Disease Prevention and Health Promotion, Office on Smoking and Health, 1994.

AUTHORS

Deborah Bowen, Ph.D.
Associate Member
Fred Hutchinson Cancer Research Center
1124 Columbia Street
Seattle, WA 98104

Lesa T. Dalton
Project Director
Division of Health Promotion Research
American Health Foundation
Fifth Floor
800 Second Avenue
New York, NY 10017

Rosemary Walker, M.Sc.
Research Associate
Department of Health Studies and
  Gerontology, MC-6081
University of Waterloo
Waterloo, Ontario N2L 3G1
CANADA

Susan Crystal
Research Assistant
Fred Hutchinson Cancer Research Center
1124 Columbia Street
Seattle, WA 98104

Mario A. Orlandi, Ph.D., M.P.H.
Chief
Division of Health Promotion Research
American Health Foundation
Fifth Floor
800 Second Avenue
New York, NY 10017

225

Involving Youth in Awareness of, Promotion of, and Political Activities for Tobacco Control

Robert J. McGranaghan, Sharon Ann Rankins-Burd, and Ted Purcell

INTRODUCTION   Despite numerous efforts to prevent youth from beginning the addictive practice of smoking, the rates of youth smoking remain alarmingly high, with the age of onset varying between 11 and 15 (U.S. Department of Health and Human Services, 1989; Johnston et al., 1991; DiFranza et al., 1987). Surveys of youth tobacco use have been conducted regularly for the past 15 years. Although the figures for smoking prevalence vary by survey and definition, one trend emerges: There has been little change since 1981 in the percentage of high school seniors who smoke cigarettes. Recent data show a statistically significant increase of 1.8 percent in high school senior daily smoking from 1992 to 1993 (Johnston et al., 1994). Almost as many young females now smoke as males, and those with no plans for higher education have higher prevalence than those with such plans (U.S. Department of Health and Human Services, 1989 and 1994). White adolescents have a higher prevalence than their African-American or Hispanic counterparts (Centers for Disease Control, 1990). The data do not capture the dropouts who are likely to have higher smoking prevalence rates (U.S. Department of Health and Human Services, 1989). The use of smokeless tobacco also is increasing, with males more likely to use this form of tobacco than females. At present, more than 1 million adolescent males use smokeless tobacco (Centers for Disease Control, 1990).

The addictive nature of tobacco is as evident in adolescents as it is in adults. Among adolescents who smoked at least half a pack of cigarettes per day, more than half had made an unsuccessful attempt to stop smoking. In addition, only a small portion (5 percent) thought they would still be smoking 5 years later; however, after 7 to 9 years, about 75 percent were still smoking (Johnston et al., 1991).

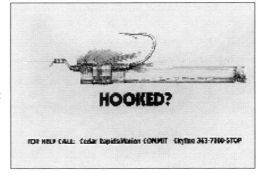

The use of tobacco by adolescents is particularly important because almost all first tobacco use occurs before graduation from high school (U.S. Department of Health and Human Services, 1994). For all adults, 89 percent began

smoking prior to age 18, and 71 percent began daily smoking by age 18 (U.S. Department of Health and Human Services, 1994). Adolescents, because of the addictive nature of nicotine, become "hooked" and are the smokers of the future. Preventing onset of tobacco use by youth will gradually result in the decline of smoking prevalence and, eventually, in the demise of all manner of tobacco use.

The Community Intervention Trial for Smoking Cessation (COMMIT) did not initially target youth in its intervention plans. The primary reason for excluding youth was that the trial was seen as being oriented toward heavy smokers (25 or more cigarettes per day), and young smokers rarely fall into that category. Nevertheless, some investigators and policy advisory committee members encouraged the inclusion of activities that targeted and included youth in intervention activities (see Chapter 12). The activities that targeted youth were primarily school based and are described in Chapter 12 (Bowen and colleagues). Activities that involved youth were important because they contributed to building awareness of smoking as a public health problem, increasing visibility of tobacco control efforts, and changing policies on youth access to tobacco.

This chapter describes some activities oriented toward youths in settings other than schools. Although Chapter 12 addresses in-school activities, it should be noted that schools were often the initial setting in which students were contacted or recruited to participate in communitywide campaigns and activities. This chapter also discusses the challenges encountered by COMMIT staff members and volunteers as they balanced a desire by volunteers for more attention to youth with COMMIT's goal of increasing cessation rates among adults. Finally, the chapter includes some key lessons learned from the COMMIT communities about this intervention channel.

GOALS, ACTIVITIES, AND PROCESS OBJECTIVES FOR YOUTH

The overall goals of this aspect of the youth channel were to:

- enlist participation of students and teachers in communitywide campaigns and intervention activities; and

- increase community interest and activity in regulations and enforcement of policies to reduce youth access to tobacco products.

The required activities involving youth in nonschool settings are discussed in Table 1.

The range of creative activities within each category demonstrates the extent to which COMMIT communities involved youth in the overall intervention beyond what was minimally required by the protocol. One recurring theme found in the records of the COMMIT communities was the lament by volunteers that COMMIT could not focus more attention on prevention and youth. Many communities reported that their community Boards or public education task forces (under which most communities coordinated youth activities) were initially inclined to put more resources into youth activities than were justified by the design of the intervention. This may be the result of a tendency of COMMIT volunteers to prevent

Table 1
Activities and process objectives for youth

Activities for Each Community	Cumulative Objectives (1988-1992)	Number Completed	Process Objectives Achieved[a] (%)
Annually Promote Participation in Magnet Events (1/2,000 of total community population)	100%		485
Annually Initiate a Youth Access to Tobacco Campaign	33 campaigns	46 campaigns	139
Establish Liaison With Tobacco-Free Young America Project	All communities	8 liaisons	73
Establish Cooperative Agreement With Tobacco-Free Young America Project	All communities	10 communities	91

[a] *Average for combined communities.*

what had not begun rather than intervening to change the behavior of adults who had already chosen to smoke. At the same time, a natural tendency to protect youth from the mistakes of their elders may have inclined volunteers to be more interested in preventing youth from smoking. This dilemma, and how COMMIT communities dealt with it, are discussed below in the "Challenges" section of this chapter.

INVOLVING YOUTH IN COMMUNITYWIDE CAMPAIGNS AND INTERVENTION ACTIVITIES

Involving Youth in Community Campaigns

Communities involved youth in a wide variety of campaigns and interventions. These campaigns focused on reframing the tobacco message to raise awareness of tobacco industry marketing tactics, especially advertising. Boards and task force members recognized that advertising of tobacco products is difficult to escape (Johnston et al., 1991; Centers for Disease Control, 1990). Despite industry disclaimers that influencing adolescents is a goal (O'Toole, 1986; Weil, 1986), there is much evidence that young people are aware of the images presented by the tobacco companies. A study of 6-year-olds showed that 91 percent were able to recognize Joe Camel (Fischer et al., 1991). A survey of 5,000 adolescents selected at random indicated that 42 percent identified Marlboro as the most advertised cigarette brand, followed by Camel at 30 percent (and also showed that Camel advertisements were most often recalled by the youngest adolescents and seldom recalled by older adult smokers) (Pierce et al., 1991). Similar results were reported in analyses of the 1992 California Tobacco Survey (McCan, 1992). In other studies amon youth, recall of cigarette advertisements is high, especially compared with recall of the U.S. Surgeon General's warning labels (Fischer and Magnus, 1981).

Tobacco advertising is seen in print media, billboards, sponsorship of events, and point-of-sale messages. Advertising and promotion are most likely to operate in an unconscious way; they provide images that support the attractiveness of smoking (U.S. Department of Health and Human Services, 1989 and 1991; Warner et al., 1992; Hensley, 1989). The images that are used are usually sexy, independent, adventure seeking, or funny (cartoon characters). Such images are often appealing to adolescents. Indirectly, adolescents may look at such advertising as evidence that it is "okay to smoke" because if smoking were not acceptable adolescent behavior, the Government would not allow the advertising of a product with such negative health consequences for adolescents (U.S. Department of Health and Human Services, 1989). For these reasons, many COMMIT communities conducted activities designed to reduce the appeal of tobacco advertising. Counteradvertising campaigns using posters developed by and targeted to youth were displayed on buses and in bus shelters in Vallejo, CA. Some antitobacco advertisements, such as those put on billboards in commercial districts, were designed by youth. Advertising of tobacco products was removed from several sporting events, including basketball in Yonkers, NY, baseball in Medford/Ashland, OR, and Bellingham, WA, and tennis in Santa Fe, NM.

Other informational and awareness programs and campaigns involving youth and targeting adults included writing letters to the editor of local newspapers. For example, letter-writing campaigns by youth supported public discussions of enforcing or enhancing policies on youth access to tobacco.

Videotape productions and slide shows, developed with creative input from youth, documented local examples of the pervasive marketing of tobacco to young people throughout the community. Theatrical events, such as puppet shows and musical plays, were produced to help youth deal with situations involving smoking and to highlight the dangers of secondhand smoke to children and adults.

Some communities trained youth to be speakers or developed peer-to-peer education to prevent smoking and to raise awareness of the problem. This strategy used students who were trained to teach their peers how to refuse cigarettes. In some cases, youth were trained to make presentations to legislators and community leaders.

Involving Youth in Magnet Events The protocol required communities to conduct community magnet events (Chapter 6). The Great American Smokeout (GASO) is a magnet event sponsored by the American Cancer Society, and every COMMIT community in the United States was involved in promoting this event. Youth played an important role in helping communities spread the message about the GASO. Some communities used youth brigades to distribute door hangers and fliers in targeted neighborhoods to advertise GASO events. Others involved youth in distributing information on quitting for the day. Many communities conducted poster contests in conjunction with the GASO. These contests were another strategy for youth to express themselves to peers and adults in creative ways, raise awareness, and spread basic information about the problem of smoking. Winning entries were displayed in shopping malls and community centers, and in Paterson, NJ, the winning entries were made into a calendar. In some cases, posters were judged by employees of companies participating in GASO activities and were displayed in their worksites.

Newspaper coverage of the contests amplified the messages of the posters to the community. Local media also publicized essay contests by printing articles about the winning writers and their tobacco control messages. Essays were reprinted in local newspapers and, in some cases, were broadcast by radio stations, providing further promotion of the no-smoking message.

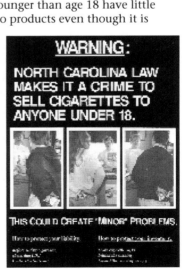

Non-Dependence Day, the fifth of July, was a summertime event sponsored by the American Lung Association allowing for more community-based involvement by youth to promote antismoking messages. For example, youth participated in local Fourth of July parades to encourage smokers to be independent by overcoming their dependence on tobacco. As with the GASO, poster contests were used to involve youth and spread the no-smoking message of this campaign.

MONITORING AND PROMOTING ENFORCEMENT OF REGULATIONS ON YOUTH ACCESS TO TOBACCO

The national health objectives for the year 2000 have targeted substantial reductions in smoking among persons younger than 20 years and reductions in smoking onset. Reducing access to cigarettes through policies or laws is an important strategy in reaching this goal. Those younger than age 18 have little difficulty in purchasing tobacco products even though it is illegal in all of the United States and Canada. With few exceptions, there is little enforcement of the laws prohibiting tobacco access by minors. Studies indicate that the vast majority of tobacco retailers sell to children (Doctors and Lawyers for a Drug-Free Youth, 1991; Altman et al., 1989). For this reason, COMMIT communities were required to develop activities to monitor and promote enforcement of regulations on youth access to tobacco.

Almost all communities used compliance checks as an initial step in the process of examining what their communities were doing about the accessibility to tobacco by youth. The compliance check was a systematic method to investigate whether merchants were adhering to local and State laws regarding the sale of tobacco to minors. In essence, a compliance check is an undercover buying operation using underage youth who have been trained in the operation to go into stores and attempt to purchase cigarettes. Prior arrangements are often made with law enforcement agencies so the youth are protected from legal action resulting from their purchasing tobacco. Accompanied by an adult driver who waits outside the retail establishment, an underage adolescent attempts to buy cigarettes or other tobacco products. The young people are trained to give truthful answers about their age if asked and to avoid any education of the retailer during the operation.

The results of compliance checks were used to educate merchants and the general public. Merchants who refused to sell to minors were usually given a certificate or a letter of commendation. Those who did sell to minors received some type of education about sales to youth. As a followup to compliance checks, interviews with store personnel about their selling behavior were sometimes conducted. Checks also documented how and where tobacco products, promotional materials, and legal age warning signs were placed.

Some communities began this activity with a merchant education campaign. Volunteers, often youth groups, visited local tobacco merchants and distributed information about local and State laws pertaining to sales to minors. Articles and letters to the editor about the dangers of smoking and the easy accessibility to tobacco by minors accompanied this outreach to merchants. Following this outreach, compliance checks were conducted to determine the extent of the problem and the effects, if any, from the merchant education campaign. Merchants were not informed at this point that a compliance check was in progress; however, some communities chose to publicize the campaign in local newspapers to warn the merchants before the youth buyers were sent out to the stores.

Initial compliance checks demonstrated that a majority of underage buyers were able to purchase cigarettes. In most communities, this outcome resulted in widespread local publicity and paved the way for public debate about enforcement and stricter laws. Youth were instrumental in promoting the importance of enforcing laws and advocating for the strengthening or changing of existing laws, such as bans on cigarette vending machines.

Young volunteers spoke at city council hearings and displayed packs of cigarettes they were able to purchase during compliance checks. Students wrote letters to the editor to encourage local lawmakers to consider tougher policies on access to tobacco by youth. The visible and enthusiastic involvement of youth in this activity was an important factor in getting communities to discuss and in some cases make policy changes restricting sales to minors.

SUCCESSFUL ACTIVITIES   The process objectives for youth activities required involving as many children as possible in smoking control activities and mounting at least one visible youth-related policy initiative each year. Success was measured primarily by meeting process objectives for the required activities, and the community measured success by the amount and frequency of media coverage, positive feedback from the community to staff members and volunteers after events, letters to the editor, attendance at public hearings, changes in local public policy, and attendance at and response to other special events that created an environment for public discussion of the issue.

ENLISTING YOUTH IN COMMUNITYWIDE CAMPAIGNS   COMMIT found many agencies eager to involve their youth groups in smoking control activities. Boy and Girl Scouts, youth activities commissions, church and synagogue youth groups, children's program directors at YMCA's and afterschool programs, Students Against Drunk Driving (SADD) chapters and Friday Night Live groups, and antidrug coalitions, such as Drug Abuse Resistance Education (DARE), were eager to incorporate COMMIT's antismoking message into their activities.

The extent to which communities became involved in youth activities was based on the priority given to youth issues by community Boards, public education task forces, and program staff. Some communities, such as Utica, NY, and Raleigh, NC, created youth subcommittees of the public education task forces. Other communities, such as Fitchburg/Leominster, MA, and Bellingham, assigned youth the status of a full task force, including direct representation on the community Board. Most communities did not separate youth from the public education task force but still devoted much time and attention to this channel.

Counteradvertising campaigns helped to reframe the message of smoking as a public health issue and provided excellent activities to involve the

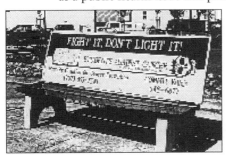

creativity and enthusiasm of young volunteers. In Vallejo, a youth group called Students Against Cancer developed a poster titled "Fight It! Don't Light It!" that was displayed in buses and bus shelters throughout the city. The Southern Oregon Drug Awareness (SODA) youth committee worked with the Medford/Ashland COMMIT community and adopted a counteradvertising billboard project. Volunteers from this group also helped place antitobacco stickers on tobacco advertisements in magazines in school libraries.

Essay contests were yet another method used to promote community campaigns and magnet events. Raleigh conducted an essay contest on the theme "Smoking Restrictions and Their Associated Benefits." Winning entries were reprinted in a local newspaper. In Fitchburg/Leominster, winning essays on no-smoking themes were read over local radio stations.

In both Santa Fe and Paterson, adults and children used their musical and dramatic talents to bring an antitobacco message to audiences. In Santa Fe, a puppet show was developed that stressed the hazards of secondhand smoke. Children were taught how to deal with situations involving smoking, including how to refuse cigarettes. Scripts were developed for both elementary and higher grades. Children who saw the show at school received brochures containing antitobacco information for their parents. In Paterson, the "Smart Moves" play also traveled to schools. The play was interactive and included a simple antitobacco song taught to the children who were encouraged to bring the song home to their parents.

A teacher and student in Fitchburg/Leominster rewrote the screenplay "Cold Turkey" as a play titled "Unfiltered Rock." The play was produced during the week of The Great American Smokeout. Advertisements were run in the newspaper and on the radio to promote the play and the GASO. Forty students participated in this theatrical venture, and 600 people attended the play.

Training youth to be speakers and active participants in events was another strategy used by communities to involve youth in educational campaigns. Utica trained young people to participate in a hypertension screening project to talk about the risks of smoking to people who have high blood pressure. Medford/Ashland sponsored two students from the SODA youth committee to attend one of the annual Stop Teen Addiction to Tobacco (STAT) conferences. These students were an important source of ideas for involving Medford/Ashland youth in more visible and active antitobacco efforts.

Vallejo's Students Against Cancer provided important help in promoting antismoking messages to adults and youth through a wide variety of campaigns and activities. This group, a youth component of the Minority Coalition for Cancer Prevention, was recruited from Vallejo high schools and the Continentals of Omega Boys & Girls Club. Students Against Cancer was routinely involved in Vallejo's community events, such as the GASO, summer antidrug block parties, and Fourth of July parades. In some cases, these youngsters helped to promote the events to their peers and adults, and in other cases, they participated actively at the events in skits and on floats that had no-smoking themes.

Santa Fe COMMIT worked with student interns who developed a presentation for other children and adults focusing on cessation. During one summer, COMMIT sought office help from student interns who were asked to make these presentations. When the students returned to high school in the fall, they worked as volunteers within the school, helping other teens to give up tobacco. By the second year of the program, funding was obtained from outside sources to continue support of the peer-to-peer program. An at-risk student, also an ex-smoker, became one of the trainers who helped reach other at-risk youth in Santa Fe, thereby lending even more credibility to his work among teens and young adults.

Vallejo's slide show "Provocative and Pervasive: Tobacco Messages Bombard Our Youth" is another example of a strategy that used youth to raise awareness among adults. The slide show depicted locations in Vallejo where tobacco products, advertisements, and tobacco-like candies and gum are placed at eye level in and near areas frequented by youth. The show included facts about smoking and health and was targeted primarily to adult audiences who attended meetings of community organizations such as the Rotary Club and church groups. The slide show drew strong reactions. Adults were indignant and sometimes outraged when they saw the extent to which the products were promoted in local stores and other locations in Vallejo. This slide show was eventually made into a short videotape starring local youth titled "Reaping Profits by Stalking Youth" and was made available to local community groups and agencies as a COMMIT legacy at the end of the project. Similarly, Bellingham adopted "Ad-libbing It" as part of its curriculum in grades 5 through 9. The videotape, developed by a physician from the Washington State affiliate of Doctors Ought to Care (DOC), shows young people how the tobacco industry manipulates them by presenting false images of smokers.

Some communities used athletic events and organizations to target both adults and youth with antismoking messages. In Medford/Ashland, a minor league baseball team sponsored a Family-No Smoking-No Drinking section for games. Medford/Ashland also purchased a billboard with an antismoking message for players and their adult supporters at a Little League field. Vallejo distributed promotional materials targeted to Little League supporters who smoke while watching the games.

Over the years, several campaigns were developed in Utica, including one for the winter holidays. A radio commercial featured a young girl who wrote to Santa asking for a Quit Kit for her dad. People were encouraged to give the kits to loved ones who smoke. One local hospital extended its heart disease prevention program to include radio advertisements using youngsters who asked their parents to quit smoking or start exercising so they will live to see their children grow up.

Vallejo offered minigrants (matched by the school district) to youth organizations, such as the Camp Fire Girls, YMCA, 4-H Club, and the Continentals of Omega Boys & Girls Club, for projects involving youth in magnet events. These grants were used as incentives to encourage youth organizations to think of creative ways to involve their members in activities targeting adults. The Boys & Girls Club used its grant to support an antidrug block party during which T-shirts with antismoking messages were distributed. The YMCA used its grant to develop a prevention curriculum for a summer day camp program. Antismoking youth groups were established through schools and community organizations and coalesced with antidrug groups. Communities reported that incorporating tobacco into their community's antidrug movements, while challenging, was a promising strategy for raising awareness of the problem of smoking and involving new groups of youth and adults.

MAGNET EVENTS   Magnet events included poster contests to promote cessation themes. In Paterson, winning posters were produced as a calendar and distributed widely throughout the community. In Cedar Rapids/Marion, IA, third-grade students were matched to local companies for the GASO. Students created posters encouraging the employees at their company to stop smoking for the day. A committee of smokers and former smokers at each company judged the posters and displayed the winner at their worksites.

In many communities, children marched in Fourth of July parades in conjunction with Non-Dependence Day or in other local parades. Young people contributed energy, enthusiasm, and much creativity during float-making enterprises for these parades. One of Vallejo's July Fourth floats featured a dinosaur theme and relied on young volunteers riding on the floats to spread the message "Smoking: The Real Reason Dinosaurs Became Extinct."

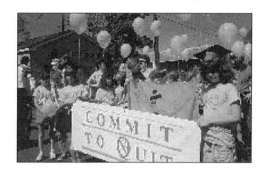

Young people were recruited to attend rallies where antismoking speakers, such as David Goerlitz (the former Winston cigarette advertising-model-turned-antitobacco advocate) or Dr. Alan Blum (of DOC), were featured. Rallies with such notable speakers as Mr. Goerlitz and Dr. Blum were held in conjunction with magnet events and received local media coverage and enhanced the promotional activities of antismoking campaigns.

In Raleigh, a local chapter of SADD was recruited to participate in a Non-Dependence Day rally at the city plaza. The students performed skits and rap songs with an antitobacco theme. As a followup to that event, Raleigh kept the SADD members involved in additional tobacco control activities. Thus, some members of this group became involved in the GASO later that year and organized a small-scale "Quit and Win" contest as part of the event. They recruited prizes; made a banner; signed up students, faculty, and staff; and learned how to use a carbon monoxide monitor to determine contest winners.

MONITORING AND ENFORCING TOBACCO ACCESS   All communities conducted compliance checks to demonstrate the easy access children have to tobacco. These compliance checks also served to raise community awareness of the problem of smoking generally and the need for enforcement of a minimum purchase age. In some communities, such as Raleigh and Vallejo, youth buys were the first step to new or additional legislation aimed at keeping children away from tobacco. In Vallejo, a concerted campaign that began with compliance checks resulted in the passage of local legislation banning cigarette vending machines and free distribution of tobacco products.

236

In Fitchburg/Leominster, youth task force members became masterful at involving other young people in activities that focused on prevention of youth access to tobacco. This activity received extensive media coverage and succeeded in moving debate forward on the need for stricter regulations at the municipal level. This activity was controversial and not always popular among adults in the community. Some felt it was a form of entrapment and that it did not set a good example to youth in the community. Nevertheless, health officials in one community moved quickly to adopt stricter regulations concerning youth access to tobacco.

Health officials in one Massachusetts COMMIT intervention community were reluctant to move as quickly because they were philosophically opposed to youth involvement in undercover operations. Board and task force members began to work with the community's youth commission, a peer leadership group with a positive image among adults. Through a series of educational sessions, the youth commission adopted protection from tobacco as one of its charges. The youth commission made a proposal to the health department asking for adoption of stricter regulations. When the health department did not act, the commission took its proposal to the city council. Members of the commission testified at hearings and succeeded in convincing the city to adopt the regulations, including provisions for monitoring enforcement using compliance checks, which had been the major stumbling block for the health department.

Youth also reminded the public and legislators about existing nonsmoking laws. Santa Fe held a major event at the State capitol building. COMMIT held a news conference in the rotunda and enlisted help and support from youth and adults. The youth issued smoking "tickets" to those who lit up in the building because New Mexico law prohibits smoking in public places. However, not every lawmaker had a sense of humor about the event. One refused to be seen on camera with his citation in hand.

For many communities, compliance checks and merchant education programs provided an excellent opportunity to involve youth in an activity that sought to protect youth and raise awareness among adults about the dangers of smoking and the pervasiveness of tobacco advertising and products in places where youth congregate. Some communities were more aggressive in their willingness to tackle this activity, especially in their use of young people to purchase cigarettes in bars or cocktail lounges. Buying operations usually resulted in media attention that kept the issue alive for public discussion, although the attention was not always favorable. The payoff for communities that successfully used compliance checks and related activities was a more powerful groundswell of support among adults for enactment of local ordinances to strengthen access laws. In addition, a cadre of dedicated youth, now schooled by COMMIT's buying operations, became involved in other COMMIT activities.

CHALLENGES   Perhaps the most significant challenge that communities encountered with this channel was the desire of many of their community Boards and public education task forces to focus more attention and resources on youth and prevention activities. Thus, COMMIT staff members were faced with the challenge of steering their volunteers away from this focus and providing consistent reminders to them that the goal of COMMIT was to increase cessation rates among adult smokers.

For some communities, the emphasis was on policy change, thought to be the only effort worth supporting in this channel. For example, in Fitchburg/Leominster, disagreement arose in the third year among youth task force members as to which activities for youth were most worthwhile. Two members of the task force, who were the major forces behind the implementation and enforcement of regulations prohibiting youth access, were adamant that these types of activities were the only effective activities for preventing youth access and that educational programs were a waste of time and money. Ultimately, task force members agreed that both educational and enforcement activities were to be part of the action plan.

In other communities, volunteers expressed many concerns and fears about involving youth in monitoring access to tobacco, resulting in much weaker compliance checks and, in some cases, cancellation of these types of operations. For example, the Paterson public education task force opposed a staff-planned compliance check because most members were concerned that it might be viewed as an attack on merchants, not on the law and its enforcement. They subsequently canceled all plans for that activity.

In Utica, concerns also were raised during plans for a second compliance check. Volunteers felt that COMMIT might receive bad publicity and were also concerned about COMMIT's liability if the local district attorney decided to file charges against merchants caught in the operation. No one wanted to risk that possibility, so the compliance check was canceled.

Another challenge facing this channel was that most at-risk youth do not belong to the kinds of organizations and groups that rallied to COMMIT's message. Targeting this hard-to-reach population, although not a primary objective of the intervention, was a challenge for project staff members and volunteers. Santa Fe used the peer-to-peer education program described above to target some of these students.

LESSONS LEARNED The youth channel was not a major priority for the intervention; the majority of COMMIT's required activities were targeted to adults. Nevertheless, most communities felt that their youth activities were among the most successful of all the interventions. In the final reports of the COMMIT intervention, 6 of the 11 communities included at least 1 youth-related intervention among their "most successful activities." That subjective evaluation by the communities provides some indication of the degree to which their volunteers were eager to focus on youth issues. Almost every community noted in its final reports that the youth channel (and its implicit message of prevention) was an important issue for volunteers. Perhaps this reflects a natural "protective" tendency on the part of adults to be concerned about creating and maintaining a safe and healthy environment for children. Such a tendency for protectiveness toward children may override the desire to intervene in the choices adult smokers have already made in their lives.

Staff members and community volunteers realized that youth could be used to heighten awareness of the problem of smoking among both adults and young people. Furthermore, youth served a critical public relations function in getting the cessation message to adults, a realization that helped communities with objectives that targeted adults and enhanced their work by involving youth and adults in magnet events and monitoring and promoting enforcement on youth access to tobacco. In fact, many communities documented that involving youth groups in monitoring youth access to tobacco became a galvanizing force for changes in local policy. For example, the Vallejo City Council ultimately responded to the strong foundation of community support given to bans on vending machines and free distribution of tobacco products. This strong foundation resulted largely from the coalescing of diverse segments of the community, a coalescing that ultimately became the "pulse" (perceived standard operating pattern) of Vallejo, to which the council responded. However, the participation of many enthusiastic, articulate, and sincere young people in the process may have been the most critical ingredient in this effort.

The linkage of tobacco use with substance abuse programs met with initial resistance (especially from the community of recovering addicts) but, in some cases, proved to be an effective strategy to merge with other groups and increase resources directed to antidrug, antismoking messages.

Young people also serve as a convenient channel from which to recruit volunteers. Youth can support program staff when adults are neither able nor willing to volunteer. As was borne out frequently with the youth-buying operations and merchant education programs, everyone seems to listen when young people deliver a message. This may be the most valuable lesson learned from COMMIT's experiences with youth activities.

REFERENCES

Altman, D., Foster, V., Rasenick-Douss, T., Tye, J. Reducing the illegal sales of tobacco to minors. *Journal of the American Medical Association* 261: 80-83, 1989.

Centers for Disease Control. Cigarette advertising—U.S., 1988. *MMWR. Morbidity and Mortality Weekly Report* 39: 261-265, 1990.

DiFranza, J.R., Norwood, B.D., Garner, D.W., Tye, J.B. Legislative efforts to protect children from tobacco. *Journal of the American Medical Association* 257: 3387-3389, 1987.

Doctors and Lawyers for a Drug-Free Youth. *Cigarettes Readily Sold to Children in 90 U.S. Communities, Tobacco Legislation Recommended.* Champaign, IL: Doctors and Lawyers for a Drug-Free Youth, 1991.

Fischer, D.A., Magnus, P. "Out of the mouths of babes . . . ." The opinions of 10 and 11 year old children regarding the advertising of cigarettes. *Community Health Studies* 5: 22-26, 1981.

Fischer, P.M., Schwartz, M.P., Richards, J.W., Jr., Goldstein, A.O., Rojas, T.H. Brand logo recognition by children aged 3 to 6 years. Mickey Mouse and Old Joe the Camel. *Journal of the American Medical Association* 266: 3145-3148, 1991.

Hensley, T. Congress considers eliminating nearly all tobacco advertising. *Journal of the National Cancer Institute* 81: 128-129, 1989.

Johnston, L., O'Malley, P., Bachman, J. "Monitoring the Future Study." Press release, University of Michigan, Ann Arbor, MI, January 31, 1994.

Johnston, L.D., O'Malley, P.M., Bachman, J.G. *National Trends in Drug Use and Related Factors Among American High School Students and Young Adults, 1975-1990*. Rockville, MD: U.S. Department of Health and Human Services, Public Health Service, Alcohol, Drug Abuse, and Mental Health Administration, National Institute on Drug Abuse, 1991.

McCan, J. Tobacco logo recognition. *Journal of Family Practice* 34: 681-684, 1992.

O'Toole, J. Testimony at the hearings on the advertising of tobacco products before the Subcommittee on Health and the Environment of the Committee on Energy and Commerce, U.S. House of Representatives, 99th Congress, 2nd Session, Serial No. 99-167, 1986.

Pierce, J.P., Gilpin, E., Burns, D.M., Whalen, E., Rosbrook, B., Shopland, D., Johnson, M. Does tobacco advertising target young people to start smoking? Evidence from California. *Journal of the American Medical Association* 266(22): 3154-3158, 1991.

U.S. Department of Health and Human Services. *Reducing the Health Consequences of Smoking: 25 Years of Progress. A Report of the Surgeon General, 1989*. DHHS Publication No. (CDC) 89-8411. Rockville, MD: U.S. Department of Health and Human Services, Public Health Service, Centers for Disease Control, Center for Chronic Disease Prevention and Health Promotion, Office on Smoking and Health, 1989.

U.S. Department of Health and Human Services. *Strategies To Control Tobacco Use In the United States: A Blueprint for Public Health Action in the 1990's*. Smoking and Tobacco Control Monographs-1. NIH Publication No. 92-3316. Washington, DC: U.S. Department of Health and Human Services, Public Health Service, National Institutes of Health, National Cancer Institute, 1991.

U.S. Department of Health and Human Services. *Preventing Tobacco Use Among Young People: A Report of the Surgeon General*. Atlanta, GA: U.S. Department of Health and Human Services, Public Health Service, Centers for Disease Control and Prevention, Center for Chronic Disease Prevention and Health Promotion, Office on Smoking and Health, 1994.

Warner, K., Butler, J., Cummings, K.M., D'Onofrio, C., Davis, R., Flay, B., McKinney, M., Myers, M., Pertschuk, M., Robinson, R., Ryden, L., Schudson, M., Tye, J., Wilkenfield, J. Report of the tobacco policy research study group on tobacco marketing and promotion. *Tobacco Control* 1(Suppl): S19-S23, 1992.

Weil, G. Testimony at the hearings on the advertising of tobacco products before the Subcommittee on Health and the Environment of the Committee on Energy and Commerce, U.S. House of Representatives, 99th Congress, 2nd Session, Serial No. 99-167, 1986.

AUTHORS

Robert J. McGranaghan, M.P.H.
Research Associate
Division of Research
Kaiser Permanente Medical Care Program
3505 Broadway
Oakland, CA 94611-5714

Sharon Ann Rankins-Burd
Box 99
North Winfield Road
West Winfield, NY 13491

Ted Purcell
Project Coordinator
Division of Preventive and Behavioral
  Medicine
University of Massachusetts Medical Center
Seventh Floor
55 Lake Avenue North
Worcester, MA 01655

What Have We Learned and Where Do We Go From Here?

Beti Thompson, William R. Lynn, and Donald R. Shopland

INTRODUCTION   The Community Intervention Trial for Smoking Cessation (COMMIT) provided unique opportunities for learning about community interventions. From the beginning of the project, when design issues played an important role in determining the extent to which communities would be involved in decisionmaking, to the final dissemination of trial data, we learned much about understanding communities, mobilizing and working with communities to implement interventions, sustaining key aspects of the intervention after the funding ended, and disseminating final results to the communities. This monograph puts together the lessons learned from the field so that future community studies can benefit from the COMMIT experience.

MAJOR LESSONS LEARNED   The individual chapters in this monograph discuss the lessons learned in specific channels and activities, but there are also overarching implications for other community projects that revolve primarily around community mobilization and the utility of the COMMIT approach for other community and social problems. This section focuses on these lessons.

The COMMIT project required communities to be heavily involved in the implementation of the intervention. This requisite led to many other demands. First, a necessary condition for intervention was that communities organize for action. Because the project was primarily a research project, the impetus for organization came from an external source rather than a ground swell within the community. Furthermore, once some community organization had been achieved, community groups had to be convinced that tobacco control was a significant problem in *their* community. Even when groups were convinced of that, mobilizing people to plan and implement interventions was not easy.

Establishing a Partnership With the Community   It is clear from the COMMIT experience that identifying and involving community members who represent the community to serve on Boards and task forces is both necessary and possible. The extensive community analysis conducted in all communities led to the involvement of appropriate individuals and organizations, as shown in a questionnaire disseminated at the end of the intervention part of the trial. Each site was asked how well the Board and task forces represented the community, and the respondents confirmed that the composition of the volunteer membership was appropriate. The process of identifying and recruiting community members to become involved in a research partnership, more fully explained in Chapter 5, resulted in structures of Boards and task forces that provided good representation of the communities. Furthermore, the process happened quickly, generally within 7 months of randomization.

We also learned that the membership of Boards and task forces was fluid, with members resigning and new individuals being recruited according to the specific project focus and the interests and availability of individuals.

Promoting the Research Agenda Initially, there were concerns that communities would not think of tobacco control as being a sufficiently important issue or as requiring the amount of volunteer time we were requesting. In the early days of the project, some community members argued that there were other compelling problems in their communities (such as alcohol, other drugs, and violence) and that those problems should be the focus of attention. As a result, there was some natural dropout in volunteer membership as individuals decided not to participate in this research. However, within a short time, all 11 intervention communities, and the individuals, groups, and organizations representing them, became heavily involved in organizing the community to help smokers achieve cessation. Thus, we learned that communities will enthusiastically embrace an externally imposed research agenda, even when that agenda is not seen as including key problems or issues facing the community. One community member stated that there were enough community problems for everyone to get involved in, and if resources were available, she was determined to make a difference where she could.

As Chapters 5 through 13 indicate, community Boards, task forces, and individual volunteers took on most of the activities with enthusiasm, which should not be construed to mean that community representatives were always pleased with the constraints of the protocol. After some practice and experience, many communities wished to rearrange the focus of the protocol, spending less time on organizations (Chapter 11) and more on preventing smoking onset (Chapter 13). Nonetheless, community volunteers regarded the protocol as being important and tried to conduct the activities in a manner congruent with the needs of their communities.

As discussed in Chapter 5, the need to put research aims before community aims was a compromise made among the investigators in the early days of COMMIT. Although every attempt was made to allow for flexibility, the intervention was set up as a "one size fits all" model, which was occasionally frustrating to investigators and community members alike. Future community intervention planners might consider ways to better incorporate the changing interests and agendas of communities into a protocol.

Planning Intervention Activities The initial task of the Boards and task forces was to develop a Smoking Control Plan, the blueprint for the 4 years of intervention activities that were to occur in a community. The plan served many purposes: It introduced the project to the community, provided an overall guide for what would be done and when it would be done, gave the community volunteers their first real opportunity to work together, and forced volunteers to agree on how the tobacco control issue would be approached in their community. Because of the research nature of the project, the timeline for producing this plan was extremely short. The community Boards and task forces were organized by the end of January 1989. By May 1989, they were expected to produce this comprehensive plan and to prepare its presentation to the community. Familiarizing the volunteers with the project and the protocol required a significant amount of learning; thus, the May deadline for developing the Smoking Control Plan was not ideal. Although staff members experienced considerable anxiety (and worked many extra hours), the volunteers put forth superb efforts, and plans were produced.

Immediately after the overall Smoking Control Plan was developed, volunteers had to begin producing Annual Action Plans, which specified the activities to be accomplished in the first intervention year. Action plan development required that Boards and task forces identify how activities would be implemented, what the activities would build on, who would do them, how much they would cost, and other details. The Boards and task forces accepted this task and devised plans that incorporated creativity in the implementation of activities, added other community groups to the intervention process, and allocated resources wisely. (Indeed, many communities used this as an opportunity to generate in-kind contributions.) Thus, it was clear that community volunteers were eager and able to become involved in planning intervention activities.

Implementing
Intervention
Activities

The final community task was to implement the intervention activities so that research objectives could be achieved. The data in Table 1 indicate that community volunteers and staff members took that task seriously, with 94 percent of process objectives achieved across COMMIT. In planning the trial, investigators outlined the percentage of intermediary groups, such as health care providers, workplaces, and schools, that had to be reached for a minimal intervention to be achieved (see Chapter 2). Community volunteers took pride in feedback that indicated they were making progress in achieving process objectives. Community volunteers participated in diverse activities, ranging from stuffing envelopes, to recruiting worksites to become involved in community promotions, to becoming media and legislative advocates, to being regular speakers at schools, and many activities in between. Some of these activities are described in Chapters 5 through 13.

Utility
for Other
Community
Projects

As COMMIT drew to a close, we began asking our community partners for input on the process. One item put forward by all communities was the relevance of the COMMIT use of community organizations to other types of community interventions. Volunteers commented that the COMMIT experience provided them with excellent skills that could be applied subsequently to other community problems. Specifically, they liked the idea of drawing on volunteers from the entire community to organize around a problem. They also liked the structures set up by COMMIT that distributed work among a Board and separate task forces. Volunteers from at least three communities stated that they had used that approach in other projects.

Table 1

Percentage of process objectives achieved trialwide by intervention channel

Intervention Channel (number of activities)	Average for All Intervention Communities Combined (%)
Mobilization of Boards and Task Forces (34)	99
Health Care Providers (30)	96
Worksites (31)	92
Organizations (13)	83
Cessation Resources (24)	92
Public Education: Media (20)	94
Public Education: Youth (15)	90
Total (167)	94

Feedback Issues   Research projects often do not have data until late in the trial. In COMMIT, a deliberate decision was made to keep everyone, including investigators, from seeing any outcome data until the project was over. More than one community representative was disturbed that outcome data were not available throughout the trial. Being blinded from outcome data made it impossible to institute midcourse corrections. Similarly, data on the attainment of impact objectives came late in the trial and were not useful for communities in planning how to direct their energies. Providing feedback during the intervention using process and outcome data can be important for motivating communities and tailoring intervention to individual communities.

Durability of Intervention Activities   Another lesson was learned late in the trial. As COMMIT ended, many investigators, community representatives, and National Cancer Institute (NCI) personnel expressed an interest in continuing tobacco control activities. The COMMIT Steering Committee developed plans for encouraging the communities to make "transition plans" for the future. Each community expressed an interest in continuing some aspects of tobacco control activities and spent considerable time on this process. Unfortunately, when intervention funding ended, the communities were left on their own to carry out their plans to institutionalize tobacco control activities. We learned that the process of ensuring longevity of intervention activities or structures needed to begin early in the trial, not in the last 18 months. Despite the problems with trying to continue intervention activities, 9 of the 11 intervention communities were still conducting tobacco control activities a year after the project ended and had dedicated staff and resources to do so. Two communities, which had received large State or provincial grants, expanded activities greatly, but the remaining communities were selective in choosing which activities to continue. Nevertheless, we learned that communities will continue tobacco control activities even after external funding ends.

**The Role
of Resources**
NCI, which funded COMMIT, perceived that resources would go to the community as "seed resources" that would generate other means to conduct activities. In many communities, the reality differed. For small communities, resources of $150,000 per year were seen as highly significant, especially because volunteers and staff members did not have to engage in fundraising to acquire those resources. This is counter to the practice in most community projects where a volunteer board is responsible for activities to generate resources. Interestingly, although the funds ended, organized, well-defined groups continued in many communities.

The following list summarizes the overall lessons learned from COMMIT field activities:

- It is possible to establish a partnership with communities so that they will organize around a community problem. The process of forming the partnership requires extensive understanding of the community and substantial input from key informants in the community regarding recruitment of appropriate individuals, organizations, and groups.

- It is possible to promote a research agenda even when that agenda is not necessarily viewed as the primary problem facing a community. The COMMIT experience indicates that external resources for addressing a problem that may not be the community's primary concern are a strong incentive for participation. Furthermore, the COMMIT communities had some existing groups and organizations that were interested in and committed to dealing with tobacco control, and those groups were able to draw other community members into the project.

- Community volunteers are willing and able to plan intervention activities that are congruent with an intervention protocol. As community volunteers gain more familiarity with projects and see other potential options for solving the problem, they may wish to change the focus of the intervention protocol. This was evident in COMMIT where, by the end of the trial, all the communities expressed a desire to spend more time and resources on prevention as opposed to cessation. Although the COMMIT project maintained the original intervention protocol to achieve its research emphasis, it may be more desirable to allow protocol changes during the intervention, as long as those changes apply to all the communities. In fact, COMMIT did allow such changes in the organizations channel (Chapter 11), and those changes were accepted by the communities.

- Community volunteers are willing to implement intervention activities. However, one cannot assume that volunteers possess all the information and skills needed to implement interventions. For that reason, ongoing training opportunities are required for individuals to learn the skills of advocating positions, presenting tobacco issues to other community sectors, and placing tobacco control on the agenda of diverse community groups and organizations. In addition, the training programs provided by COMMIT (i.e., training for physicians, dentists, other health care professionals, worksites, organizations, cessation services providers, and educators) were generally well received and left a substantial legacy in the communities.

- The COMMIT model of community organization and a structure of Boards and task forces was well received and has utility for other community problems. Board and task force members also found it a good structure to distribute COMMIT's work activities.

- As noted above under "Feedback Issues," community volunteers would have liked outcome data during the trial so that they could have made midcourse corrections, if necessary. Formative evaluation methodology requires continuous feedback to revise interventions. Availability of process and early outcome data also would have provided opportunities to sell the project to other groups and organizations in the community. Process data on events, contests, and new strategies to recruit heavy smokers also would have allowed for changes to be made the next time those activities were conducted. Community volunteers felt hampered by lack of data.

- Communities were interested in maintaining tobacco control activities. Unfortunately, the COMMIT protocol did not include durability as one of its goals or intervention objectives. Despite this, all 11 communities discussed the issue and developed plans for sustaining at least some project activities. An earlier planning period for transition and assistance in obtaining resources would have been useful for the communities. The plan for durability and transition from a funded research project to a community-supported project should have been an explicit COMMIT goal, and steps to achieve that should have been incorporated from the beginning of intervention activities.

- Resources are important in maintaining tobacco control; however, organized groups can undertake tobacco control. The COMMIT experience suggests that a foundation was laid by the project, considerable enthusiasm and energy were developed, and avenues were found for maintaining many project activities. Although these results differed by community, 9 of the 11 communities continued some form of activity for a year after the project ended, and 2 expanded activity with new funding.

IMPLICATIONS OF COMMIT RESULTS ON LESSONS LEARNED Although COMMIT data continue to be assessed, especially in terms of impact objectives, the outcomes of the trial have been published (COMMIT Research Group, 1995a and 1995b). A statistically significant difference in the proportion of light-to-moderate smokers who quit during the 4 years of the intervention was noted in the intervention communities (30.6 percent) compared with control communities (27.5 percent). However, there was no difference in smoking cessation between intervention and control communities among heavy smokers.

Cessation among light-to-moderate smokers was associated with educational level, with most of the beneficial effect of the intervention seen in the less educated subgroup (no college education). This is contrary to other studies that indicate cessation is more likely to occur among more educated groups (Pierce et al., 1989). It may be that less educated smokers benefit more from a community-based intervention.

Receipt indices were calculated from questions regarding respondents' experiences in the various intervention channels; for example, individuals were asked whether their physician had talked with them about stopping smoking, whether there were any antismoking activities in their worksite, and whether they had participated in any stop-smoking contests. Separate indices were devised for cessation resources, health care, worksites, public education and media, religious organizations, programs and materials, contests and events, and perceived unacceptability of smoking. Summary standardized scores of those indices for heavy smokers were 0.695 for the intervention communities and 0.118 for the control communities (p = .012). For light-to-moderate smokers, the summary scores were 0.386 for the intervention communities and -0.178 for the control communities (p = .004). These scores indicate that cohort members in the intervention communities were more aware of and had participated in more smoking control activities than their counterparts in the control communities. There also was a significant rank order correlation between community receipt indices and the quit rate for the light-to-moderate cohort (rank order correlation = .75, p = .01). In addition, an examination of the observed quit rates over time shows an emerging difference between intervention and control communities for light-to-moderate smokers.

Quitting was measured in 1990, 1991, 1992, and at the end of the trial in 1993. Heavy and light-to-moderate smokers showed an increase in quitting over time in both the intervention and control communities. However, Figure 1 suggests an emerging difference in quit rates for light-to-moderate smokers, one that could perhaps attest to the durability of the community intervention approach if smoking cessation were to be measured again (COMMIT Research Group, 1995a). One of the primary considerations in selecting a community-based approach for the COMMIT intervention was the potential for a sustained intervention effect.

The COMMIT findings regarding heavy smokers and cessation are consistent with other studies (Luepker et al., 1994; Dwyer et al., 1986). The difference detected in light-to-moderate smokers is consistent with those reported earlier in eight community studies in seven different countries. Furthermore, the difference observed in COMMIT is greater than that in the Minnesota Heart Health Program, where a difference was seen only among women (Luepker et al., 1994), and the Pawtucket Heart Health Program, where there was no significant difference in cessation rates (Carleton et al., 1995). Based on their cohort sample, the Stanford Five-City Project observed a greater decline in prevalence in treatment cities compared with controls, and light-to-moderate smokers did better than heavy smokers; however,

Figure 1
Observed quit rates over time for heavy and light-to-moderate smoker cohorts

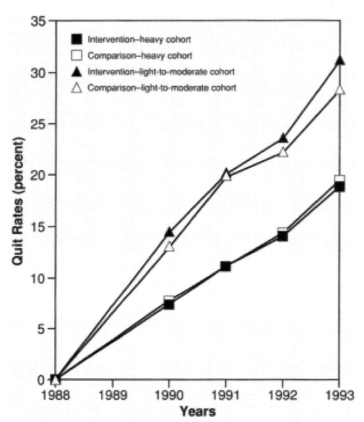

nearly half the cohort could not be followed (Fortmann et al., 1993). No difference was detected between treatment and controls based on cross-sectional data in the Stanford Five-City Project (Fortmann et al., 1993).

Although process objectives were achieved and the intervention receipt indices were favorable for reaching smokers, they had an influence on the quit rates of only light-to-moderate smokers. These outcomes, although significant in terms of potential public health benefit, are more modest than the investigators had hoped to achieve and should be interpreted in light of the successful implementation of the intervention protocol. Several possible reasons for this limited impact of community organization on smoking behavior exist.

First, the project may not have lasted long enough to realize the link between process objectives and impact objectives or between impact objectives and outcomes. This has been the case in other studies, such as the North Karelia Project, where significant results were not seen until the 10-year followup (Puska et al., 1983). Conversely, the Stanford Three Community Study saw results in the 2nd and 3rd years of intervention, although that study did not focus on heavy smokers. It may be that heavy smokers take longer to move from awareness and participation to cessation than do light-to-moderate smokers. Second, the group of interventions, although efficacious in specific settings, may not have been the right ones for a community trial. Clearly, the interventions did not reach heavy smokers who are strongly addicted to nicotine, so it is possible that they need more individualized and clinical attention to quit. Third, COMMIT did not emphasize policy and media interventions; there is some evidence that these could be more effective, especially if done in conjunction with the other COMMIT activities (Flora and Cassidy, 1990; Sorensen and Pechacek, 1989).

Other investigators believe that behavioral outcome measures may not be the only appropriate outcome for a community trial. Mittelmark and colleagues (1993) argue that problems of secular trend, sampling, economic patterns that can contribute to migration, difficulty of measuring outcomes, need to follow cohorts, and need to repeatedly survey large cross-sections of the population make it unreasonable to rely on behavioral change outcomes as indicators of success; rather, they argue that assessing participation may be the most important measure of success. Although COMMIT investigators were not willing to give up the behavioral outcome, they did believe it necessary to collect enough process data so that outcomes could be better understood. Only a few of those process data have been published to date. The process objectives indicate that interventions targeting heavy smokers were conducted. The intervention receipt indices described above indicate heavy smokers received the intervention. Other process measures, such as those documenting policy changes in worksites, organizations, and schools, remain to be analyzed. Similarly, we do not know yet whether there was an impact on the intermediary agencies (e.g., health care providers, cessation resources) that serve smokers. Those analyses are being conducted.

FUTURE DIRECTIONS FOR COMMUNITY TOBACCO CONTROL Increasingly, community intervention programs for tobacco control are being funded and implemented. Sponsorship varies from support from public health departments, to grants and contracts from Federal agencies (e.g., NCI's American Stop Smoking Intervention Study for Cancer Prevention [ASSIST] and the Centers for Disease Control and Prevention's Initiatives To Mobilize for the Prevention and Control of Tobacco Use [IMPACT] program), to foundation support (e.g., the Robert Wood Johnson Foundation Program for Smokeless States). However, fiscal resources for these projects vary considerably. In ASSIST, NCI has committed $20 million annually to support smoking interventions in 17 States, whereas 33 States are due to receive approximately $5 million annually under the IMPACT program. Staff members who are charged with implementing the programs seek information from COMMIT and other previously implemented community tobacco control projects to determine how best to address tobacco control. Given the limited resources of an implementation project compared with a research project, important decisions must be made as to project emphasis.

The cornerstone of COMMIT and any other community intervention project is community organization. Community representatives know how their communities operate and how to reach individuals or groups who practice unhealthy behaviors such as smoking. Although community organization may require a considerable amount of work at the beginning of a project, it is effective in mobilizing a community because a variety of volunteers can be recruited to participate in the project and the diversity of representatives will ensure that all community sectors are involved.

Community organization requires a careful and thorough community analysis. All sectors of the community must be analyzed for their potential contribution to reaching project goals within the community. This analysis is the basis for forming community structures to take on tobacco control or other community problems. For some communities, a small coalition may work best; for others, one existing community agency may be prepared to take on the implementation role while involving others in the decisionmaking processes. The importance of community analysis cannot be overemphasized; an incomplete or erroneous analysis can omit the very groups or individuals who are most necessary to reach a target population.

Community tobacco control projects must be clear as to their specific aims. For example, Fisher (1995) has argued that what needs to be tested in community studies is a defined approach to community organization, not a defined intervention. Such an approach would require considerable flexibility for program planning, development, and implementation. Funding agencies may need to accept that greater flexibility and community freedom are necessary for effective community interventions. On the other hand, ASSIST embraces coalitions as a defined organizational structure (Shopland, 1993) but requires an intervention that focuses on policy and media (National Cancer Institute, 1991). The defined intervention has some general components but is not as regulated as COMMIT. Perhaps that approach will be more suitable to coalitions and the groups they represent.

Community groups must consider many factors when deciding on tobacco control activities. Are there particular subgroups that must be reached? How can they best be reached? Is addiction a major issue for the intervention the community groups wish to implement? If so, is a community study the best avenue for dealing with addiction? Is prevention the primary goal? If so, a focus on policy and media is probably most appropriate. Community projects that are not part of research have the advantage of picking their area of emphasis and then using the best knowledge available to tackle that problem. Community projects involved in research have less latitude.

Future tobacco control activities must be seen as part of a comprehensive national agenda. In COMMIT, most communities did not have the concurrent stimulus from Federal, State, county, and local regulations and ordinances that could form a synergy between local efforts and broader efforts. Although it is well known that the price of cigarettes is a major factor in consumption (Warner, 1986; Sweanor et al., 1993), only recently have substantial increases in tobacco taxation been instituted. Both Canada and California saw significant decreases in smoking prevalence after such tobacco tax increases. Environmental restrictions also have an impact on decreasing prevalence (Borland et al., 1990; Brighan et al., 1994). Taxation, environmental restrictions, and government-funded mass media campaigns are necessary elements for a comprehensive, synergistic approach to tobacco tax control. Communities do not operate independently of the broader political and social systems, and sources of future community projects may be limited without support from those broad sectors.

The tobacco problem is likely to continue for some time. Community projects are ways to organize entire communities to combat this problem, and all the evidence from COMMIT indicates that communities will organize and implement many activities to fight tobacco use. The lessons learned from the field in the COMMIT project can and should be used to help communities develop and implement their own tobacco control activities.

REFERENCES

Borland, R., Chapman, S., Owen, N., Hill, D. Effects of workplace smoking bans on cigarette consumption. *American Journal of Public Health* 80: 178-180, 1990.

Brighan, J., Gross, J., Stizer, M.L., Felch, L.J. Effects of a restricted worksite policy on employees who smoke. *American Journal of Public Health* 84: 773-778, 1994.

Carleton, R.A., Casater, T.M., Assaf, A.R., Feldman, H.A., McKinlay, S., and the Pawtucket Heart Health Program Writing Group. The Pawtucket Heart Health Program: The community changes in cardiovascular risk factors and projected disease risk. *American Journal of Public Health* 85: 777-785, 1995.

COMMIT Research Group. Community Intervention Trial for Smoking Cessation (COMMIT): I. Cohort results from a four-year community intervention. *American Journal of Public Health* 85: 183-192, 1995a.

COMMIT Research Group. Community Intervention Trial for Smoking Cessation (COMMIT): II. Changes in adult smoking prevalence. *American Journal of Public Health* 85: 193-200, 1995b.

Dwyer, T., Pierce, J.P., Hannam, C.D., Burke, N. Evaluation of the Sydney "Quit for Life" anti-smoking campaign: 2. Changes in smoking prevalence. *Medical Journal of Australia* 144: 344-347, 1986.

Fisher, E.B. Editorial: The results of the COMMIT trial. *American Journal of Public Health* 85: 159-160, 1995.

Flora, J.A., Cassidy, D. Roles of media in community-based health promotion. In: *Health Promotion at the Community Level*, N.F. Bracht (Editor). Newbury Park, CA: Sage, 1990, pp. 143-157.

Fortmann, S.P., Taylor, C.B., Flora, J.A., Jatulis, D.E. Changes in adult smoking prevalence after 5 years of community health education: The Stanford Five-City Project. *American Journal of Epidemiology* 137: 82-96, 1993.

Luepker, R.V., Murray, D.M., Jacobs, D.R., Mittelmark, M.B., Bracht, N., Carlaw, R., Crow, R., Elmer, P., Finnegan, J., Folsom, A.R., Grimm, R., Hannan, P.J., Jeffrey, R., Lando, H., McGovern, P., Mullis, R., Perry, C.L., Pechacek, T., Pirie, P., Sprafka, M., Weisbrod, R., Blackburn, H. Community education for cardiovascular disease prevention: Risk factor changes in the Minnesota Heart Health Program. *American Journal of Public Health* 84(9): 1383-1393, 1994.

Mittelmark, M.B., Hunt, M.K., Heath, G.W., Schmid, T.L. Realistic outcomes: Lessons from community-based research and demonstration programs for the prevention of cardiovascular diseases. *Journal of Public Health Policy* 14(4): 437-462, 1993.

National Cancer Institute. "ASSIST Program Guidelines." Internal document prepared for the National Cancer Institute, 1991.

Pierce, J.P., Fiore, M.C., Novotny, T.E., Hatziandreu, E.J., Davis, R.M. Trends in tobacco smoking in the United States: Educational differences are increasing. *Journal of the American Medical Association* 261: 56-60, 1989.

Puska, P., Nissinen, A., Salonen, J.T., Toumilehto, J. Ten years of the North Karelia Project: Results with community-based prevention of coronary heart disease. *Scandinavian Journal of Social Medicine* II: 65-68, 1983.

Shopland, D.R. Smoking control in the 1990's: A National Cancer Institute model for change. *American Journal of Public Health* 83(9): 1208-1210, 1993.

Sorensen, G., Pechacek, T.F. Implementing nonsmoking policies in the private sector and assessing their effects. *New York State Journal of Medicine* 89: 11-15, 1989.

Sweanor, D., Martial, L., Dossetor, J. *The Canadian Tobacco Tax Increase: A Case Study*. Ottawa, Ontario, Canada: The Non-Smokers' Rights Association (Canada) and the Smoking and Health Action Foundation (Canada), 1993.

Warner, K. Smoking and health implications of a change in the federal excise tax. *Journal of the American Medical Association* 255: 1028-1032, 1986.

AUTHORS

Beti Thompson, Ph.D.
Associate Professor
University of Washington School of
   Public Health and Community Medicine
Associate Member
Fred Hutchinson Cancer Research Center,
   MP-702
1124 Columbia Street
Seattle, WA 98104

William R. Lynn
COMMIT Project Officer
Public Health Applications Research Branch
Cancer Control Science Program
National Cancer Institute
National Institutes of Health
Executive Plaza North, Room 241
6130 Executive Boulevard, MSC-7337
Bethesda, MD 20892-7337

Donald R. Shopland
Coordinator
Smoking and Tobacco Control Program
National Cancer Institute
National Institutes of Health
Executive Plaza North, Room 241
6130 Executive Boulevard, MSC-7337
Bethesda, MD 20892-7337